T0258268

Practical Colonoscopy

The authors would like to dedicate the book to Marguerite (JDW), Suzanne (JA) and Liz, Jessica and Fern (PHR).

Practical Colonoscopy

Jerome D. Waye, MD
Director of Endoscopic Education
Clinical Professor of Medicine
Mount Sinai Medical Center
New York, NY, USA

James Aisenberg, MD
Clinical Professor of Medicine
Mount Sinai Medical Center
New York, NY, USA

Peter H. Rubin, MD
Associate Clinical Professor of Medicine
Mount Sinai Medical Center
New York, NY, USA

With the assistance of Shannon Morales, MD

WILEY Blackwell

WEO
World Endoscopy Organization

This edition first published 2013 © 2013 by John Wiley & Sons, Ltd.

Wiley-Blackwell is an imprint of John Wiley & Sons, formed by the merger of Wiley's global Scientific, Technical and Medical business with Blackwell Publishing.

Registered office: John Wiley & Sons, Ltd., The Atrium, Southern Gate, Chichester, West Sussex, PO19 8SQ, UK

Editorial offices: 9600 Garsington Road, Oxford, OX4 2DQ, UK
The Atrium, Southern Gate, Chichester, West Sussex, PO19 8SQ, UK
111 River Street, Hoboken, NJ 07030-5774, USA

For details of our global editorial offices, for customer services and for information about how to apply for permission to reuse the copyright material in this book please see our website at www.wiley.com/wiley-blackwell

The right of the author to be identified as the author of this work has been asserted in accordance with the UK Copyright, Designs and Patents Act 1988.

All rights reserved. No part of this publication may be reproduced, stored in a retrieval system, or transmitted, in any form or by any means, electronic, mechanical, photocopying, recording or otherwise, except as permitted by the UK Copyright, Designs and Patents Act 1988, without the prior permission of the publisher.

Designations used by companies to distinguish their products are often claimed as trademarks. All brand names and product names used in this book are trade names, service marks, trademarks or registered trademarks of their respective owners. The publisher is not associated with any product or vendor mentioned in this book. This publication is designed to provide accurate and authoritative information in regard to the subject matter covered. It is sold on the understanding that the publisher is not engaged in rendering professional services. If professional advice or other expert assistance is required, the services of a competent professional should be sought.

The contents of this work are intended to further general scientific research, understanding, and discussion only and are not intended and should not be relied upon as recommending or promoting a specific method, diagnosis, or treatment by physicians for any particular patient. The publisher and the author make no representations or warranties with respect to the accuracy or completeness of the contents of this work and specifically disclaim all warranties, including without limitation any implied warranties of fitness for a particular purpose. In view of ongoing research, equipment modifications, changes in governmental regulations, and the constant flow of information relating to the use of medicines, equipment, and devices, the reader is urged to review and evaluate the information provided in the package insert or instructions for each medicine, equipment, or device for, among other things, any changes in the instructions or indication of usage and for added warnings and precautions. Readers should consult with a specialist where appropriate. The fact that an organization or Website is referred to in this work as a citation and/or a potential source of further information does not mean that the author or the publisher endorses the information the organization or Website may provide or recommendations it may make. Further, readers should be aware that Internet Websites listed in this work may have changed or disappeared between when this work was written and when it is read. No warranty may be created or extended by any promotional statements for this work. Neither the publisher nor the author shall be liable for any damages arising herefrom.

Library of Congress Cataloging-in-Publication Data

Waye, Jerome D., 1932–
Practical colonoscopy / Jerome D. Waye, James Aisenberg, Peter H. Rubin ; With the assistance of Shannon Morales.
p. ; cm.
Includes bibliographical references and index.
ISBN 978-0-470-67058-3 (hardback : alk. paper)
I. Aisenberg, James. II. Rubin, Peter H. III. Title.
[DNLM: 1. Colonoscopy–methods. 2. Colonic Diseases–diagnosis. 3. Colonic Diseases–surgery. WI 520]

616.3'407545–dc23
2012044841

A catalogue record for this book is available from the British Library.

Wiley also publishes its books in a variety of electronic formats. Some content that appears in print may not be available in electronic books.

Cover image: Micrograph © iStockphoto/beholdingEye; all other images courtesy of the authors.
Cover design by Meaden Creative

Set in 8.5/13 pt Meridien by Toppan Best-set Premedia Limited

1 2013

Contents

List of Video Clips, vii
Preface, x
About the companion website, xii

Section 1: Pre-procedure

1 The Endoscopy Unit, Colonoscope, and Accessories, 3
2 The Role of the Endoscopy Assistant during Colonoscopy, 16
3 Indications and Contraindications for Colonoscopy, 24
4 Preparation for Colonoscopy, 30

Section 2: Basic Procedure

5 Sedation for Colonoscopy, 39
6 Colonoscopy Technique: The Ins and Outs, 46
7 Colonoscopic Findings, 69
8 Diagnostic Biopsy, 83

Section 3: Operative Procedures

9 Thermal Techniques: Electrosurgery, Argon Plasma Coagulation, and Laser, 91
10 Basic Principles and Techniques of Polypectomy, 99
11 Difficult Polypectomy, 116
12 Management of Malignant Polyps, 132
13 Therapeutic Colonoscopy, 140
14 Complications of Colonoscopy, 147

Section 4: Current and Future Considerations

15 Quality in Colonoscopy, 161
16 Teaching and Training in Colonoscopy, 167
17 Computed Tomographic Colonography ("Virtual" Colonoscopy), 175
18 Advanced Imaging Techniques, 178
19 The Future of Colonoscopy, 186

Index, 191
Plate section can be found facing page 52

List of Video Clips

All videos are accompanied by audio commentary.

Video Clip 7.1 Melanosis coli with polyp see page 69
An adenoma is hidden behind the ileocecal valve in the setting of melanosis coli.

Video Clip 7.2 Squamous papillomas in the rectum see page 70
Multiple diminutive papules are seen near the dentate line during careful retroflex examination.

Video Clip 7.3 Diverticular colitis see page 71
Prominent polypoid red folds seen in a patient with sigmoid colon diverticular disease.

Video Clip 7.4 Segmental colonic ischemia see page 72
A segment of sigmoid colon is involved with moderate to severe ischemia.

Video Clip 7.5 Solitary rectal ulcer syndrome see page 72
Endoscopic findings of solitary rectal ulcer syndrome include ulceration, erythema, edema, and exudate.

Video Clip 7.6 Radiation proctopathy see page 72
Angioectasias in the rectum treated with argon plasma coagulation therapy.

Video Clip 7.7 Cobble-stoning in chronic ulcerative colitis see page 73
Severe edema, erythema, and ulceration in a patient with active ulcerative colitis.

Video Clip 7.8 Small carcinoma in chronic ulcerative colitis see page 74
Small carcinoma detected during surveillance in chronic ulcerative colitis. Extensive mucosal scarring is also seen.

Video Clip 7.9 Large carcinoma in chronic colitis see page 74
Large carcinoma in colitis, mucosal bridging is seen and snare biopsy technique is used.

Video Clip 7.10 Dysplasia in ulcerative colitis see page 74
The spray catheter is used for chromoendoscopy, which reveals a dysplastic plaque.

Video Clip 7.11 Nodular carcinoma arising in ulcerative colitis see page 74
Small, nodular carcinoma detected during surveillance in patient with chronic ulcerative colitis.

Video Clip 7.12 Chromoendoscopy in colitis surveillance see page 74
Areas of flat dysplasia are detected during chromoendoscopy in colitis surveillance.

Video Clip 7.13 Sessile dysplasia in chronic ulcerative colitis see page 74
Large area of villiform, sessile dysplasia is seen in chronic ulcerative colitis.

Video Clip 7.14 Giant inflammatory polyp see page 76
Giant inflammatory polyp identified in chronic colitis.

Video Clip 7.15 Dysplastic polyp in ulcerative colitis see page 76
Identification and snare resection of flat, dysplastic polyp in chronic ulcerative colitis.

Video Clip 7.16 Bleeding angioectasia see page 78
Detection and cauterization of ascending colon, bleeding angioectasia.

Video Clip 7.17 Pinworms see page 79
Live pinworms seen during colonoscopy.

Video Clip 7.18 *Ascaris* see page 79
Live *Ascaris* worm seen during colonoscopy.

Video Clip 7.19 Flat adenoma in microscopic colitis see page 80
Large flat adenoma seen in ascending colon in a patient with microscopic colitis. The colitis has caused edema and a mosaic pattern, which is atypical for this disease.

Video Clip 10.1 Sessile serrated adenoma/polyp see page 101
Multiple examples of identification and resection of sessile serrated adenomas/polyps are provided.

Video Clip 10.2 Resection of sessile serrated polyp see page 101
Sessile serrated adenoma/polyp identified and resected with saline lift followed by piecemeal snare polypectomy.

Video Clip 10.3 Giant lipoma see page 101
Giant, pedunculated lipoma with erythema related to trauma.

Video Clip 10.4 Ileal carcinoid see page 101
Intubation of the ileum reveals a 1.5-cm submucosal carcinoid.

Video Clip 11.1 Detachable loop and pedunculated polypectomy see page 117
The detachable loop is used to promote hemostasis before resection of this large, pedunculated polyp.

Video Clip 11.2 Piecemeal polypectomy, argon plasma coagulation, and net retrieval of fragments see page 120
The sequence of saline injection, piecemeal polypectomy, and argon plasma coagulation and net retrieval of polyp fragments is used to eradicate this 3-cm adenoma.

Video Clip 11.3 Piecemeal resection of sessile adenoma see page 120
Large sessile adenoma removed piecemeal following saline lift.

Video Clip 11.4 Saline-assisted polypectomy see page 122
Multiple injection sites are used to elevate the polyp with methylene blue and saline.

Video Clip 11.5 The non-lifting sign see page 123
This polyp does not lift with saline injection, suggesting the presence of malignancy.

Video Clip 11.6 Giant villous adenoma see page 126
This enormous sigmoid adenoma occupied the entire lumen and is debulked. Water immersion is used to examine the defect for signs of residual polyp, which are ablated with the argon plasma coagulator.

Video Clip 11.7 Cecal retroflexion with polypectomy see page 127
A large, right-colon polyp is hidden behind a fold and identified and removed in retroflexion.

Video Clip 11.8 Flat right colon polyp see page 127
A flat right-colon polyp is seen and resected in retroflexion.

Video Clip 12.1 Familial adenomatous polyposis see page 133
Innumerable adenomas seen in a patient with familial adenomatous polyposis.

Video Clip 12.2 The Non-Lifting Sign see page 134
3 cm malignant polyp in ascending colon which exhibits the non-lifting sign upon sub-mucosal saline injection.

Video Clip 12.3 Malignant sessile polyp see page 134
A 2-cm sessile malignant polyp removed with saline injection and snare polypectomy.

Video Clip 13.1 Dilation of strictured anastomosis see page 142
Strictured ileocolic anastomosis dilated with a through-the-scope balloon.

Video Clip 13.2 Foreign body in sigmoid see page 145
A chicken bone is identified embedded in the colon wall, and is removed with the snare.

Video Clip 14.1 Giant rectal polyp with bleeding see page 154
Snare resection of giant rectal polyp complicated by post-polypectomy hemorrhage, managed colonoscopically.

Video Clip 14.2 Immediate postpolypectomy bleeding: sessile polyp see page 154
Arterial bleeding seen following snare polypectomy. Clip placement used to achieve hemostasis.

Video Clip 14.3 Immediate postpolypectomy bleeding: pedunculated polyp see page 154
Bleeding from pedicle of polyp is controlled with compression and with clip placement.

Video Clip 14.4 Delayed postpolypectomy bleeding see page 155
Unprepped colonoscopy used for identification and treatment of bleeding site several days following ascending colon polypectomy.

Video Clip 18.1 Narrow band imaging see page 181
Narrow band imaging is used extensively to enhance visualization during resection of this minimally elevated adenoma.

Preface

Approximately 15 million colonoscopies are conducted annually in the USA. This widespread uptake, mirrored in other nations, reflects the power of colonoscopy as a diagnostic and therapeutic tool. Most notably, it is the leading means of preventing death from colorectal cancer, the second leading cause of cancer-related deaths in the USA, and is a first-line test in the management of gastrointestinal bleeding and colitis.

Colonoscopy continues to evolve, owing to enhancements in scope design, image processing, and data management that are offshoots of the modern technology revolution. Novel insights into colonic diseases from contemporary molecular and cell biology are also rapidly advancing the field.

Despite its attributes, colonoscopy remains imperfect. It is a costly, inconvenient, and unpopular procedure that carries some risk. In the USA, at least 50% of adults for whom screening colonoscopy for colon cancer is recommended never receive it, whereas others undergo colonoscopy more frequently than is recommended in expert guidelines. And "interval" colorectal cancer—i.e. cancer detected within 3 years of a "clearing" colonoscopy—is reported in some analyses to occur in as many as 1 in 150 individuals.

Recent studies have underscored the inconvenient truth that colonoscopy quality (safety and effectiveness) varies considerably among practitioners. Accordingly, leaders in the field are promoting quality enhancement measures such as mid-career provider education, implementation of validated quality benchmarks, continuous peer review, and implementation of financial incentives such as pay-for-performance.

Practical Colonoscopy is written with this context in mind. Our goal is to create a succinct, easily readable volume, enhanced by drawings, photos, and videos, which communicates the "nuts and bolts" of high-quality colonoscopy practice. Drawing from our collective experience of over 100 years in the private practice of colonoscopy and gastroenterology, we share the principles and "pearls" we have found most useful. We integrate ideas presented in the recently published, comprehensive, second edition of *Colonoscopy: Principles and Practice*. We share insights derived from our teaching and research as Professors of Medicine at The Mount Sinai Medical Center in New York. Finally, we present our expectations for forthcoming developments in colonoscopy. Of course, our ultimate hope is that readers will gain an enhanced ability to prevent and treat colonic diseases.

Practical Colonoscopy provides an overview of colonoscopy, while focusing on the practical aspects of quality, indications, and technique. Our objective during the planning and writing of this book was to bring new, practical information to trainees, mid-career colonoscopists, endoscopy assistants, nurses, pathologists, anesthesiologists, and to the motivated lay person who is curious about the science and art of our craft.

The authors wish to acknowledge the use and adaptation of images from Colonoscopy: Principles and Practice, edited by Jerome D. Waye, Douglas K. Rex, Christopher B. Williams. 2nd edition. Blackwell Publishing Ltd; 2009. We thank our medical and surgical colleagues, from whom we have learned so much, and especially the endoscopy staff at the Gastrointestinal Endoscopy Unit at The Mount Sinai Hospital in New York, the staff in our office endoscopy units, our practice partners, patients, and students. Ms. Rebecca Sweeney and Ms. Jennifer Kolb (Icahn School of Medicine at Mount Sinai, Class of 2014) provided invaluable assistance with preparation of the manuscript and videos. We are also grateful to our expert collaborators at Wiley-Blackwell, in particular Ms. Elisabeth Dodds, Mr. Oliver Walter, and Ms. Rebecca Huxley. We thank Jane Fallows and Roger Hulley who have expertly redrawn all line drawings; and Aileen Castell for the help she provided during the production stage. Dr. Shannon Morales, then a 4th-year medical student, was a full collaborator in every aspect of the book, and maintained order in the input submitted at the weekly meetings of the three authors during the many months of drafts, discussions, and eventual agreements. We owe Shannon a special degree of gratitude.

Jerome D. Waye, MD
James Aisenberg, MD
Peter H. Rubin, MD

New York, NY
May 2013

About the companion website

Companion website

This book is accompanied by a website:

www.wiley.com/go/waye/practicalcolonoscopy

The website includes:

- 41 videos showing procedures described in the book
- All videos are referenced in the text where you see this logo

SECTION 1
Pre-procedure

CHAPTER 1

The Endoscopy Unit, Colonoscope, and Accessories

Introduction

Colonoscopy is performed in the hospital, the ambulatory surgical center, or the physician office. Endoscopy units range in size from 1 to 10 or more procedure rooms, and in staffing from one or two to over 50 persons. Regardless of size, staffing, and location, the endoscopy unit must promote safe, efficient, cost-effective, high-quality patient care. A pleasant, comfortable endoscopy facility promotes staff productivity and alleviates patient anxiety. The modern gastrointestinal endoscopy unit is constructed specifically for endoscopic procedures. Specific design concerns include: smooth patient flow; patient privacy; patient safety, spacious procedure rooms; adequate preparation and recovery space; and a pleasant, reassuring environment. The materials must be durable and sanitary, yet aesthetically attractive.

In broad terms, the facility is divided into the administrative area—which is used for patient intake, scheduling, billing, and record maintenance—and the clinical area—which contains the dressing rooms, the pre-procedure area, the procedure rooms, a clean equipment storage area, a cleaning and disinfection zone, and a recovery room. Amenities such as physician–patient consultation rooms, a procedure reporting area, and staff lounge and dressing rooms enhance the quality of the unit.

When building a facility, careful planning and close collaboration between the endoscopists and an architect who possesses expertise in endoscopy unit design is encouraged. The unit design should conform to the practice styles of the endoscopists and the procedure mix and demographics of the practice. Unit construction requires patience (it may take a year to design and construct a new unit), attention to detail, experience, foresight, and cost-sensitivity. As modern endoscopy units are increasingly digitized, specialized expertise in information technology, cabling, and connectivity is essential.

If the facility is built as an ambulatory surgical center or within a hospital, many of the specifics, such as the size of the rooms and

Practical Colonoscopy, First Edition. Jerome D. Waye, James Aisenberg, and Peter H. Rubin.
© 2013 John Wiley & Sons, Ltd. Published 2013 by John Wiley & Sons, Ltd.

Optimizing the work environment

- Proper ventilation
- Appropriate temperature
- Adjustable lighting
- Free of trip hazards
- Workspace fastidiously cleaned between cases and especially at the end of the day
- Free of distractions such as sounds from other rooms
- Adequate workspace for each member of the team

corridors, will be regulated. Office-based endoscopy in many states must now meet the criteria of one of the national accrediting organizations. In general, a circular flow of patients works well: the patient moves from the waiting and intake area to the pre-procedure assessment/changing area, to the procedure room, to the recovery/dressing area, and then back to the intake area, where billing and/or new appointment scheduling is completed. The interdependent areas (e.g. procedure and recovery, procedure and scope washing) should be located close to each other. The number of procedure rooms should be projected from the procedure volume of the practice, and will drive the number of overall square feet and all other architectural decisions. The procedure rooms contain the complex, expensive equipment and are the most heavily staffed rooms in the unit. Therefore, the entire facility must be designed to keep the procedure rooms busy with active procedures, rather than also having to serve as recovery rooms.

The procedure rooms

In the USA, licensing laws generally mandate that the procedure room have a net area of at least 19 m^2. This excludes areas occupied by built-ins, such as cabinets or equipment towers, but not area occupied by movable equipment, such as an endoscopic equipment tower. The room must accommodate the equipment and the patient stretcher, and still allow free movement and clear sight lines for the physician, assistant, anesthesiologist and other participants. Because of the amount of equipment required for endoscopy, vertical arrangement of components on towers or carts or in built-in cabinets is generally desirable.

In a modern video-endoscopy room, the central architectural design point is the "physician tower," which holds the endoscopic light source and image processor. The endoscope is plugged into the processor, and the endoscopist stands immediately in front of the tower. The patient stretcher must be within easy reach of the endoscopist. The distance from the front of the tower to the edge of the patient stretcher should be between 66 and 81 cm, as determined by the length of the scope's universal cord (Fig 1.1). It

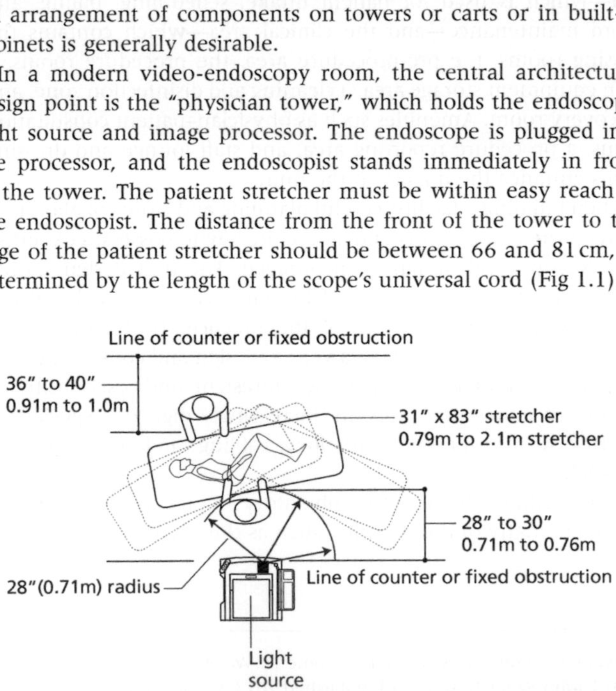

Fig 1.1 Basic clearances in the procedure room.

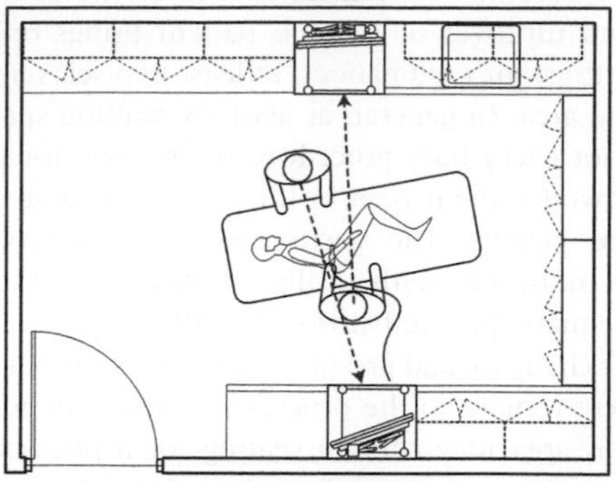

Fig 1.2 Position of monitors for the colonoscopist and assistant.

is most efficient for the assistant to stand on the opposite side of the stretcher from the endoscopist (Fig 1.2); this location promotes easy access to the patient (e.g. to give abdominal pressure and to monitor respirations), the endoscopist (e.g. to provide a snare for polypectomy), and the other equipment (e.g. the cautery device).

Once the positions of the tower and stretcher are established, then the other equipment is located. One video monitor is situated directly across from the endoscopist, establishing a comfortable, clear sight line. The monitor should be mounted at least 1.8 m above the floor. A second endoscopy video monitor is positioned behind the endoscopist for the assistant. The assistant should have clear visual access to the patient, the monitor, and the cardiopulmonary monitoring equipment.

An endoscopic reporting system is often integrated into the room design. This allows nurses and physicians to chart immediately, increasing both accuracy and efficiency. The equipment and electrical cabling must be laid out with forethought: it is unsafe and unkempt to have wires running across the floor. Often an overhead cabling conduit will keep the room tidy but a series of floating ceiling booms will also (expensively) solve the problem. The ancillary equipment should be carefully positioned and handy for the endoscopy assistant. Lighting must be purposeful: the patient's face and chest should be visible, allowing the assistant to monitor the patient's color and respiratory pattern, but the ambient lighting should be minimal, to encourage the team to focus on the endoscopic image. The room must be well ventilated with continuous air exchange and adequately soundproofed, and the temperature must be controlled by an independent thermostat.

Ancillary equipment and built-ins

- Suction machine (unless wall suction is available)
- Water irrigation pump
- Location to place the scope before and after the case
- Counter space for gloves, lubricant, and other accessories
- Cabinetry for accessories, medications, and miscellaneous small equipment such as catheters and saline
- Counter space for the assistant to process specimens and perform charting
- Ancillary monitoring devices, such as machines for obtaining vital signs (blood pressure and pulse), and perhaps capnography
- At least one sink
- Oxygen and perhaps CO_2 tanks

The non-procedure areas

The waiting and recovery areas also merit careful planning. The total number of required seats in the waiting area depends on the projected case volume of the unit, as well as the procedure and recovery room turnover time. Each patient brings one or more companions; thus, for each patient, at least two seats are required in the waiting area. In general, at least six waiting spaces should be provided for every busy procedure room—two for the patient in recovery, two for the patient in the procedure, and two for the pre-procedure patient. The gastrointestinal endoscopy patient waiting area must be aesthetically pleasant, comfortable, and served by adequate, private bathroom facilities.

The patient changing and pre-procedure areas should be private, secure, and convenient to the procedure area. Depending on the workflow, this area may contain seating for a physician or staff member to perform the pre-procedure interview and obtain informed consent. In some units, the patient walks to the procedure room; in others, the patient lies on a stretcher in the pre-procedure room and intravenous access is obtained in this area.

The recovery bed capacity is a notorious bottleneck in endoscopy units. If colonoscopy takes 45 minutes and recovery takes 45 minutes, one recovery bed will be required per procedure room. In general, this ratio is desirable. The recovery room must permit close patient monitoring and be adequately served by restroom facilities. In some units, patients recover in individual rooms, whereas in others, patients recover in separate "bays" within a larger recovery room.

The administrative area should accommodate all reception, scheduling, filing and record-keeping, and billing/insurance functions. The reception area should promote face-to-face interactions between patients and staff, but also accommodate private conversations regarding sensitive matters. Adequate, well-marked toilet facilities must be nearby. Many waiting rooms include artwork, wi-fi access, telephones, television monitors, water coolers, reading materials, or music. Computer- and telephone-equipped staff workstations should be available. Staff foot traffic should move unimpeded. Cabinets for patient record storage should be adequate, although the transition to electronic records may diminish this requirement. Depending on the characteristics of the practice, an on-site billing area may be included.

The colonoscope

The modern video colonoscope combines state-of-the-art electronic imaging technology and sophisticated mechanical engineering. Its fragile components—glass illumination fibers, angulation cables, and suction and air/water channels—are packed within a water-tight tube that is 130–168 cm in length but only 9–13 mm in diameter. The column must be strong enough to permit the endoscopist to push it through the 1.8-m-long colon, flexible enough to bend around the sharp turns, and elastic enough to return to a straight shape when the scope is pulled back. It must transmit the hand actions of the endoscopist from the proximal shaft down to

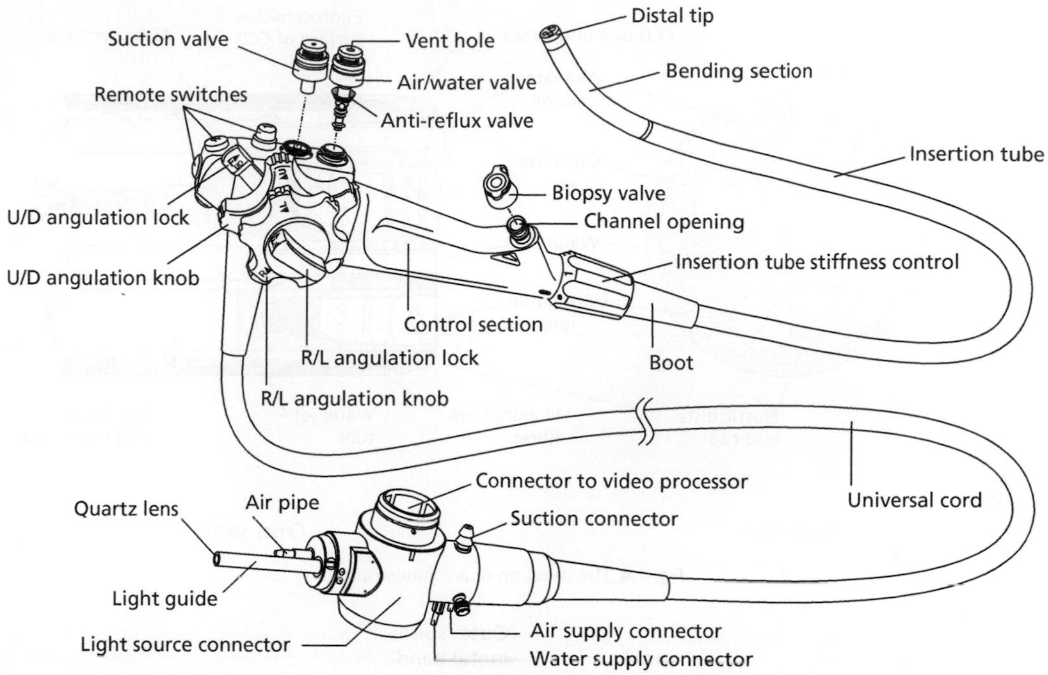

Fig 1.3 The design and parts of a typical video colonoscope.

the tip. The scope must be sturdy enough to withstand the repetitive and diverse stresses that occur during thousands of procedures and cleaning cycles, yet delicate enough to provide impeccable tip control and visualization.

The scope is divided into several sections (Fig 1.3). The long connector tube that runs from the scope head to the light source is called the "universal cord." The universal cord is plugged into the light source, which also has connections to the video processor, the suction, and the air/water supplies. The head of the instrument contains endoscopist-operated switches and valves that control many scope functions. The "insertion tube" is the long, straight tube that intubates the colon. At the distal end of the insertion tube is a 10-cm bending section, which is controlled by the angulation wires using two control wheels. The variable stiffness control, if present, is located at the junction where the control section meets the insertion tube. The distal scope tip contains the channel openings, the air–water nozzle that allows insufflation and lens cleaning, the objective lens, and the light guide lens. The charge-coupled device (CCD) is a small chip (camera) that is located just behind the objective lens and that electronically captures the images and transmits them through electrical wires to the video processor

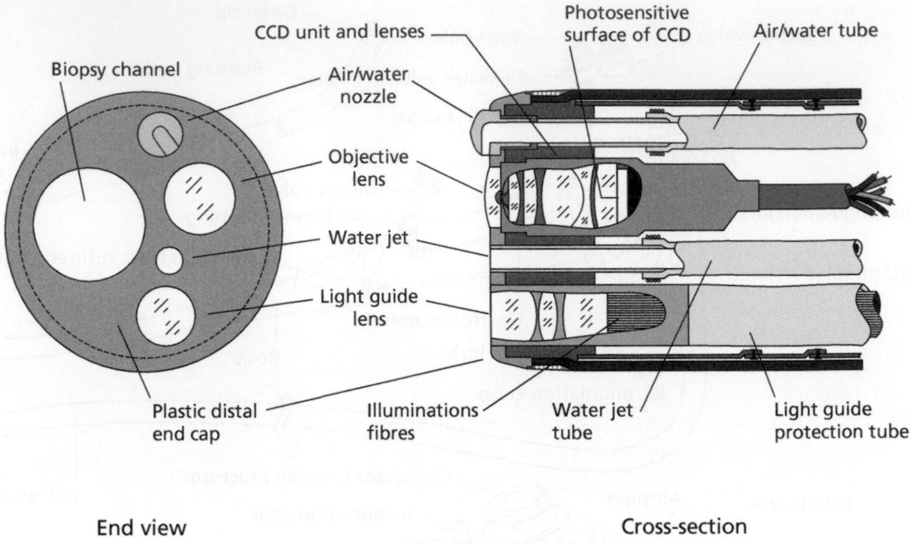

Fig 1.4 The distal tip of a colonoscope.

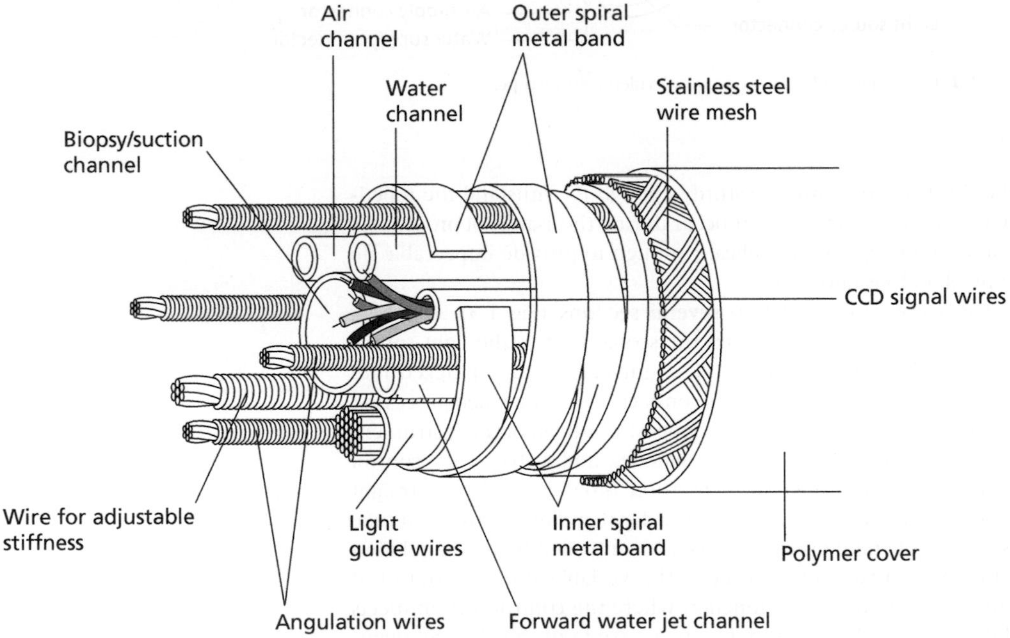

Fig 1.5 Internal cutaway view of a colonoscope shaft.

(Fig 1.4). The control section contains: the angulation dials and locks for up/down and right/left tip deflection; the air–water and suction valves; and the remote switches that control photography, illumination light type (e.g. white light versus narrow band), and zoom.

Although the control section has the greatest visible complexity, the insertion tube is a marvel of modern engineering (Fig 1.5).

The insertion tube must carry: three hollow tubes (channels) for suction/biopsy, air and water (to wash the lens), and water (for the forward-directed jet); four angulation cables, positioned at 3, 6, 9 and 12 o'clock, which connect the right/left and up/down controls to the distal bending section of the instrument; the variable-stiffness cable; the fine electrical wires that carry the signals from the CCD to the image processor; the fiber-optic bundles—containing thousands of hairlike, 30-μm-wide, glass fibers—which transmit the light from the xenon lamp to the distal end of the instrument; the outer casings of metal that provide the scope with its mechanical properties; and the polymeric outer casing, which is smooth, durable, biocompatible, and watertight. The insertion tube must responsively transmit torque from the external shaft of the instrument, through the bends in the colon, to the instrument's tip. Mechanically, this is accomplished by oppositely spiraled flat metal bands that run the length of the instrument. These bands are arranged so that a twist of the scope in one direction will tighten one set of bands and maintain torque integrity, whereas a twist in the opposite direction will tighten the other spiral bands. The stiffness of the insertion tube is determined principally by the formulation of the outer polymeric layer and an outer wire mesh.

The distal 40 cm of the insertion tube is more flexible than the proximal portion. This allows the distal segment to snake around the convolutions of the colon without the proximal portion forming loops. Some instruments have a variable stiffness capability activated by a ring on the proximal end of the insertion tube. Rotation of the ring pulls a wire and adds rigidity to the insertion tube. The tip deflection capability of most colonoscopes is 180° up/down and 160° right/left. The angle of view of most scopes is 140°, although one manufacturer has recently introduced a scope that has a 170° viewing angle. Most modern video colonoscopes contain "high-resolution" optics that can distinguish two lines or points that are located only fractions of a millimeter apart. The image resolution increases as the scope tip moves closer to the mucosal surface, until a critical distance is reached (<1 cm) when focus is no longer achieved and the image degrades. Modern instruments also offer "high-definition" image sensors, which can feed to densely pixilated monitors.

Preventing scope damage between cases

- After washing scopes, hang them vertically (for drainage) in a protected, ventilated, dedicated cabinet
- When transferring the scope from person-to-person or person-to-storage-location, hold the scope tip carefully so it cannot drop to the floor
- Leak-test scopes between cases
- Train dedicated individuals for scope cleaning and maintenance
- Quality control all reprocessing reagents
- Adhere strictly to established scope reprocessing methods
- Educate all clinical staff regarding proper scope handling
- Service scopes at appropriate intervals

Preventing scope damage during the case

- When passing an ancillary device through a working channel, use gentle thrusts and never force
- Whenever possible, do not pass ancillary devices through a channel when the scope tip is in a retroflexed position
- Avoid hyper-deflection of dial controls, which strains cables
- Avoid suctioning large seeds and debris
- If scope malfunction occurs, switch scopes and inform staff of the problem

Mucosal imaging can be further enhanced with magnification or with alteration of the light that is delivered to the mucosal surface. The electronic magnification feature on most commercially available scopes simply enlarges the image, sacrificing the outer portion of the image, without increasing resolution. True optical zoom technology increases resolution, but is not widely commercialized. The white light typically used for illumination can also be selectively filtered. In narrow band imaging (NBI), filters transmit wavelengths of light that are highly absorbed by hemoglobin, thus producing a brownish color to the surface with intensity related to mucosal blood flow. Some manufacturers use image-processing technology to "bring out" characteristics and contrasts in the image after it has been acquired.

Endoscopic accessories

The endoscopy unit must stock a variety of accessories, including snares, forceps, retrieval devices, clips, and injector needles. The unit must stock an adequate inventory and a variety of devices needed to solve the commonly encountered colonoscopic predicaments. Many accessories are available in disposable and reusable versions. The disposable variety increases the up-front cost, but saves labor (no reprocessing and reassembly required) and ensures case-to-case sterility. Reusable devices must be sturdy enough for repeated use and sterilization cycles. Reusable snares require disassembly for cleaning. Most accessories are available from a variety of manufacturers, with small differences in engineering and cost.

Polypectomy snares

The polypectomy snare consists of a thin wire loop attached by a long connector wire to the control handle. The wire is enclosed within a 7-French plastic sheath, which is passed through the working channel of the scope. The wire loop is opened and closed by the endoscopy assistant, using the control handle. The snare handle connects to an electrosurgical unit, and the connector wire conducts electrical current to the loop. Although bipolar snares have been developed (one wire positive and the other negative), most snares are monopolar, requiring a remote return electrode (grounding pad) to complete the electrical circuit.

The wire loop is typically fashioned from braided stainless steel wire, which combines favorable strength, configurational memory, and electrical conductance. Stiffer monofilament wires promote transection over coagulation. The loop configuration is usually oval or elliptical, although "D" and hexagonal shapes are available

(Fig 1.6). Rotatable snares and combination injector/snares are available but are not essential. Some colonoscopists believe that tiny wire protrusions (barbs) on the wire snare loop facilitate flat polyp capture. The large loop snares are 5 × 3 cm, whereas the "mini-loop" is 3 × 1 cm. As most polyps are less than 1 cm in diameter, the smaller loop is adequate for most polypectomies.

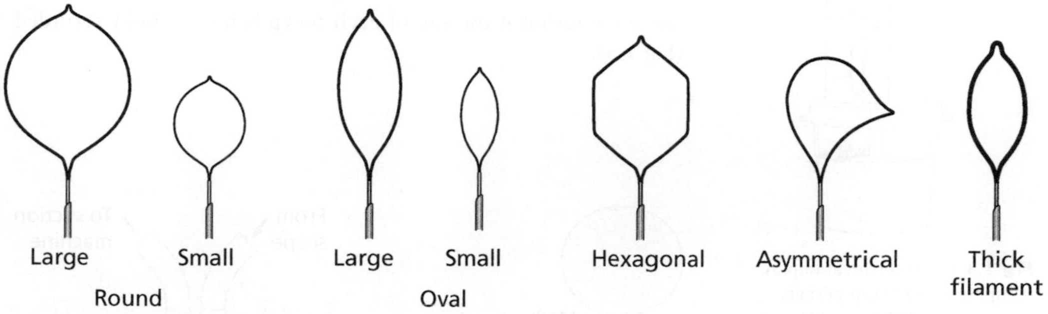

Fig 1.6 Polypectomy snares. Snares differ in loop diameter, shape, and filament diameter. After it is embedded in the mucosa, the pointed tip can act as a fulcrum.

> **Polypectomy snares**
> - Stock small-loop and large-loop snares
> - Maintain an appropriate-sized inventory of snares, so that the "right" snare is available at all times
> - Disposable or multiple-use varieties are acceptable
> - Multi-use snares require careful (time-consuming) reprocessing
> - Specialty snares (e.g. barbed snares) are not necessary for almost all polypectomies
> - Train endoscopic assistants and endoscopists regarding the differences among snares

Polyp retrieval devices

A resected polyp can usually be retrieved from the lumen by suctioning it through the working channel into a specimen trap, or by grasping it within the snare loop and pulling out the scope. Most metal grasper-type retrieval devices can only capture one or two fragments of a resected polyp. The synthetic fiber mesh baskets (such as the "Roth Net" or "Spider Net") function like a butterfly net, and can collect multiple pieces of tissue during one pass; they are useful for retrieving multiple fragments of a large polyp after a piecemeal resection in the proximal colon (Fig 1.7a,b).

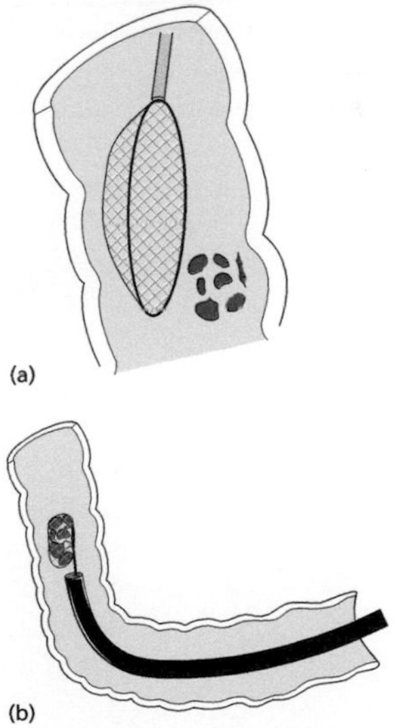

Fig 1.7 **(a)** Use of retrieval net. The net is placed above the fragments and closed. **(b)** Fragments are captured, and the assembly is withdrawn out of the colon.

Specimen traps

Several types of specimen traps are available (Figs 1.8 and 1.9). The single bucket type is best for obtaining a fluid/stool for microbiology; it is adequate for polyp entrapment, but can overflow, causing the polyp to travel into the main suction canister (Fig 1.10). The single chamber, filter type cannot overflow, but cannot collect fluid for microbiology (Fig 1.11). The four chamber type allows polyps from several locations to be caught within one device, but can cause confusion if the site of each polyp is not carefully recorded (Fig 1.8).

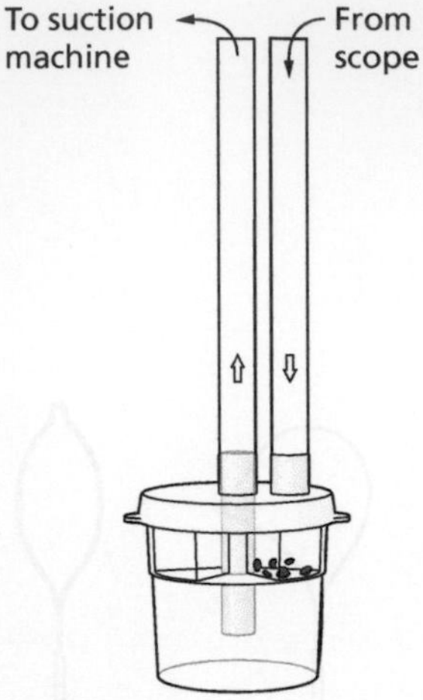

Fig 1.8 Polyp retrieval trap. A compartmented trap permits capture of polyp from different areas of the colon. Even samples taken by biopsy forceps will be caught within the small grid that collects polyps.

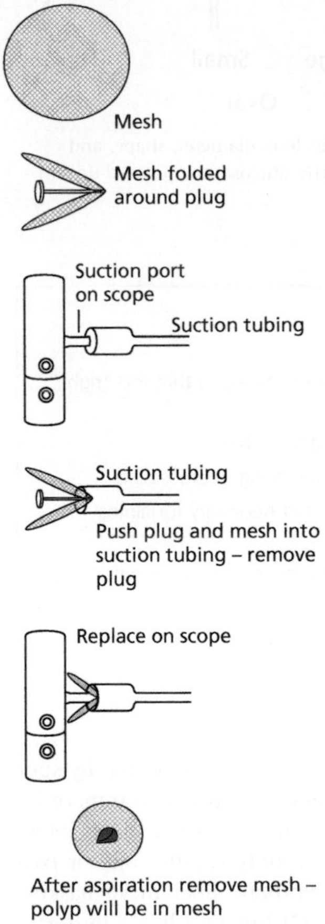

Fig 1.9 Using simple mesh to retrieve polyp specimens. A mesh pad can be inserted between the suction port on the scope and the suction tubing. This will function as a filter, trapping a resected specimen when it is suctioned through the system.

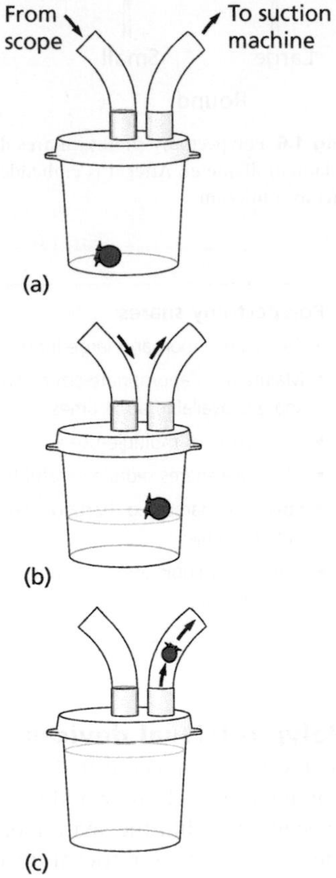

Fig 1.10 The canister-type traps can overflow. This can cause a polyp to be lost (c).

Biopsy forceps

Biopsy forceps are discussed in Chapter 8.

Injection needles

During colonoscopy, there are multiple indications for tissue injection, including elevation of sessile polyps, hemostasis, and tattooing. Injection is accomplished using disposable metal injection needles. These needles have a stiff outer sheath of 2.3–2.8 mm diameter, with a smaller inner channel for fluid passage. The tip of the needle is beveled and the needle size is 21–25 G. The needles are retractable, and must be passed through the working channel in the retracted position in order to avoid an expensive puncture injury to the scope. The needles can be locked in their extended position during introduction of the tip into target tissue. Fluid is pushed from a syringe connected to the sheath. In general, if the tiny needle punctures the full thickness of the colon wall, there is no untoward effect.

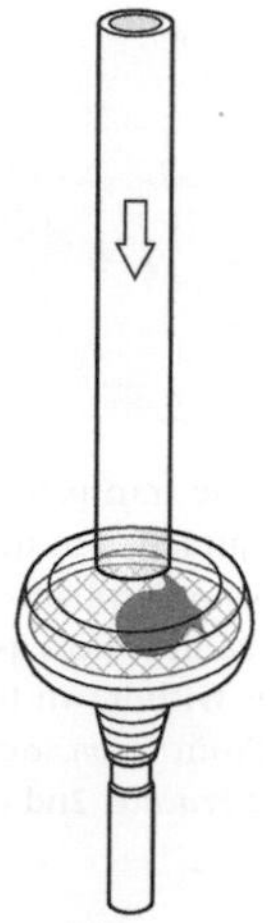

Fig 1.11 Simple filter-type specimen trap. Unlike the canister-type traps, this device cannot overflow with fluid, causing specimen to be lost. However, fluid/stool cannot be captured for microbiological analysis.

Spray catheters

When fluid is pushed through a spray catheter, it is dispersed through multiple fine apertures in the metal nozzle at the catheter's tip, producing a fine mist in a 360° arc. The technique is useful for chromoendoscopy, because it can cover the mucosal surface efficiently and relatively evenly. Spray catheters may be disposable or reusable.

Endoscopy clips

Clipping devices contain two stainless steel, detachable, tweezer-like prongs that are attached by a long delivery catheter to an external control handle. Clips can be used to close a polypectomy site, seal a perforation, mark a lesion (they are radiopaque, and are palpable by a surgeon), clamp a bleeding vessel, or anchor a decompression tube. Numerous clips can be placed on a lesion. Clips can be deployed with the colonoscope in the retroflexed position. Most clip applicators are for single use. Some are applied and fired without the ability to reposition the device, whereas others may be repeatedly opened and closed. Some devices are rotatable, which may help achieve a favorable orientation. The outer plastic sheath is the same diameter as a snare sheath. Once fired, the clip remains attached to the target tissue for 2–4 weeks, after which it sloughs.

Detachable loops

These plastic, non-conductive loops close like a noose around a polyp pedicle and strangulate the large blood vessels that course through the stalk. Their main use is for prevention of bleeding when removing a large pedunculated polyp, but they can also be applied to a bleeding pedicle after polypectomy. Once positioned, the loop is tightened, and then locked shut with a plastic collar controlled by an external handle. In practice, these ligatures have a limited role, partly because the loop has little tensile strength and can become enmeshed in the head of a polyp during attempts to encircle the stalk.

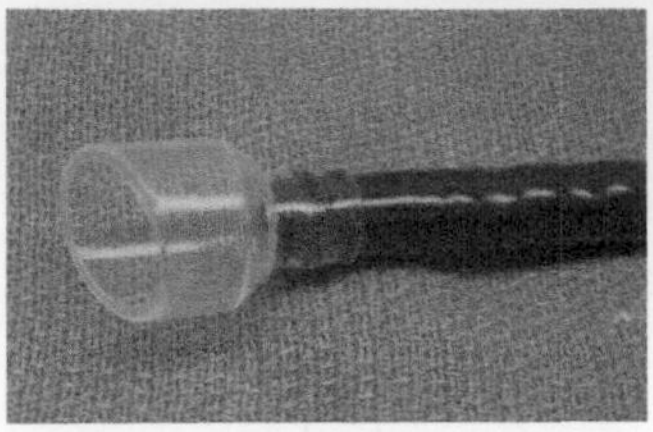

Fig 1.12 Plastic transparent cap. This may be attached to the end of an endoscope and enhance observation behind folds as the instrument is withdrawn through the colon. (From *Colonoscopy: Principles and Practice*, 2nd edition.)

Thermal devices

Thermal devices are discussed in Chapter 9.

Transparent caps

Affixed to the tip of the colonoscope and extending several millimeters beyond the faceplate, these clear plastic cylinders are designed to enhance visualization of the valleys between the haustral folds (Fig 1.12). Several reports suggest that they may increase detection of small polyps, with no decrease in the maneuverability of the scope. A special cap may be used during endoscopic mucosal resection, in a method analogous to variceal banding. Here the mucosal target is suctioned into the cap, and then a snare seated in a small ridge at the tip of the device is closed around the tissue.

Overtubes

Overtubes slide over the scope after it has been straightened in the sigmoid and restrict loop formation and facilitate advancement of the instrument. Overtubes should not be used to straighten a loop, as it may damage the colon wall. Overtubes must be placed on the colonoscope before it is inserted into the colon, effectively shortening the instrument until they are deployed. Originally, overtubes were inserted under fluoroscopic control to ensure that the scope was straight, but "feel" may also be relied upon to deploy this device. With enhancements in scope engineering, overtubes are not commonly used today.

Summary

The modern endoscopy suite should promote safety, efficiency, hygiene, and comfort. Electronic procedure reporting represents an important advance. Careful attention to practice characteristics during the planning phase is essential. The scope is a platform for numerous diagnostic and therapeutic procedures. Improvements in optics and mechanical engineering have enhanced all clinical functions, and further improvements are forthcoming. Multiple accessories are available that support colonoscopic practice.

Further reading

1. Barlow DE. The video colonoscope. In: Waye JD, Rex DK, Williams CB, editors. *Colonoscopy: Principles and Practice*. 2nd ed. Chichester: Wiley-Blackwell; 2009.
2. Croffie J, Carpenter S, Chuttani R, *et al.* ASGE Technology Status Evaluation Report: disposable endoscopic accessories. *Gastrointest Endosc* 2005;62:477–9.
3. Kaltenbach T, Watson R, Shah J, *et al.* Colonoscopy with clipping is useful in the diagnosis and treatment of diverticular bleeding. *Clin Gastroenterol Hepatol* 2012;10:131–7. Epub 2011 Nov 2.
4. Luigiano C, Ferrara F, Ghersi S, *et al.* Endoclip-assisted resection of large pedunculated colorectal polyps: technical aspects and outcome. *Dig Dis Sci* 2010;55:1726–31. Epub 2009 Aug 6.

5. Marasco JA, Marasco RF. Designing the ambulatory endoscopy center. *Gastrointest Endosc Clin N Am* 2002;12:185–204, v.
6. Pike IM. Outpatient endoscopy possibilities for the office. *Gastrointest Endosc Clin N Am* 2002;12:245–58.
7. Schembre DB, Ross AS, Gluck MN, Brandabur JJ, McCormick SE, Lin OS. Spiral overtube-assisted colonoscopy after incomplete colonoscopy in the redundant colon. *Gastrointest Endosc* 2011;73:515–9.
8. Technology Assessment Committe, Barkun A, Liu J, *et al*. Update on endoscopic tissue sampling devices. *Gastrointest Endosc* 2006;63:741–5.
9. Technology Assessment Committee, Chuttani R, Barkun A, *et al*. Endoscopic clip application devices. *Gastrointest Endosc* 2006;63:746–50.
10. de Wijkerslooth TR, Stoop EM, Bossuyt PM, *et al*. Adenoma detection with cap-assisted colonoscopy versus regular colonoscopy: a randomised controlled trial. *Gut* 2012;61:1426–34. Epub 2011 Dec 20.
11. Waye JD, Rex DK, Williams CB, editors. *Colonoscopy: Principles and Practice*. 2nd ed. Chichester: Wiley-Blackwell; 2009.

CHAPTER 2
The Role of the Endoscopy Assistant during Colonoscopy

Introduction

A well-trained endoscopy assistant is crucial to a successful colonoscopy. By providing an additional set of eyes and hands, anticipating the next step in the procedure, and understanding the preferences of the endoscopist, the assistant enhances the efficiency and thoroughness of the procedure, and the safety and comfort of the patient. Perhaps most importantly, the assistant creates an atmosphere that is reassuring to the patient, family, and endoscopist.

Certification and training

Different professional societies provide varying recommendations. The certification of endoscopy assistants reflects the requirements of the hospital, ambulatory endoscopy center, or medical office employing the assistant. In addition, the assistant's training reflects the requirements of national accrediting agencies. Regardless of certification and educational level, proper training of endoscopic assistants is essential. Training may be acquired through didactic courses, written materials, formal testing, or an apprenticeship with observation of procedures. The skills required of an endoscopy assistant are highly specialized and not taught in most general nursing or medical technician educational programs. One reasonable approach is to provide a new recruit with a minimum of a 2-week training period to study didactic materials and observe procedures. After this, a graduated introduction into participation during the procedures is begun, with experienced personnel available to observe, to mentor, and to step in when challenging situations arise. Continuing education programs and competency evaluation should be required of all endoscopic assistants, regardless of seniority.

The endoscopy assistant should wear personal protective equipment. This universally includes gloves, which should be

Practical Colonoscopy, First Edition. Jerome D. Waye, James Aisenberg, and Peter H. Rubin.
© 2013 John Wiley & Sons, Ltd. Published 2013 by John Wiley & Sons, Ltd.

well-fitting, as well as surgical scrubs or a gown. In some cases, a protective mask and/or protective eyewear may be appropriate.

Pre-colonoscopy tasks

• Setting up the procedure room, including readying the stretcher, the endoscopic equipment, the monitoring equipment, the accessories (e.g. irrigation syringes, biopsy forceps, polypectomy snares), and the electrosurgical equipment.
• Preparing the materials for intravenous sedation, including medications and supplies required for intravenous access.
• Turning on and testing the endoscopic equipment.
• Conducting a pre-procedure assessment regarding the patient's medical history, medications, most recent oral intake, drug and food allergies, bowel preparation protocol and its results, answering any last-minute questions, and availability of a post-procedure escort. The assistant should remind the endoscopist immediately before the procedure of immediate issues, such as relevant allergies, systemic anticoagulant, antiplatelet drug utilization, or the presence of a defibrillator or prosthetic cardiac valves.
• Escorting the patient to the changing room, and/or restroom.
• Reassuring and calming the patient.
• Escorting the patient into the procedure room, and applying the hemodynamic and respiratory monitoring equipment.
• Obtaining and recording initial blood pressure, oxygen saturation, and pulse readings.
• Preparing all documents or electronic records to record intraprocedural data.
• Notifying the colonoscopist and/or anesthesiologist when the patient is ready.
• Positioning the patient in the left lateral decubitus position.
• Adjusting and securing a safety belt around the patient's waist (Fig 2.1).
• In some endoscopy centers, the assistant obtains informed consent, but many experts recommend that the colonoscopist performs this task.

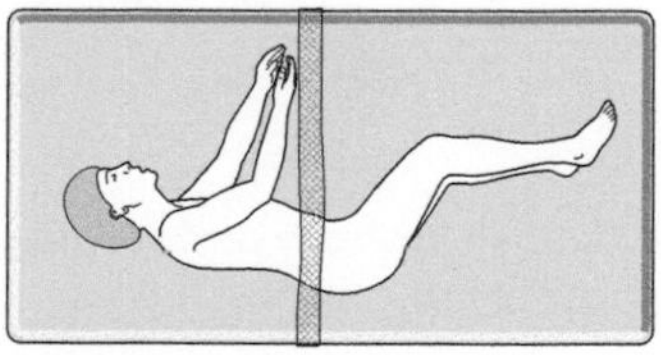

Fig 2.1 The safety strap. This is attached snugly around the patient's waist in order to prevent falls. It is detached or loosened as needed when the patient is repositioned.

Intra-colonoscopy tasks

1. Assisting with sedation

Dosing amount, drug choice, and bolus timing is determined by the colonoscopist; the endoscopic assistant may, in some instances, be instructed to inject sedative medications under observation, although some endoscopists prefer to inject them personally.

During the examination, the colonoscopist's visual attention is focused principally on studying the colonoscopic image. Therefore, the assistant monitors the patient's depth of sedation, by observing the patient, and by observing the cardiopulmonary monitors. The assistant should be vigilant for evidence of undersedation, such as restlessness or pain, or of oversedation, such as loss

Clinical signs monitored by assistant during case

- Cardiopulmonary status
  - Direct observation of patient
  - Observation of monitors
- Depth of sedation
- Adequacy of analgesia
- Level of abdominal distension
- Patient position on stretcher
- Functionality of intravenous access

of responsiveness to voice and touch, pallor/cyanosis, hypoxia, hypotension, tachycardia, or decreased chest excursions. If evidence of over- or undersedation appears, the assistant should immediately inform the colonoscopist and, if appropriate, take other actions.

2. Assisting with advancing the colonoscope

The endoscopic assistant performs maneuvers that promote safe and efficient cecal intubation. The most common is application of manual pressure to the anterior abdominal wall, which creates resistance to looping. The site of compression is generally selected by the colonoscopist, and reflects the location of the loop or a site where the scope advances. Successful pressure is required usually for less than 30 seconds, until the problem is solved or another tactic is selected. If the first abdominal compression site does not help with scope advancement, other sites on the abdominal wall can be compressed. Usually the sites of compression correspond to colonic anatomic turns (sigmoid, splenic, or hepatic flexures). On occasion, a two-handed (or "sandwich") technique may be useful.

A second useful maneuver is to reposition the patient. This is most commonly performed when the instrument fails to advance through the ascending colon to the cecum. In this situation, the supine position is usually most helpful. When the sedated patient is supine, the right knee must be flexed in order to allow the colonoscopist to maneuver the colonoscope. If the patient is awake enough to cooperate, the patient will be able to maintain a flexed-knee position. If not, the assistant holds the knee in the proper position. Alternatively, the safety belt from around the patient's waist can be repositioned around the knee to maintain the flexed position. Once examination of the cecum and ascending colon is complete, it is generally best to return the patient to the left lateral position.

The assistant may be requested to hold the shaft of the colonoscope briefly to prevent the scope slipping back while both the endoscopist's hands are manipulating the controls for tip deflection. The assistant is responsible also for ensuring that surgical lubricant and gauze sponges are handy throughout the case.

3. Enhancing mucosal inspection

Fecal debris, fluid, and bubbles often obscure visualization of parts of the colon. Many newer colonoscopes accommodate an integrated irrigation system. However, often the assistant will need to manually flush fluid through the working channel of the colonoscope to help clean the mucosa, to dislodge large particle debris that can clog the channel, and/or to deliver anti-foaming agents. An additional pair of trained eyes directed at the colonoscopic monitor can increase polyp detection. Endoscopic assistants should therefore look for polyps during the colonoscopy when they are not occupied with other tasks. A physician's narration of the procedure during the examination is a valuable teaching tool, and helps to engage the assistant in the colonoscopy and to promote the assistant's professional satisfaction.

4. Monitoring the abdomen

A small degree of abdominal distension during colonoscopy is inevitable and clinically insignificant. However, excessive distension of the abdomen can impair respiratory function, cause pain, prolong recovery, impact hemodynamic function, and even cause perforation. The assistant must monitor the patient for over-distension, palpating the abdomen before the procedure begins in order to establish the baseline and periodically during the examination. If the assistant detects over-distension, the colonoscopist should be notified immediately.

5. Assisting with biopsy, polypectomy, and other interventions

Colonoscopic interventions require close coordination between the colonoscopist and the assistant. An adjustment in the snare position of one or two millimeters may represent the difference between complete and incomplete polypectomy, or between perforation and safe resection. If during a procedure an assistant is not comfortable with a particular intervention, then the endoscopist should be informed or a more experienced assistant summoned.

The assistant must be certain that the procedure room is stocked with the appropriate ancillary equipment, and know the location of each item. Upon request, the assistant is responsible for testing the accessory and making all necessary preparations such as priming an injection catheter or marking a snare. Once the tool is prepared and tested, the assistant should place it into the outstretched fingertips of the colonoscopist into a pencil-grip position. "No-look" technique allows transfer to occur without the endoscopist's eyes leaving the monitor (Fig 2.2). All tools should be transferred closed, with any sharp points concealed, to prevent inadvertent provider injury or damage to the colonoscope. If electrocautery usage is planned, the assistant is responsible for placing the grounding pad on the patient's leg or hip, and adjusting the current delivery. If the team plans to retrieve a specimen by suction, the assistant should place a tissue trap before the resection is performed.

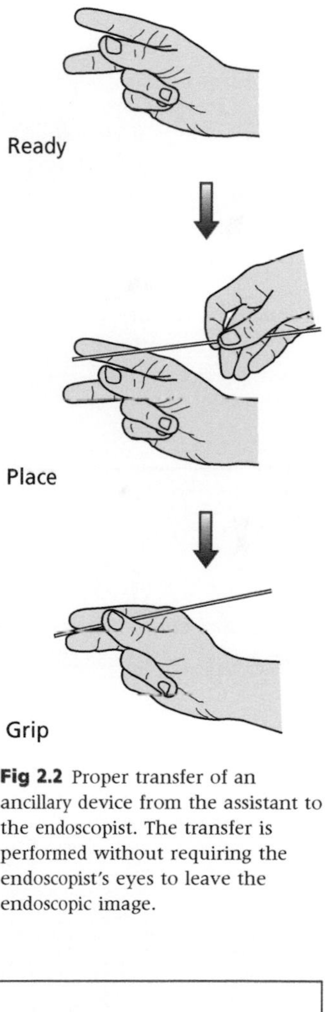

Fig 2.2 Proper transfer of an ancillary device from the assistant to the endoscopist. The transfer is performed without requiring the endoscopist's eyes to leave the endoscopic image.

"No-look" transfer of forceps/snare

- Endoscopist extends right hand in "dart-throw" position (Fig 2.2)
- Assistant places tool between thumb and index finger of endoscopist's right hand, with approximately one inch of tool extending to left of endoscopist's hand
- Using right hand and tactile sense only, endoscopist locates suction cap, punctures cap with tool, and advances tool through working channel
- Endoscopist's gaze never leaves image on video monitor
- Assistants must be trained in nuances of tool transfer

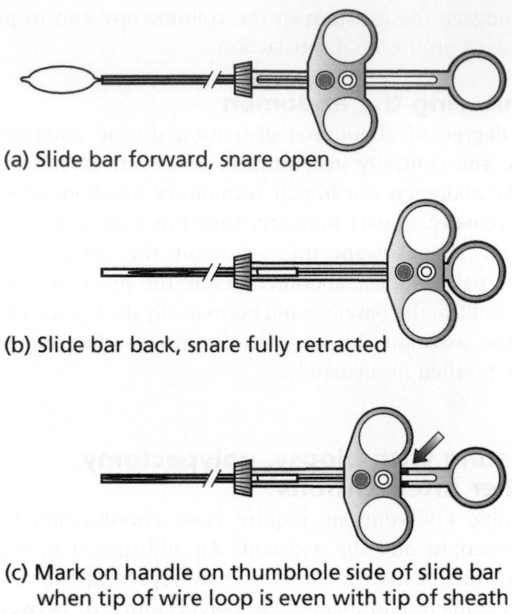
(a) Slide bar forward, snare open
(b) Slide bar back, snare fully retracted
(c) Mark on handle on thumbhole side of slide bar when tip of wire loop is even with tip of sheath

Fig 2.3 Marking the snare handle.

Once the device has been passed through the entire working channel and the tip appears in the colonoscopic image, the assistant must execute precisely the endoscopist's requests. The assistant must be familiar with the nuances of snare control, such as how far to open the snare, how rapidly the snare should be closed, and how tight to squeeze the snare around a polyp (Fig 2.3). Occasionally during difficult polypectomy or biopsy, it is useful for the assistant to function as the colonoscopist's "third hand," either by advancing the ancillary tool through the working channel (thus allowing the colonoscopist to use two hands to maintain a precise colonoscope tip position), or by gripping the colonoscope insertion tube near its entry into the anal canal and maintaining axial pressure and torque (thus freeing the colonoscopist's right hand for advancing the ancillary tool). Some colonoscopists prefer to take the snare handle and to guillotine the polyp themselves as they simultaneously apply electrocautery current.

After the intervention is completed, the assistant is responsible for placing the accessory in an appropriate receptacle for additional use, reprocessing, or discarding. When tissue is retrieved via suction, the assistant is responsible for checking the trap and confirming when the polyp has been successfully retrieved. This may involve delicately sifting through debris in order to identify small fragments of tissue. The endoscopy assistant is responsible for transferring tissue into formalin and for proper labeling of the specimen container. The assistant records the location and size of the lesion.

When the injection catheter is used, the assistant is responsible for preparing and drawing up the injection fluid, priming the needle, and retracting it before it is handed to the doctor. Once the catheter is deployed, the assistant extends the needle and injects the fluid, following the colonoscopist's direction regarding the timing and volume.

6. Troubleshooting

Like any complex mechanical/electronic system, colonoscopy equipment is subject to malfunctions, which may occur during the procedure. Many procedural snags can be solved by simple maneuvers, such as rebooting the computer or unclogging the working channel of the colonoscope.

Trouble shooting air/water failure

Cause	Solution
Nozzle at tip of scope clogged	• Flush with water, air, pull out scope and manually clean nozzle, or change scope
Air/water button malfunctions	• Reattach or replace air/water button
Water bottle malfunctions	• Add/remove water from bottle • Ensure bottle top is screwed on tightly • Ensure bottle is properly connected to scope • Change water bottle • Change O-ring
Scope incompletely inserted into light source	• Firmly push scope into light source
The air control on light source set to "off"	• Push "on" control

Troubleshooting suction failure

Cause	Solution
Suction button channel clogged	• Clean or replace button
Cap on working channel not providing adequate seal	• Readjust or replace cap
Colonoscope working channel clogged	• Flush channel with water • Remove suction button and then seal suction port with index finger, creating stronger suction force • "Back-suction" channel (remove suction cap and place end of suction tube over suction port at scope handle) • Mechanically unclog by passing cleaning brush through handle antegrade and retrograde suction port in scope • Change colonoscopes
Suction failure "proximal" to scope	• Ensure pump turned on • Ensure tubing not clogged, kinked, or compressed • Empty suction waste container • Increase suction force with dial control on pump • Replace pump filter • Change pump

When to recruit additional personnel into endoscopy room

- Equipment malfunction despite basic troubleshooting
- Clinically unstable patient
- Assistant unfamiliar with specialized intervention
- Complex procedure that requires "extra pair of hands"
- Hard-to-sedate patient
- Difficult intraprocedure decision
- Difficult colonic intubation

7. Assisting with intraprocedural decision-making

Ideally, the colonoscopist and assistant are experienced and skilled and enjoy mutual trust. In this situation, the endoscopy assistant often serves as a useful sounding board or source for ideas and approaches to a colonoscopic problem. If the endoscopist is inexperienced, a thoughtful, experienced endoscopy assistant is particularly helpful. If the assistant is inexperienced, the endoscopist should narrate the decision-making thought process to educate the assistant.

Post-procedure tasks

In a large facility with one large central recovery room, the recovering patient is "handed off" to a recovery team, whereas in a smaller facility with individual recovery rooms, the endoscopic assistant may also be responsible in assisting the patient after the procedure.

Most endoscopists use room air to distend the large bowel. This can cause some abdominal discomfort after the procedure. Excess gaseous bowel distention can often be rapidly decompressed by changing the position from left lateral (when air rises and is trapped in the right colon) to the right lateral so that the air will rise into the sigmoid and be expelled (Fig 2.4).

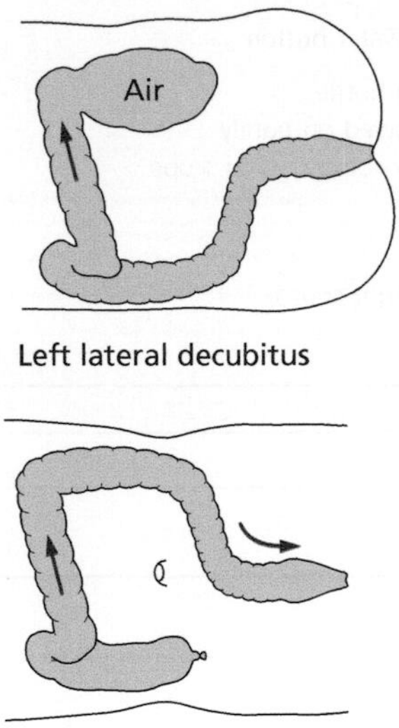

(a) Left lateral decubitus

(b) Right lateral decubitus

Fig 2.4 Rotating the patient from the left lateral position (a) into the prone or right lateral position (b) after colonoscopy will help the air to "rise" out of the colon.

Post-procedure tasks required of the endoscopic assistant may include:

- detaching the patient from the intravenous and/or monitoring equipment;
- transporting the patient to the recovery room;
- connecting post-procedure monitoring equipment;
- monitoring the post-procedure recovery of the patient, including vital signs and alertness score;
- bringing the patient juice or a snack once the level of consciousness permits;
- obtaining the patients' consent for discharge;
- reviewing discharge instructions with the patient;
- discharging the patient from the endoscopy area;
- recording all intraprocedural medication usage, including maintaining a narcotic log;
- documenting all elements of the procedure;
- recording any adverse events or incidents;
- transporting the endoscopic and ancillary equipment to the dirty utility room for reprocessing;
- cleaning the procedure room, including discarding all biohazardous materials;
- discarding all unused medication;
- reprocessing the colonoscope and ancillary equipment.

Further reading

1. Aisenberg J. Endoscopic sedation: equipment and personnel. *Gastrointest Endosc Clin N Am* 2008;18:641–9, vii.
2. ASGE Standards of Practice Committee, Jain R, Ikenberry SO, *et al.* Minimum staffing requirements for the performance of GI endoscopy. *Gastrointest Endosc* 2010;72:469–70. Epub 2010 Jun 26.
3. Bohlander S, Grand A, Kelsey L, *et al.* Standards of professional performance and standards of practice for the gastroenterology and/or endoscopy setting. *Gastroenterol Nurs* 2005; 28:422–7.
4. Dykes CA. The gastrointestinal assistant during colonoscopy. In: Waye JD, Rex DK, Williams CB (eds). *Colonoscopy. Principles and Practice.* 2nd ed. Chichester: Wiley-Blackwell; 2009.
5. Herron-Rice L, Girard D, Anderson P, *et al.* SGNA Guideline. Guideline for performance of flexible sigmoidoscopy by registered nurses for the purpose of colorectal cancer screening. *Gastroenterol Nurs* 2009;32: 427–30.
6. McAloose B, Gruber M. SGNA standards for practice for gastroenterology nurses and associates. *Gastroenterol Nurs* 1990;12:229–31.
7. Society of Gastroenterology Nurses and Associates (SGNA). *Minimum registered nurse staffing for patient care in the gastrointestinal endoscopy unit.* Available at: http://www.sgna.org/Portals/0/Education/Position%20Statements/MinimumStaffingPositionStatement.pdf (accessed November 22, 2012).
8. Society of Gastroenterology Nurses and Associates (SGNA). *Joint Position Statement: Role of GI registered nurses in the management of patients undergoing sedated procedures.* Available at: http://www.sgna.org/Portals/0/Education/Position%20Statements/ASGESGNASedationPositionStatement.pdf. (accessed November 22, 2012).
9. Society of Gastroenterology Nurses and Associates (SGNA) Practice Committee. Role delineation of unlicensed assistive personnel in gastroenterology. *Gastroenterol Nurs* 2006;29:64–5.
10. Society of Gastroenterology Nurses and Associates (SGNA). SGNA guidelines for nursing care of the patient receiving sedation and analgesia in the gastrointestinal endoscopy setting. *Gastroenterol Nurs* 2000;23:125–9.
11. Society of Gastroenterology Nurses and Associates (SGNA). *SGNA Position Statement: Role delineation of Assistive Personnel.* Available at: http://www.sgna.org/Portals/0/Education/Position%20Statements/NAP2010PositionStatement.pdf (accessed November 22, 2012).
12. Voynarovska M, Cohen LB. The role of the endoscopy nurse or assistant in endoscopic sedation. *Gastrointest Endosc Clin N Am* 2008;18:695–705, viii.

CHAPTER 3

Indications and Contraindications for Colonoscopy

Introduction

Because colonoscopy is generally safe and allows both mucosal visualization and therapeutic intervention (biopsy, resection, cauterization), it has numerous indications and few contraindications. The yield of a colonoscopy performed for an accepted indication is higher than for a non-accepted indication. Several gastrointestinal professional societies have published guidelines regarding appropriate indications for colonoscopy.

Specific indications

Investigation of overt or occult bleeding

In the setting of gastrointestinal bleeding of undetermined origin, colonoscopy may be both diagnostic and therapeutic. Evidence of bleeding may be in the form of bright red blood per rectum (BRBPR), a positive fecal occult blood test (FOBT), or an unexplained anemia and/or iron deficiency. These signs may portend the presence of a potentially curable colon neoplasm. BRBPR often arises from hemorrhoids or other anal pathology, especially if sporadic, separate from or only on the surface of the bowel movement, seen dripping into the bowl, or only on the tissue after wiping. Blood on the surface of the stool may also arise from a neoplasm in the left colon. Although false-positive FOBT is common, when it is found without visible bleeding, particularly if associated with an iron-deficiency anemia, it raises the possibility of a neoplasm in the more proximal colon.

Abnormal radiological imaging

Radiology may detect colonic abnormalities incidentally or during imaging directed specifically at the colon. The abnormalities may be diffuse, such as colonic thickening on computed tomography (CT) scan or increased uptake on a positron emission tomography (PET) scan, or localized, such as a discrete mass. Any significant colonic mass should be investigated by colonoscopy. The best approach to small polyps found during CT colonography is a matter of debate. Some experts advocate radiographic surveillance, whereas others promote colonoscopy. If wall thickening or other diffuse abnormalities are detected, the approach is based on the clinical context. If the finding reflects under-distension of the colon during imaging, then usually colonoscopy can be avoided. However, if there is suspicion of a clinically significant process, then colonoscopy can be diagnostic. Abnormal imaging can contraindicate colonoscopy if it indicates acute diverticulitis, toxic colonic distension, or gastrointestinal obstruction.

Irritable bowel syndrome

In general, long-standing symptoms that are highly suggestive of irritable bowel syndrome do not warrant colonoscopy. However, the diagnosis of irritable bowel syndrome may require excluding infection, mechanical obstruction, inflammatory bowel disease, or microscopic colitis. If the symptoms are pronounced, the pattern is changing, or the patient describes "warning signs," such as weight loss, anorexia, nocturnal symptoms, or bleeding, then colonoscopy is indicated.

Diarrhea

Colonoscopy is rarely indicated for acute, non-bloody diarrhea, which is usually infectious, self-limited, and can be managed symptomatically. If the diarrhea is bloody, the differential diagnosis also includes idiopathic colitis and ischemic colitis, for both of which colonoscopy with biopsy may be diagnostic. For chronic non-bloody diarrhea, colonoscopy is used to rule out inflammatory bowel disease (particularly

Practical Colonoscopy, First Edition. Jerome D. Waye, James Aisenberg, and Peter H. Rubin.
© 2013 John Wiley & Sons, Ltd. Published 2013 by John Wiley & Sons, Ltd.

Crohn's disease) and to search for microscopic colitis. If Crohn's disease is being considered, the terminal ileum should be inspected. As the macroscopic appearance of microscopic colitis is often normal, the diagnosis requires random biopsies from the proximal and distal colon, which may reveal infiltration of lymphocytes in the lamina propria or a thickened collagen band beneath the epithelium.

Constipation

In general, colonoscopy is not useful in the evaluation of stable mild or moderate chronic constipation. If the patient's constipation is worsening, colonoscopy may be worthwhile to look for a narrowed sigmoid diverticular segment, an atonic colon, a tumor (either intrinsic or extrinsic), or a twist (e.g. volvulus). If mechanical obstruction is a possibility, care must be taken not to overinflate the colon, as the blockage may act as a one-way valve and trap the insufflated air, resulting in perforation. If severe constipation is related to colonic inertia, the colon may appear dilated and flaccid, and melanosis coli from chronic laxative use may be noted.

Inflammatory bowel disease

Colonoscopy is commonly used to evaluate the activity, severity, and extent of inflammatory bowel disease. Colonoscopic findings can guide therapy; for instance, if the disease is primarily distal, a topical approach may be indicated; if the disease is diffuse and severe, an immediate "step up" in therapy may be required. Colonoscopy also allows assessment of the effectiveness of treatment and mucosal healing.

Individuals who have chronic idiopathic colitis are at increased risk for colorectal cancer (CRC). Colonoscopy with biopsy is used as a surveillance tool for precancerous changes (dysplasia) in this setting. The optimal intervals and techniques for colitis surveillance are subject to debate. It is generally believed that the CRC risk is influenced by the duration (8–10 years of greater) and anatomical extent of the colitis (one-third or more of the colon). Thus, a patient with chronic proctosigmoiditis is considered to be at relatively low risk whereas a patient with long-standing pan colitis is at higher risk. Colonoscopy with biopsy is recommended beginning 8–10 years after the onset of symptoms in patients with extensive ulcerative or Crohn's colitis, and is repeated annually or every 2 years. There is some consideration that after 20 years of disease the interval for surveillance should be reduced. Most colonoscopists obtain four-quadrant biopsies approximately every 10 cm from the cecum to rectum, corresponding to eight different segments of the colon (cecum, ascending, hepatic flexure, transverse colon, splenic flexure, descending colon, sigmoid, and rectum). The addition of chromoendoscopy and targeted biopsy during surveillance examinations may increase the yield for dysplasia.

Idiopathic colitis surveillance recommendations

- Risk arising from ulcerative colitis and Crohn's colitis is similar
- Perform in extensive (>35 cm) ulcerative colitis or Crohn's colitis after 8–10 years' disease duration
- Where possible, perform surveillance when colitis is in remission
- Obtain four-quadrant biopsies every 10 cm throughout affected colon; for pan colitis, at least 32 biopsies recommended
- Obtain targeted biopsy from any suspicious area
- Repeat colonoscopy/biopsy every 1–3 years depending on patient's risk status
- Consider pan-colonic chromoendoscopy to enhance mucosal discrimination
- For dysplastic polyps that can be removed completely, perform colonoscopic polypectomy and obtain biopsies around polyp rim to ensure no contiguous dysplasia
- Consider colectomy if polyp is not amenable to complete colonoscopic resection, if dysplasia is multifocal, or if polyp does not resemble a typical adenoma
- Intensify surveillance if:
  - previous dysplasia;
  - concurrent primary sclerosing cholangitis;
  - family history of colorectal cancer in first-degree relative;
  - chronic moderate or severe inflammation;
  - stricture in ulcerative colitis.

Colonoscopy to assess early post-operative recurrence of Crohn's disease

- Often recommended in high-risk individuals 6–12 months after ileocolic resection
- Findings often guide drug treatment decisions
- When possible, perform deep ileal intubation and biopsy
- Report extent and severity of recurrence
- Ulceration at the rim of the anastomosis may be post-surgical and not reflective of recurrent Crohn's disease

Factors that increase colon cancer risk in chronic colitis

- Duration of disease
- Anatomic extent of disease
- Family history of CRC
- Degree of endoscopic and histologic activity
- Previous dysplasia
- Early age of onset
- Primary sclerosing cholangitis

Colorectal cancer screening

Screening for CRC and its precursors is the most common indication for colonoscopy. Optical colonoscopy remains the gold standard. The goal of screening is to detect polyps, neoplasia and cancers before they progress to a stage at which colonoscopic and surgical therapies are no longer curative. Early intervention in the step-wise progression toward colon cancer is crucial. Usually any dysplastic polyp detected during screening is resected.

CRC screening guidelines

Risk profile	Age when screening begins (years)
• Average-risk	• 50*
• One first-degree relative with CRC/advanced adenoma diagnosed <60 years • Two first-degree relatives with CRC or advanced adenoma	• 40, or • 10 years younger than age at diagnosis of the youngest affected relative
• Family history of polyposis syndrome (e.g. hereditary non-polyposis colon cancer or familial adenomatous polyposis)	• Screening begins in childhood/early adulthood depending on syndrome • Refer for genetic counseling/testing

*consider age 45 years in African Americans, heavy smokers, morbidly obese

Unfortunately, a large number of individuals who could benefit from screening never undergo it. There are significant barriers to screening, and marked disparities in adherence rates among different cultural and socioeconomic groups continue to exist. Some progress toward adherence to screening guidelines has occurred over the past decade.

Screening guidelines have been published by expert task forces and gastroenterology societies. Average-risk adults who are asymptomatic and who have no first-degree family history of colon polyps or cancer should receive CRC screening by age 50 and every 5–10 years thereafter. Patients with a positive family history in a first-degree relative with colonic neoplasia should undergo colonoscopic screening examination at age 40, or 10 years before the proband was diagnosed with CRC. If there is a history of a familial colorectal cancer syndrome such as hereditary non-polyposis colon cancer (HNPCC) or familial adenomatous polyposis, screening should begin earlier and be more frequent. In this setting, genetic counseling and gene testing may be helpful.

Post-polypectomy surveillance

Colon polyps tend to recur. Recurrence may be either at the site of polypectomy or, more commonly, a new polyp may arise *de novo* at another site. Once a premalignant polyp is resected, surveillance colonoscopy is performed at an interval shorter than every 10 years. These intervals are based on expert guidelines. The recommended surveillance intervals depend on the number, size, and histology of the index polyps. Multiple polyps, large polyps, and polyps with advanced histology require more frequent or earlier follow-up examinations.

Post-polypectomy surveillance guidelines

Adenomatous polyps

Lesion(s) found	Surveillance interval (years)
none	10
1 or 2 adenomas <1 cm with only low-grade dysplasia	5
3–10 adenomas Adenoma with villous features Adenoma with high-grade dysplasia	3
>10 adenomas	Shorter interval (<3) at discretion of physician; consider genetic evaluation
Sessile adenomas removed piecemeal	Bring back in 2–6 months to verify complete removal
HNPCC confirmed	1

Post-polypectomy surveillance

Serrated polyps

Lesion(s) found	Surveillance interval (years)
Diminutive hyperplastic polyps in recto-sigmoid	10
1 or 2 serrated polyps <1 cm proximal to splenic flexure	5
Serrated lesion with cytological dysplasia >3 serrated lesions proximal to splenic flexure Serrated lesion >1 cm	3
Serrated lesion removed piecemeal	2–6 months (to inspect site)
Serrated polyposis	1

The most commonly accepted guidelines call for surveillance: in 5 years if one to two small adenomas are removed; in 3 years if three to ten adenomas are removed, or with adenomas >1 cm, or with villous components; and with shorter intervals at the discretion of the colonoscopist if the resection was performed piecemeal, of if more than ten polyps were removed. Guidelines for surveillance intervals for serrated lesions have not yet been published, but will probably parallel the adenoma guidelines.

If the colonoscopist is uncertain that the polypectomy was complete, then follow-up in 3–6 months to reexamine the site is reasonable. If a polyposis syndrome is suspected, genetic testing and shorter surveillance intervals should be considered, as well as screening of other organs (including the upper gastrointestinal tract) where indicated.

Post-colon-cancer resection surveillance

Post-cancer-resection surveillance recommendations

- If colon not cleared of synchronous lesions before CRC surgery, perform colonoscopy 3–6 months after surgery (unless metastatic disease)
- If no metastatic disease at surgery, perform colonoscopy 1 year after surgery
- If year 1 examination is negative, perform next exam 3 years later
- If year 3 exam is normal, extend interval to 5 years
- Special circumstances when shorter intervals may be appropriate:
  - polyposis syndrome (e.g. HNPCC);
  - rectal lesions (to screen for local recurrence—rigid or flexible proctosigmoidoscopy may be adequate);
  - multiple adenomas detected on post-surgery surveillance.

Once a CRC has been surgically resected, the recurrence rate at the anastomosis is low and will occur usually within a few years of the resection. Most recurrences of the primary tumor occur in the liver or abdominal cavity, and cannot be diagnosed colonoscopically. Thus the main indication for colonoscopy after cancer resection is to detect metachronous cancers or polyps. Recent guidelines suggest that a follow-up colonoscopic examination should be performed 1 year after surgical resection of a colorectal carcinoma. If this procedure reveals no new lesions, the next examination should follow 3 years later. Surgical resection of rectal cancer may require more frequent follow-up examinations, as the risk of local recurrence in this area is higher than in the more proximal colon.

Miscellaneous diagnostic indications

- Rectal bleeding (overt or occult)
- Iron-deficiency anemia
- Chronic diarrhea
- New or worsening constipation
- Abnormality on CT scan, PET scan, or barium enema
- Surveillance after removal of neoplasm
- Surveillance in chronic ulcerative or Crohn's colitis
- Unexplained abdominal/pelvic pain
- CRC screening
- Idiopathic colitis: determination of disease extent/activity and/or response to therapy
- Intraoperative identification of a previously identified lesion not apparent at surgery

Miscellaneous therapeutic indications
- Removal of foreign body
- Excision of polyp
- Treatment of acute or chronic colonic bleeding
- Decompression of colonic pseudo-obstruction (Ogilvie syndrome)
- Decompression of volvulus
- Intramucosal injection of drug
- Dilation/stenting of symptomatic colonic stricture
  - Benign
  - Malignant
- Marking (tattooing) site of lesion before surgical resection

Absolute contraindications to colonoscopy
- Toxic megacolon
- Fulminant colitis
- Free colonic perforation
- Patient refuses consent
- Patient cannot cooperate with the procedure

Relative contraindications to colonoscopy
- Acute diverticulitis
- Inadequate colonic cleansing
- Recent myocardial infarction, pulmonary embolism, or clinical instability for any other cause
- Immediately post-colonic surgery (recent anastomosis)
- Severe coagulopathy

Colonoscopy during pregnancy

Colonoscopy is relatively contraindicated during pregnancy, but it may be performed if benefits outweigh the risks. There are few data, particularly during the first trimester. The theoretical risk to the fetus is least during the second trimester: in the first, the risk of teratogenicity is believed to be highest, and in the third the risk of premature labor is highest. Most reports suggest that the procedure is fairly well tolerated by both fetus and mother, that cecal intubation can be achieved, and that the procedure confers important benefits in the majority of well-selected cases. Sedation with propofol by an anesthesiologist is generally recommended, although the alternative of benzodiazepine/opioid-based sedation is safe as well. A polyethylene glycol (PEG)-based colon cleansing preparation is recommended.

The most common indications in pregnancy are lower gastrointestinal bleeding, active colitis, or unexplained obstruction. The gastroenterologist should collaborate with the obstetrician. The lightest acceptable sedation should be used, and the scope tip should be advanced the minimum distance needed to achieve the goal of the procedure.

Pediatric colonoscopy

Pre-procedure considerations

Colonoscopy in the infant or child differs from adult colonoscopy in the spectrum of diseases and the technical challenges. In communities in which pediatric gastroenterologists are available, colonoscopy for infants and toddlers may be performed by an individual with this subspecialty training. The colonoscopist and assistant should be familiar with the potential peculiarities of pediatric anatomy and physiology.

The pediatric colonoscope should be used for patients younger than 3–5 years of age. It has a smaller diameter than the adult colonoscope (11.3 mm versus 12.8 mm) and a shaft that is more flexible. The tip of the scope can be deflected at more acute angles to facilitate navigation of the pediatric bowel. An adult colonoscope can be used in older pediatric patients.

Bowel preparation in the pediatric patient is normally uncomplicated. In the infant, substituting clear liquids for breast or bottle feedings for 12–24 hours and administering small-volume saline enemas is usually effective. In older children, osmotic agents such as PEG-electrolyte are recommended, with the dosage adjusted for the patient's weight. If the oral solution cannot be tolerated, administration via nasogastric tube can be considered, as can a prolonged fasting period (48–72 hours) followed by oral magnesium citrate and enemas.

In general, deeper sedation is required because children are less likely than adults to cooperate with the exam. In many instances, general anesthesia is preferred. When conscious sedation is utilized, an additional endoscopy assistant may be required solely to attend to the sedation. Personnel must be experienced in the sedation and resuscitation of the pediatric patient, and pediatric-sized resuscitation equipment must be available.

Indications and contraindications

The major indications for pediatric colonoscopy are rectal bleeding, chronic unexplained diarrhea or constipation, an abnormal radiographic finding, abdominal pain, and abnormal growth.

Common scenarios in the pediatric patient include the following.

- Suspicion of inflammatory bowel disease or infectious colitis. These entities may appear similar colonoscopically and histologically. Stool culture may be useful.
- Colonic tuberculosis, schistosomiasis, and amebiasis can be definitively diagnosed on colon biopsy, even in the setting of negative stool cultures.
- Pinworm infection can be diagnosed via direct colonoscopic visualization of motile parasites.
- Lymphonodular hyperplasia in the terminal ileum is an incidental finding in pediatric patients but can be confused with Crohn's disease.
- In patients who have undergone a small bowel transplant, regular surveillance ileoscopy with biopsy will allow for assessment of graft rejection.
- Flexible sigmoidoscopy with biopsy is used in infants presenting with bleeding due to a suspected cow's milk or soy protein allergy. Biopsies may reveal high numbers of eosinophils in the lamina propria and muscularis mucosa.
- Therapeutic applications of colonoscopy include polypectomy, ablation of bleeding vessels, retrieval of a foreign body, decompression of megacolon, balloon dilation of strictures, and placement of a percutaneous cecostomy tube.
- In the pediatric population, dysplasia screening and surveillance colonoscopy may be indicated with unusual cancer risk factors, such as chronic colitis (in older pediatric patients) or a familial polyposis syndrome.

As in adults the contraindications to pediatric colonoscopy include toxic colitis and suspected bowel perforation. Relative contraindications include bleeding disorders and recent bowel surgery.

Summary

The risks, benefits and alternatives to colonoscopy should be considered and discussed with each patient. When appropriately indicated and carefully performed, colonoscopy is a widely indicated, safe, and effective diagnostic and therapeutic tool.

Further reading

1. ASGE Standards of Practice Committee, Lee KK, Anderson MA, *et al.* Modifications in endoscopic practice for pediatric patients. *Gastrointest Endosc* 2008;67:1–9.
2. ASGE Standards of Practice Committee, Shen B, Khan K, *et al.* The role of endoscopy in the management of patients with diarrhea. *Gastrointest Endosc* 2010;71:887–92. Epub 2010 Mar 25.
3. Cappell MS. Risks versus benefits of gastrointestinal endoscopy during pregnancy. *Nat Rev Gastroenterol Hepatol* 2011;8:610–34.
4. Chan G, Fefferman DS, Farrell RJ. Endoscopic assessment of inflammatory bowel disease: colonoscopy/esophagogastroduodenoscopy. *Gastroenterol Clin North Am* 2012;41:271–90.
5. Rex DK, Johnson DA, Lieberman DA, Burt RW, Sonnenberg A. Colorectal cancer prevention 2000: screening recommendations of the American College of Gastroenterology. *Am J Gastroenterol* 2000;95:868–77.
6. Goddard AF, James MW, McIntyre AS, Scott BB; British Society of Gastroenterology. Guidelines for the management of iron deficiency anaemia. *Gut* 2011;60:1309–16. Epub 2011 May 11.
7. Kiesslich R, Fritsch J, Holtmann M, *et al.* Methylene blue-aided chromoendoscopy for the detection of intraepithelial neoplasia and colon cancer in ulcerative colitis. *Gastroenterology* 2003;124:880–8.
8. Lieberman DA. Clinical practice. Screening for colorectal cancer. *N Engl J Med* 2009;361:1179–87.
9. Lieberman DA, Rex DK, Winawer SJ, Giardiello FM, Johnson DA, Levin TR. Guidelines for colonoscopy surveillance after screening and polypectomy: a consensus update by the US Multi-Society Task Force on Colorectal Cancer. *Gastroenterology* 2012;143:844–57. Epub 2012 Jul 13.
10. Minoli G, Meucci G, Bortoli A, *et al.* The ASGE guidelines for the appropriate use of colonoscopy in an open access system. *Gastrointest Endosc* 2000;52:39–44.

CHAPTER 4

Preparation for Colonoscopy

Introduction

In order to achieve the best outcome, the patient and the colonoscopist must accomplish several objectives before the colonoscopy begins. These include a comprehensive medical history, managing the patient's standing medications, cleansing the colon, and achieving informed consent.

Management of standing medications

When the patient makes the colonoscopy appointment, a medical and medication history must be obtained. This can occur in the office, by telephone, or in an Internet-based encounter. Decisions regarding medication management must sometimes be made weeks in advance of the colonoscopy. Office personnel must be instructed in the nuances of clinical history-taking, and patient intake templates should be formulated that guide these interactions.

Anticoagulants and antiplatelet agents

Many patients take medications that inhibit clotting, including warfarin, the newer direct coagulation factor inhibitors, oral antiplatelet agents, and platelet glycoprotein IIB/IIIA inhibitors. Colonoscopic interventions confer a spectrum of bleeding risks, ranging from virtually none in a purely diagnostic procedure to significant when a large polyp is resected. In most cases, it is unknown beforehand whether a colonoscopy will require tissue removal. Antithrombotic drug management must be considered prior to each colonoscopic examination and should reflect the relative risks of thrombotic versus bleeding events. Guidelines exist and reflect expert opinion. Partly because of the paucity of data, clinicians vary widely in their management of pre-colonoscopy antithrombotic agents.

The following comments reflect commonly encountered scenarios and routine colonoscopy.

- Unlike stroke or myocardial infarction, colonic bleeding is rarely fatal or results in long-term debility. This fact should govern decision-making in patients at high risk for serious thromboembolic events.
- In patients with prosthetic heart valves, recently placed drug-eluting intracoronary stents, or other pathology that places them at high risk for serious adverse thromboembolic events, the antithrombotic drugs should be managed collaboratively by the gastroenterologist, cardiologist, and sometimes hematologist.
- Daily low-dose prophylactic aspirin and other nonsteroidal anti-inflammatory agents (NSAIDs) are often stopped 5 days before colonoscopy. However, most experts and guidelines state that polypectomy and other colonoscopic interventions are safe in the presence of NSAIDs and aspirin.
- In general, colonic biopsy is safe in the setting of systemic anticoagulation. Resection of diminutive and small polyps is generally also low risk for bleeding. However, medium-sized and large polyps confer greater bleeding risk because of the presence of larger and more numerous feeding blood vessels.
- If tissue removal is performed in a patient receiving anticoagulants or antiplatelet agents, it is prudent to observe the site after polypectomy to ensure hemostasis and to inform the patient of signs of post-procedural bleeding and the steps that should be taken if it occurs.
- If the patient takes dual antiplatelet therapy for a fresh intracoronary stent, options include: deferring

Practical Colonoscopy, First Edition. Jerome D. Waye, James Aisenberg, and Peter H. Rubin.
© 2013 John Wiley & Sons, Ltd. Published 2013 by John Wiley & Sons, Ltd.

the colonoscopy; continuing the dual therapy through the colonoscopy period, with an understanding that if a large polyp is encountered, resection may not be reasonable and will require a second colonoscopy after appropriate adjustments in anticoagulation; discontinuing one of the two antiplatelet agents. Typically, the cardiologist will be involved in the decision-making.

• If the patient takes warfarin for atrial fibrillation and has not had a cerebral vascular accident (stroke), most cardiologists view the thromboembolic risk related to stopping the drug for several days as acceptable. The drug is generally stopped approximately 5 days before the colonoscopy. The patient's international normalized ratio (INR) may be checked the morning of the procedure at the discretion of the team, but that is optional.

• If the patient takes warfarin for stroke or systemic anticoagulant prophylaxis related to a mechanical heart valve, "bridging" anticoagulation is typically recommended. This entails the use of short-acting subcutaneous, injectable anticoagulants, such as low-molecular-weight heparin, or the inpatient administration of intravenous heparin, which can be discontinued at an appropriate interval before the colonoscopy.

• Guidelines regarding management of the new oral, direct clotting-factor inhibitors, such as dabigatran, are limited. These drugs are shorter-acting (cleared in 12–24 hours), and the principles governing their management around the time of colonoscopy are similar to those governing the management of low-molecular-weight heparin.

• There are few studies regarding when to re-institute antithrombotic agents following colonoscopic interventions. Most experts recommend resuming the antithrombotic treatment within a day or two of the polypectomy—despite the risk of "late" bleeding—as the risk of a serious cardiovascular event is thought to outweigh the risk of colonic bleeding. If "bridging" anticoagulation is recommended, then it should generally be resumed for a few days post-polypectomy even after warfarin has been resumed, as it takes time for the INR to reach therapeutic levels.

• In patients who are at high thromboembolic risk receiving systemic anticoagulation, an acceptable option is to continue anticoagulation with the foreknowledge that if a significant polyp is detected, a second procedure will be required for resection.

When to resume anticoagulation after polypectomy

- Discuss with patient's cardiologist/internist
- No "hard-and-fast" rules
- Estimate risk of post-polypectomy bleeding (from characteristics of polyp and polypectomy)
- Estimate risk of patient's thromboembolism
- Make best judgment regarding net clinical benefit of resuming/withholding anticoagulation
- In general a stroke/other cardiovascular event results in a worse long-term outcome than post-polypectomy bleed

Antibiotics

Colonoscopy confers an extremely low risk of systemic infectious complications, which presumably could result from sustained bacteremia induced by breaching the colonic mucosal barrier. Several case reports suggest a possible association of colonoscopy with infective endocarditis, and traditionally colonoscopists administered pre-procedural antibiotics to patients considered to be at high risk. However, it is uncertain whether antibiotic prophylaxis during colonoscopy is even effective, or whether the risks associated with colonoscopy are any greater than those associated with brushing or flossing of teeth, and most expert guidelines do not currently recommend the use of antibiotics around the time of colonoscopy. At times, a discussion among patient, gastroenterologist, and relevant subspecialist (cardiac surgeon, orthopedic surgeon) is helpful.

Summary of current guidelines regarding antibiotic prophylaxis during colonoscopy

- American Heart Association:
  - does not recommend antibiotics for infective endocarditis prophylaxis.
- American Society for Gastrointestinal Endoscopy (ASGE):
  - use of prophylactic antibiotics in patients at high risk for infective endocarditis is optional;
  - for endovascular grafts <1 year old, consider antibiotic prophylaxis on a case-by-case basis, but inadequate evidence to recommend routine use;
  - for new prosthetic joints, routine antibiotics are not recommended.

Insulin and oral hypoglycemic agents

The physiological stresses that accompany colonoscopy may influence blood sugar levels. There are no guidelines for management of insulin or oral hypoglycemic drugs prior to colonoscopy; the approach must be individualized. Typically, the medication adjustments will be supervised by the diabetologist. One common approach is for the patient to take one-half of the usual dosage of long-acting insulin but no short-acting insulin on the morning of the colonoscopy. This decreases the risk of ketosis, while minimizing the risk of hypoglycemia. Generally, oral hypoglycemic agents are held the morning of colonoscopy in the belief that there is more to fear from hypo- than hyperglycemia. In diabetic patients careful pre-procedural review of dietary restrictions is helpful. Notably, the complete fasting period (no solids or fluids) may be altered in individual circumstances. It is prudent to obtain a pre-procedural finger-stick blood glucose level. Intravenous fluids can be administered as needed during the procedure and a light snack offered immediately after colonoscopy.

Colon cleansing

Among patients, the bowel preparation before colonoscopy is notorious and dreaded—"the worst part of the procedure." But a well-cleansed colon is fundamental to a high-quality examination. It decreases the risks of an incomplete procedure and missed lesions. It also spares the colonoscopist the onerous task of irrigating the colon. This "low-tech" aspect of colonoscopy retains an outsize influence on its safety, efficiency, and effectiveness.

Diet and timing of the cathartic preparation

There are few trials examining how diet affects colon cleansing, especially when the newer lavage and cathartic agents are utilized. Thus, recommendations about oral intake are generally based on experience and common sense. The preparation often begins with a 24-hour liquid diet. Puddings, custards, ice-creams, or yogurts that contain no nuts or fruit pieces are often permitted. Some endoscopists advise patients to avoid red foods or beverages that could in theory be confused with blood during the colonoscopy.

The presence of intraluminal seeds is particularly problematic during colonoscopy, because they can clog the suction channel of the colonoscope. Some endoscopists prohibit ingestion of foods containing seeds (e.g. wholegrain breads, fruits) for 5 days prior to the colonoscopy; other protocols mandate a low-residue diet for 3 days.

The preparation instructions must stress the importance of consuming large quantities of electrolyte-containing fluids during the 24 hours before the exam. The well-hydrated patient arrives at the colonoscopy stronger, tolerates the anesthesia better, has more hemodynamic stability during the colonoscopy, and recovers more quickly.

The current standard of care is to use a "split-dose" approach, whereby one-half or one-third of the cathartic is administered the day before the colonoscopy in one or two doses, and the remaining portion is administered closer (4 to 6 hours) to the beginning of the procedure. When compared to single dosing, split dosing results in improved colon cleansing and improved polyp detection. It is generally acceptable to patients and carries no increased risks.

The cathartic agents

There are a number of acceptable, widely used alternatives for colon cleansing. The addition of enemas is usually not necessary.

Per oral gut lavage with an osmotically balanced solution is widely used, safe, and effective. The most commonly used osmotically active solute is polyethylene glycol (PEG) 3350, a large, inert, non-fermentable, non-absorbable polymer. Because PEG-based lavage solutions do not induce significant fluid or electrolyte absorption or secretion, they are relatively safe, even in individuals with heart, liver, or kidney failure. Patients should be informed that they cannot ingest any glucose-containing product (e.g. gum, candy, flavoring additives, juice) during the phase of active drinking because the glucose will activate the small bowel sodium pump and start the cascade that results in water absorption. A disadvantage of this preparation is that it requires the patient to ingest a large volume of fluid that tastes quite salty. Traditionally, PEG 3350 was marketed in a 1 gallon (~4 L) formulation. More recently, 2-quart (~2 L) preparations, supplemented with adjunctive agents such as bisacodyl or ascorbic acid have been marketed. These appear to be equally effective and better tolerated. A smaller-volume preparation using an over the counter PEG 3350 product (MiraLax) is available in the USA. However, this preparation is not balanced osmotically and may result in electrolyte disorders and, rarely, seizures.

Until recently hypertonic phosphate-based cathartics were utilized widely because they achieved excellent cleansing with small-volume liquid or pill formulations. However, these agents confer a risk of renal failure due to deposition of calcium phosphate crystals, greatest in patients with preexisting underlying kidney injury from diabetes or hypertension, in patients who take medications that inhibit the renin–angiotensin system or diuretics, and in patients who do not follow the hydration instructions. Renal failure can also occur idiosyncratically. Because these agents contain large quantities of sodium, they are contraindicated in individuals with cardiac, renal, or liver disease. For all these reasons, phosphate-based cathartics have generally fallen out of favor among patients and providers.

A cathartic preparation that utilizes sulfates rather than phosphates ("SUPREP") has recently become available. It results in cleansing comparable to the PEG-based products, while avoiding the toxicities related to the sodium phosphate salts. The preparation requires a smaller volume of oral intake (two 180-ml bottles) than the PEG-based methods. Split dosing the sulfate-based regimen (see below) achieves better cleansing than a single dose.

Some colonoscopists prefer traditional cathartics such as citrate of magnesia, often combined with a pill laxative such as bisacodyl or senna. This approach is inexpensive, widely available, and effective.

Preparing for colonoscopy with a restricted diet and enemas without an oral cathartic is usually unsatisfactory, because even "high-colonic" enemas do not adequately clean the cecum and ascending colon.

Drinking the agent through a straw and chilling the agent may increase the tolerability of the various solutions.

Contraindications to bowel preparation

- Gastrointestinal tract obstruction
- Gastrointestinal tract perforation
- Severe gastroenteritis/diarrhea
- Dysphagia/pulmonary aspiration risk*
- Inability to drink preparation*
- Hemodynamic instability

*consider administering via nasogastric tube

Bowel preparation: Instructing the patient

- Emphasize that suboptimal cleansing can cause missed lesions and repeat procedures
- Provide preparation instructions well in advance in hard copy and/or in electronic format; include a list of frequently asked questions, and simple visual aids such as videos or images of "clean" and "dirty" colons
- Write preparation instructions in clear lay language
- Provide non-English language instructions if needed
- Confirm that patient received and understood preparation instructions and prescriptions; a convenient time to do this is when appointment is confirmed
- Educate office staff so they can answer patient questions in a clear and reassuring manner
- Inform patient that customized preparation instructions from the endoscopist supersede commercial instructions
- Reassure patient that cathartics may take a number of hours to work
- Emphasize that patient must consume entire preparation, even if initial dose caused diarrhea
- If smaller/older patients request a reduced cathartic dosage, explain that in general the potency of the cleansing agent depends on colon physiology and function rather than on size or age so dose should not be reduced

The "difficult-to-prepare" patient

At the time the colonoscopy is scheduled, ask the patient about risk factors for inadequate cleansing. These include prior inadequate preparation for colonoscopy, chronic constipation, or inability to tolerate the standard bowel preparations. In these situations, the approach to bowel cleaning may need to be modified.

In the chronically constipated patient, a 2-day liquid diet may be utilized, with an extra dose of a cathartic (such as citrate of magnesia) administered 48 hours before the procedure. The standard preparation protocol then follows. This approach, augmented by enemas as needed, is generally effective. Consider scheduling the "difficult-to-prepare" patient early in the week, so that if the preparation is inadequate more time and cathartics can be taken. In elderly or infirm patients or those who are otherwise unable to adhere to the preparation, the involvement of a family member or other "sponsor" may result in success. Some patients "just cannot take" the preparation because the solution is not palatable for them. A reassuring discussion of different preparation strategies is an important first step in this situation. On rare occasions it may be useful to coadminister an antiemetic agent (e.g. ondansetron) or an anxiolytic medication (e.g. diazepam) with the oral cathartic.

The character of the rectal effluent on the morning of the exam may not accurately reflect the quality of colon cleansing, so an inadequate preparation may not be apparent until colonoscopy is begun. If the cleansing is grossly inadequate, the colonoscopist should abort the exam. After the patient awakes, the colonoscopist should determine the cause of the incomplete preparation and respond accordingly.

The purgative agents can be administered to patients with colostomies. If the colostomy is of the ascending colon, the oral dose may be reduced. If a bypassed segment of rectum and colon is to be inspected then gentle enemas may be required.

To achieve an excellent bowel preparation: six recommendations

1. Only use split-dose preps
2. Screen patients for history of inadequate bowel preparation or chronic constipation; if present, consider a 2-day preparation
3. Provide clear instructions in native language of patient using several formats (hard copy, video, Internet-based, photographs)
4. Teach patient that "a clean colon = a high-quality exam"
5. Designate staff member for handling pre-procedural questions
6. If during colon intubation preparation is found to be inadequate:
   - terminate case;
   - recommend that patient take more laxative and return;
   - reschedule procedure with 2-day preparation.

Informed consent

Colonoscopy confers a legal and ethical requirement that patients be provided with sufficient information about the procedure so that they can participate in the decision to proceed. The informed consent discussion affords the colonoscopist an opportunity to address the patient's concerns, strengthens the alliance with the patient, and confers some medicolegal protection. In an era of "open access" colonoscopy, where patient and colonoscopist may not meet until minutes before the exam, sharing of information is particularly important. An appropriate discussion in most cases requires only a few minutes but should involve dialogue. The first step can occur weeks before the colonoscopist has met the patient, when the patient reviews video or documentary materials that explain colonoscopy. These materials can be created internally by the practitioner, or obtained through professional societies. They can be posted online, mailed to the patient, or provided at the office.

What to review during informed consent

- Benefits of colonoscopy
- Alternatives to colonoscopy
- Major risks of colonoscopy, including bleeding, perforation, and adverse cardiopulmonary events with some indication of their frequency
- The less serious but common risks, such as intravenous infiltration or post-colonoscopy bloating
- The limitations of colonoscopy (e.g. missed lesion despite technically adequate exam)
- The risks, benefits and alternatives to the sedation
- What the patient should expect during and after
- Proper post-procedure management (including need for escort)

Ideally, informed consent is achieved by a face-to-face conversation between the colonoscopist and the patient, who has the capacity to provide consent. The colonoscopist should allow the patient to verbalize concerns, and have questions answered. Legally, the colonoscopist is obligated to reveal the risks that a "reasonable patient" would want to know. The patient is responsible for disclosing any personal information that may influence the risks and benefits of the procedure. The informed consent document should enumerate the important risks and limitations of colonoscopy, and document that the conversation has occurred and that the patient's questions have been answered. The document should be signed by both parties and entered in the permanent medical record.

Summary

There are important choices to be made before the day of colonoscopy. Decisions may require the input of other consultants, and must be individualized and shared with the patient and family. In the modern era, pre-procedure communication of information relevant to colonoscopy may be achieved through Internet-based resources. An appropriate informed consent discussion protects both patient and colonoscopist.

Further reading

1. ASGE Standards of Practice Committee, Levy MJ, Anderson MA, *et al.* Position statement on routine laboratory testing before endoscopic procedures. *Gastrointest Endosc* 2008;68:827–32.
2. Belsey J, Crosta C, Epstein O, *et al.* Meta-analysis: the relative efficacy of oral bowel preparations for colonoscopy 1985-2010. *Aliment Pharmacol Ther* 2012;35: 222–37. Epub 2011 Nov 24.
3. Cohen LB. Split dosing of bowel preparations for colonoscopy: an analysis of its efficacy, safety, and tolerability. *Gastrointest Endosc* 2010;72:406–12. Epub 2010 Jul 1.
4. Fordtran JS, Santa Ana CA, Cleveland MvB. A low-sodium solution for gastrointestinal lavage. *Gastroenterology* 1990;98:11–16.
5. Hassan C, Fuccio L, Bruno M, *et al.* A predictive model identifies patients most likely to have inadequate bowel preparation for colonoscopy. *Clin Gastroenterol Hepatol* 2012;10:501–6. Epub 2012 Jan 10.
6. Kao D, Lalor E, Sandha G, *et al.* A randomized controlled trial of four precolonoscopy bowel cleansing regimens. *Can J Gastroenterol* 2011;25:657–62.
7. Kelly NM, Rodgers C, Patterson N, Jacob SG, Mainie I. A prospective audit of the efficacy, safety, and acceptability of low-volume polyethylene glycol (2 L) versus standard volume polyethylene glycol (4 L) versus magnesium citrate plus stimulant laxative as bowel preparation for colonoscopy. *J Clin Gastroenterol* 2012;46:595–601.
8. Lai, EJ, Calderwood AH, Doros G, Fix OK, Jacobson BC. The Boston bowel preparation scale: a valid and reliable instrument for colonoscopy-oriented research. *Gastrointest. Endosc* 2009;69:620–625.
9. Markowitz GS, Stokes MB, Radhakrishnan J, D'Agati VD. Acute phosphate nephropathy following oral sodium, phosphate bowel purgative: an under recognized cause of chronic renal failure. *Am Soc Nephrol* 2005;16:3389–96.
10. Wexner SD, Beck DA, Baron TH, *et al.* A consensus document on bowel preparation before colonoscopy: prepared by a task force from The American Society of Colon and Rectal Surgeons (ASCRS), the American Society for Gastrointestinal Endoscopy (ASGE), and the Society of American Gastrointestinal and Endoscopic Surgeons (SAGES). *Gastrointest Endosc* 2006;63:894–909.

SECTION 2

Basic Procedure

CHAPTER 5
Sedation for Colonoscopy

Introduction

Sedation and analgesia improve the quality of the colonoscopy and increase patient satisfaction. However, sedation accounts for 75% of the total in-office time of a colonoscopy, 40% of the costs, and 50% of the serious adverse events. In the USA, sedation is used routinely during colonoscopy by >98% of practitioners, but in other countries unsedated colonoscopy is common. Anesthesiologists currently participate in approximately one-half of the colonoscopies performed in the USA. Colonoscopists must have a complete understanding of the principles and practice of sedation.

Levels of sedation

1. *Minimal sedation* is a drug-induced relief of apprehension with minimal effect on consciousness. The patient is awake and alert.
2. *Moderate sedation,* previously termed conscious sedation, is a depression of consciousness in which the patient can respond purposely to verbal or light tactile stimuli. Airway reflexes, spontaneous ventilation, and cardiovascular function are maintained.
3. *Deep sedation* is a depression of consciousness in which the patient cannot be aroused by voice or light touch but responds purposefully to repeated or painful stimuli. The patient may not be able to maintain airway reflexes or spontaneous ventilation, but cardiovascular function is usually maintained.
4. *General anesthesia* is a state of unconsciousness. Airway intervention is often required and cardiovascular function may be impaired.

The lines of distinction among these levels are not clearly delineated, and during colonoscopy a patient may rapidly go from one to another. Moderate to deep sedation is generally recommended for colonoscopy procedures.

Pharmacology of drugs

Opioids

The opioids possess potent analgesic but minimal sedative properties.

Meperidine

Compared with fentanyl, meperidine has many disadvantages, including: a longer biologic half-life; production of toxic metabolites; increased risk of tachycardia and hypotension; increased histamine release; higher risk of nausea and vomiting; and increased risk of drug–drug interactions. For these reasons, meperidine has been abandoned in many institutions for routine use. Dosage: 25–100 mg intravenously followed by boluses of 25 mg titrated to effect.

Fentanyl

A synthetic, high-affinity opioid agonist, fentanyl is 75–125 times more potent than morphine. Its high lipid solubility allows rapid onset of action (1–2 minutes) and short duration of effect (30–60 minutes). Fentanyl depresses respiratory drive and may cause vomiting and nausea. Unlike meperidine, fentanyl's metabolites are inactive. Further, fentanyl does not produce vasodilation, facial flushing, depressed myocardial contractility, or idiosyncratic adverse drug interactions. Dosage: 25–100 μg intravenously followed by 25–50 μg as needed.

Benzodiazepines

Benzodiazepines enhance the action of γ-aminobutyric acid (GABA). They produce anxiolysis, sedation, amnesia, and at higher doses, hypnosis and respiratory depression. Opioids potentiate the sedative and circulatory depressant effects of benzodiazepines.

Diazepam

Thrombophlebitis is common with intravenous administration of diazepam. Diazepam should be

Practical Colonoscopy, First Edition. Jerome D. Waye, James Aisenberg, and Peter H. Rubin.
© 2013 John Wiley & Sons, Ltd. Published 2013 by John Wiley & Sons, Ltd.

avoided in patients with glaucoma. Dosage reduction is required in the elderly, individuals with limited pulmonary reserve, and those receiving opioids or other sedatives. Dosage: 2–10 mg intravenous dose with additional 2–5 mg boluses titrated to effect.

Midazolam

Intravenous midazolam does not cause phlebitis, and has rapid onset and short duration of effect. Midazolam is 1.5–3.5 times more potent than diazepam. Because of these advantages, it is has replaced diazepam in many settings. The clearance of midazolam is reduced in the elderly and patients with hepatic or renal dysfunction. Dosage: 0.5–2 mg intravenous bolus followed by 0.5–2 mg doses titrated to effect.

Narcotic and benzodiazepine antagonists

Naloxone

Naloxone competitively blocks the opioid receptor, reversing analgesia, respiratory depression, and hypotension. The initial dose is 0.2–0.4 mg intravenously, which may be repeated at 2–3 minute intervals.

Flumazenil

Flumazenil, a competitive benzodiazepine antagonist, reverses sedation, amnesia, anxiolysis, and respiratory depression. Its onset of action is 2 minutes. The initial dose is 0.2 mg, which may be repeated at 20-minute intervals and titrated to effect. Caution should be exercised when administering these drugs to patients who are opioid- or benzodiazepine-dependent, as this may precipitate serious symptoms of withdrawal, such as seizures. Additionally, patients treated with an antagonist should be monitored for re-sedation, as the duration of antagonist effect is shorter than that of the agonists.

Propofol

Propofol is an ultra-short-acting hypnotic. It has been called the "on–off switch" of human consciousness. The dosage of propofol must be carefully titrated to clinical effect. It is ideal for a short procedure such as colonoscopy, permitting quick induction and recovery. Like benzodiazepines, propofol works through the GABA receptor, but by a different mechanism. Patients differ widely in their sensitivity to the drug. Factors that influence dosage requirements include age, weight, preexisting medical conditions, and concomitant pharmacologic therapy. Propofol has no pharmacological antagonist. Propofol is typically administered with an initial bolus (e.g. 20–100 mg intravenously), followed by 5–20 mg boluses titrated to effect, or by a continuous infusion provided via a pump. Because it is so potent, propofol can depress consciousness from moderate sedation to general anesthesia within seconds; therefore careful monitoring and fastidious dosing are essential.

Approaches to sedation for colonoscopy

Unsedated colonoscopy

Unsedated colonoscopy reduces complications and costs. However, in most settings the pain associated with colonoscopy is not considered acceptable, and unsedated colonoscopy has achieved limited application. Its popularity may grow if new technologies that reduce pain prove viable. Predictors of successful unsedated colonoscopy include male gender, college education, and low pre-procedural anxiety. The success of unsedated colonoscopy can be optimized by good colonoscopist–patient communication both before and during the procedure.

Benzodiazepine/opioid sedation

Traditionally, gastroenterologists sedate their patients using an opioid combined with a benzodiazepine. No anesthesiologist is present and moderate ("twilight" or "conscious") sedation is targeted. Today, approximately half of the colonoscopy in the USA is being performed using this strategy. The therapeutic synergy between opioids and the benzodiazepines is widely appreciated, as is the increased risk of respiratory depression when the agents are combined. Conventionally, a starting dose of each agent (e.g. fentanyl 50–75 mg plus midazolam 1–2 mg) is administered, and then additional small boluses of each are added every 3–5 minutes as needed. The average time required to achieve therapeutic effect is 6–12 minutes, and it is often not necessary to administer additional drug after the colonoscopy is begun. Oversedation may occur if boluses are added before the peak effect of the previous dose has been achieved. Following colonoscopy, on-site recovery averages 30–60 minutes. Full recovery requires up to 16 hours, so patients are generally unable to resume normal activities until the next day.

The majority of patients sedated with a benzodiazepine and an opioid for colonoscopy are satisfied. Individuals who have high levels of pre-procedural anxiety, a history of alcohol or substance abuse, and a history of being difficult to sedate are more likely to have unsatisfactory analgesia. Although benzodiazepine/opioid combinations are generally safe, adverse or fatal cardiopulmonary events have occurred. Respiratory depression is the greatest risk, requiring extra caution in the elderly, patients with preexisting neurological disease, and those with high-risk airways.

Propofol sedation

Compared with benzodiazepine/opioid regimens, propofol use during colonoscopy is associated with improved patient and physician satisfaction and more rapid induction and recovery. Although there is abundant data suggesting that propofol may be safely administered by well-trained colonoscopists, this strategy has not achieved widespread adoption in the USA. Induction of sedation averages 2–3 minutes, and recovery may take 15–20 minutes. Propofol can be administered as monotherapy or in combination with a narcotic and a benzodiazepine ("balanced propofol sedation"). Because propofol possesses little intrinsic analgesic activity, higher doses and deep sedation are generally required with monotherapy. Routine capnography, which provides a real-time measurement of the concentration of carbon dioxide in the patient's expired breath depicted as a number and a waveform, is recommended. Despite the rapid metabolism of propofol, patients should be discharged after colonoscopy in the presence of a responsible companion and refrain from driving or vigorous exercise for the balance of that day.

Patient-controlled sedation

Several systems permit the patient to self-administer medication during colonoscopy in response to pain. Propofol, due to its rapid-on, rapid-off properties, is the drug most often used.

Pre-colonoscopy management

A sedation-focused history should elicit: prior difficulties during anesthesia/sedation; major medical problems; airway abnormalities including excessive snoring and sleep apnea; significant alcohol or drug use; diabetes or hypoglycemia; medication and food allergies; last food intake; concurrent medications; and the possibility of pregnancy. The physical exam should evaluate the general robustness of the patient (Is the patient dehydrated or lethargic?); the physical habitus (Is the patient obese?); the anxiety level; vital signs and weight; and the mouth, head, and neck anatomy. Routine laboratory or electrocardiogram testing is not required. Pregnancy testing should be performed where appropriate. An American Society of Anesthesiology (ASA) physical status classification (Table 5.1) should be documented. Because sedation during colonoscopy has risks, benefits, and alternatives, it should be discussed with the patient during the pre-procedure informed consent.

Table 5.1 The American Society of Anesthesiology Physical Status Classification (adapted from http://www.asahq.org/for-members/clinical-information/asa-physical-status-classification-system.aspx).

ASA physical status classification system	
Class	**Characteristics**
1	A normal healthy patient
2	A patient with mild systemic disease
3	A patient with severe systemic disease
4	A patient with severe systemic disease that is a constant threat to life
5	A moribund patient who is not expected to survive without the operation
6	A declared brain-dead patient whose organs are being removed fo rdonor purposes

Post-colonoscopy management

The effects of sedative drugs persist, and therefore careful monitoring of the patient during recovery is essential. Validated recovery scores can confirm readiness for discharge. Patients may experience prolonged amnesia and cognitive impairment, and therefore should leave accompanied by a companion and with written instructions regarding post-procedure precautions. Patient recovery must be documented. In many units, a nurse calls the patient the day after a procedure.

Equipment for sedation

The colonoscopy room must permit free movement of staff and comfortably house the required monitors.

Sedation is delivered through a well-secured intravenous line. The catheter must be immediately replaced if it ceases to function properly. In general, use the smallest syringe appropriate for the drug being administered; this helps to minimize the risk for accidentally administering more drug than intended. All syringes must be appropriately labeled with the name of the medication.

Emergency resuscitative equipment (adapted from Cohen et al., 2007)

- Assorted syringes, tourniquets, adhesive tape
- Intravenous access equipment including fluid
- Basic airway management equipment
  - Oxygen supply
  - Suction machine and catheter
  - Nasal cannulae and face-masks
  - Bag–mask ventilation device
  - Oral and nasal airways (all sizes)
- Advanced airway management equipment
  - Laryngoscope handles and blade*
  - Endotracheal tubes and stylets*
  - Laryngeal mask airway*
- Cardiac equipment
  - Pulse oximeter
  - Cardiac defibrillator
- Emergency medications
  - Atropine
  - Diphenhydramine
  - Epinephrine
  - Ephedrine
  - Flumazenil
  - Glucose, 50%
  - Hydrocortisone
  - Lidocaine
  - Naloxone
  - Sodium bicarbonate

*All appropriate sizes should be available

Many colonoscopists utilize supplemental oxygen, although studies have not established a benefit. A nasal cannula designed to deliver oxygen and simultaneously sample expired gases is useful for real-time capnography. When supplemental oxygen is provided from a tank, a spare oxygen tank and regulator should be available. Blood pressure monitoring and pulse oximetry are generally recommended. Oximeters provide visual and auditory feedback and electronically store data. Electrocardiography during colonoscopy is of unproven benefit but is widely utilized. "Side-stream" capnography, which provides a real-time waveform reflecting the patient's respiration, is a more sensitive indicator of hypoventilation than either pulse oximetry or visual inspection. Resuscitation equipment must be immediately available. The colonoscopy room must have a communication system that can be used to summon personnel in case of a sedation-related emergency. Sedation-related emergency equipment must be inspected and inventoried regularly.

Hypoventilation during colonoscopy: Management

- Recognize promptly
- Call for help if needed
- Consider whether appropriate to discontinue colonoscopy
- Identify cause
  - Central
  - Upper airway
    - Collapse of soft tissues
    - Laryngospasm
  - Lower airway
    - Pulmonary aspiration
    - Bronchospasm
    - Other
- Initiate treatment
  - Oxygen
  - Suction
  - If colon distended, aspirate air (may restrict diaphragm)
  - Sedative/analgesic drug antagonists
  - Simple airway maneuvers (jaw thrust, chin lift, oral airway)
  - Advanced airway maneuvers (bag–mask ventilation, etc.)

Staffing and colonoscopic sedation

In the USA currently, an anesthesiologist participates in approximately 50% of colonoscopies. This reflects the benefits of propofol, as well as the added value of a dedicated sedationist. Some colonoscopists consider that an anesthesia specialist should always participate during colonoscopy when the patient is high risk or when the procedure is especially complex (e.g. an advanced polypectomy).

In the absence of an anesthesia specialist, the colonoscopy assistant generally: prepares the medications; sets up the infusion and monitoring equipment; monitors patient ventilation and hemodynamic parameters; administers the drugs (under the direction of the gastroenterologist); performs all documentation; and initiates and participates in support/resuscitation measures. The number and qualifications (licensure) of the assistant(s) utilized during colonoscopy vary depending upon local regulations and norms. The ASA has stated that when deep sedation is intended, an individual dedicated to sedation and monitoring should be present, but during moderate sedation the assistant involved in sedation and monitoring may assist with "minor interruptible tasks."

Both the colonoscopist and the endoscopy assistant should understand the continuum of sedation, the pre-procedural assessment, the basic pharmacology of the drugs in use, the signs of cardiopulmonary complications, simple rescue maneuvers (such as the chin lift), the use of the monitoring equipment, and the action plan in the event of an adverse event. Each colonoscopy center should implement a sedation-related quality-improvement program, including analysis of "near misses," and adhere to institutional and local regulations regarding sedation. The colonoscopist should be certified in advanced cardiac life support or its equivalent.

Sedation and analgesia: Optimizing safety

- Use minimal necessary drug doses required for comfort
- Target moderate (versus deep) sedation
- For higher-risk patients (ASA 3 or 4), consider dedicated anesthesia provider
- Obtain sedation-related history prior to starting colonoscopy
  - Sleep apnea
  - Prior difficulties with anesthesia
  - Cardiopulmonary comorbidities
- Maintain intravenous access throughout case
- Train assistants in signs of cardiopulmonary compromise
- Utilize appropriate monitoring devices
- Maintain required resuscitation equipment and protocols

Pain after colonoscopy

- Usually related to gaseous distension
- Insufflation of CO_2 rather than room air causes less pain due to faster clearance of gas
- Decompress the colon during scope withdrawal (suction out air)
  - Particularly important with narrowed diverticular sigmoid, which can "trap" air above
- If abdomen very distended at end of colonoscopy, consider rapid re-intubation to transverse colon to aspirate air from colon
- Less gas in colon decreases recovery time

Pain during colonoscopy

- Related to stretch on mesentery or colon wall
- Caused by:
  - large loops;
  - overdistended with air.
- If the patient expresses pain:
  - reduce loops;
  - remove air if possible;
  - then increase sedation/analgesia as needed.
- Titrate short-acting sedation agents (e.g. propofol) so that sedation and analgesia are greatest during intubation when pain potential is greatest

Sedative/analgesic drugs: Pharmacokinetics during colonoscopy

- Bowel cathartics may alter drug pharmacokinetics, due to:
  - altered serum electrolytes;
  - dehydration.
- "Start low, go slow"
  - Allow adequate time for drugs to take effect before adding additional dose
  - 3–5 minutes for benzodiazepines/opioids
  - Titrate to patient age, comorbidities, and body mass

Monitoring cardiopulmonary function during colonoscopy

- Colonoscopist positioned behind patient
  - Limited visualization of patient's face/anterior chest wall
- Endoscopy assistant (or anesthesiologist) in front of patient
  - Monitors face and chest wall
  - Requires unimpeded sight lines and adequate lighting
- Cardiopulmonary monitors
  - Continuous monitoring of O_2, blood pressure, electrocardiogram, and pulse
  - Real-time side-stream capnography
  - Must be:
    - in clear sight line;
    - well-maintained.

Hypotension during colonoscopy: Causes

- Dehydration related to procedure preparation:
  - cathartics;
  - *Nil per os* status.
- Vagotonic responses to:
  - colon instrumentation;
  - sedation/analgesic drugs;
  - colonic distension;
  - nausea.
- Direct hypotensive effects of sedative/analgesic drugs
- Primary cardiac cause (unusual):
  - ischemic;
  - arrhythmia.
- Intra-abdominal (rare):
  - colon perforation;
  - hemorrhage.

Hypotension during colonoscopy: Management

- Recognize promptly
- Call for help, if needed
- Consider whether appropriate to discontinue colonoscopy
- Identify cause
- Initiate treatment
  - IV fluids
  - IV vasopressor agents
  - Sedative/analgesic drug antagonists
  - Treatments geared to underlying cause (e.g. treatment of arrhythmia or cardiac ischemia)

Summary

Sedation and analgesia improve the quality of the colonoscopy and increase patient satisfaction. However, sedation increases the risks and costs associated with colonoscopy. Worldwide, widespread variations in sedation practices exist. The individual colonoscopist must understand the options, and select and master a sedation approach that works for his/her practice style, patient population, and work setting.

Further reading

1. Aisenberg J, Cohen LB. Sedation in endoscopic practice. *Gastrointest Endosc Clin N Am* 2006;16:695–708.
2. American Association for the Study of Liver Diseases, American College of Gastroenterology, American Gastroenterological Association Institute, *et al.* Multisociety sedation curriculum for gastrointestinal endoscopy. *Gastrointest Endosc* 2012;76:e1–25. Epub 2012 May 22.
3. Cohen LB, DeLegge M, Kochman M, *et al.* AGA Institute review on endoscopic sedation. *Gastroenterology* 2007;133:675–701.
4. Cohen LB, Wecsler JS, Gaetano JN, *et al.* Endoscopic sedation in the United States: results from a nationwide survey. *Am J Gastroenterol* 2006;101:967–974.
5. Froehlich F, Harris JK, Wietlisbach V, Burnand B, Vader JP, Gonvers JJ. Current sedation and monitoring practice for colonoscopy: an International

Observational Study (EPAGE). *Endoscopy* 2006;38: 461–469.
6. McQuaid KR, Laine L. A systematic review and meta-analysis of randomized, controlled trials of moderate sedation for routine endoscopic procedures. *Gastrointest Endosc* 2008;67:910–23.
7. Petrini J, Egan JV. Risk management regarding sedation/analgesia. *Gastrointest Endosc Clin N Am* 2004;14:401–414.
8. Sharma VK, Nguyen CC, Crowell MD, Lieberman DA, De Garmo P, Fleischer DE. A national study of cardiopulmonary unplanned events after GI endoscopy. *Gastrointest Endosc* 2007;66:27–34.
9. Silverman WB, Chotiprasidhi P, Chuttani R, *et al.* Monitoring equipment for endoscopy. *Gastrointest Endosc* 2004;59:761–765.
10. Vargo JJ, Ahmad AS, Aslanian HR, *et al.* Training in patient monitoring and sedation and analgesia. *Gastrointest Endosc* 2007;66:7–10.

CHAPTER 6

Colonoscopy Technique: The Ins and Outs

Introduction

The goals of scope insertion and withdrawal are to traverse the serpentine colon safely and efficiently, and to inspect the mucosa thoroughly. During insertion, most colonoscopists focus on the technical demands of intubation; during scope withdrawal, the focus shifts to examining the colon lining. Most expert colonoscopists use a similar technique.

Preparation for scope insertion

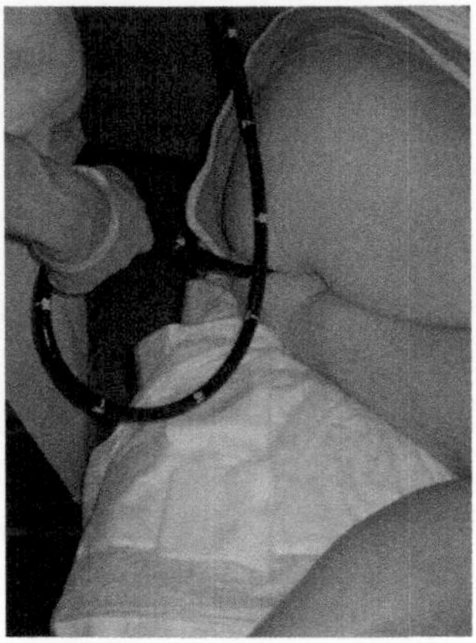

Fig 6.1 Correct patient positioning. With the patient in the left lateral decubitus position, the buttocks are near the edge of the stretcher. The right leg is in front of the left leg. Extra gauze pads are on the examination table within easy reach, and an absorptive pad has been placed under the buttocks.

It is easier to position the patient before sedation is given, as the alert patient can participate in turning. The patient is positioned comfortably in the left lateral decubitus position with the buttocks at the edge of the examining table (Fig 6.1). Typically, the knees are slightly flexed, and the right knee is positioned in front of the left knee. Some endoscopists prefer that the patient be supine with the right leg crossed over the left.

The stretcher is elevated to the height that permits the endoscopist's arms to move most comfortably. The patient's buttocks are positioned an inch or two from the side of the stretcher.

The colonoscopist confirms scope functionality before every examination, even if the assistant has checked it during set-up, as it is easier, safer, and more time-efficient to troubleshoot equipment when the scope is outside the patient.

Sedation is administered (see Chapter 5) and then the digital rectal examination is performed, to evaluate anal pathology, the effectiveness of the cathartic preparation, sphincter tone, the prostate gland or gynecologic organs, and the wall of the distal rectum. In addition, it lubricates and relaxes the anal sphincter in preparation for scope entry.

Proper technique for holding the scope

Colonoscopy is physically demanding, and places repetitive, sustained stresses on the endoscopist's musculoskeletal system.

Practical Colonoscopy, First Edition. Jerome D. Waye, James Aisenberg, and Peter H. Rubin.
© 2013 John Wiley & Sons, Ltd. Published 2013 by John Wiley & Sons, Ltd.

Maneuvers such as torquing exert unusual forces on the joints, and musculoskeletal injuries involving the hands, arms, back, and neck are not uncommon. The colonoscopist should remain cognizant of posture, arm position, hand tension, and neck position throughout the case. In general, colonoscopy should proceed without a need for much force. If significant force seems to be required, it is time to pull back the scope and consider a new tactic. Although specifics of colonoscopy technique vary from operator to operator, certain principles are followed. Colonoscopy is almost always performed with the endoscopist standing. The viewing monitor should be positioned near eye level, 1.8 to 2.5 m directly in front of the endoscopist. The stretcher should be elevated to the height of the endoscopist's hip.

The stretcher must be positioned far enough away from the equipment tower to provide adequate space to work. The light source is situated behind the endoscopist and the scope umbilicus is usually positioned on the left side of the endoscopist. The foot pedals for irrigation or cautery must be positioned conveniently for left foot access.

The head of the scope is held in the left hand (Fig 6.2), gripped securely between the palm and the middle, ring, and little fingers. The large up/down dial is manipulated with the left thumb, which remains in contact with this dial throughout most of the procedure. This thumb also stabilizes the scope head. In order to facilitate dial rotation, the thumb is aligned in the same plane as the dial control (Fig 6.3). The smaller, right/left control is often locked so that it does not need to be constantly attended to by the endoscopist. Many endoscopists use the right hand to turn the right/left dial, whereas others use the left thumb to move the smaller dial as well. The advantage of the second option is convenience; the disadvantages are that the large dial may slip when the thumb is taken off, and the stretched left thumb cannot maximally deflect the small dial.

The index finger is extended in front of the air/water and suction trumpet valves, so that it can depress either of them easily. Alternatively, the index finger is deployed over the suction valve with the middle finger over the air/water valve (Fig 6.3). The dial control locks are manipulated by the right hand, and either hand can use the smaller buttons on the head of the scope required for magnification, photo capture, or switching from the white light view.

The shaft of the colonoscope is held between the thumb and fingers of the right hand, in a screwdriver grip. If the entire insertion tube is left on the examining table, torque or twisting maneuvers may be difficult to perform; therefore many experts allow the insertion tube to drape over the edge of the examining table closest to the endoscopist and held in place by the examiner's right leg. The scope is gripped with a small gauze pad about 30 cm from the anus. During the times when the right hand is removed from the shaft, some practitioners ask the assistant to grip the shaft to stabilize the position. Many experts find it easier and more efficient to stabilize the scope themselves by securing the shaft against the

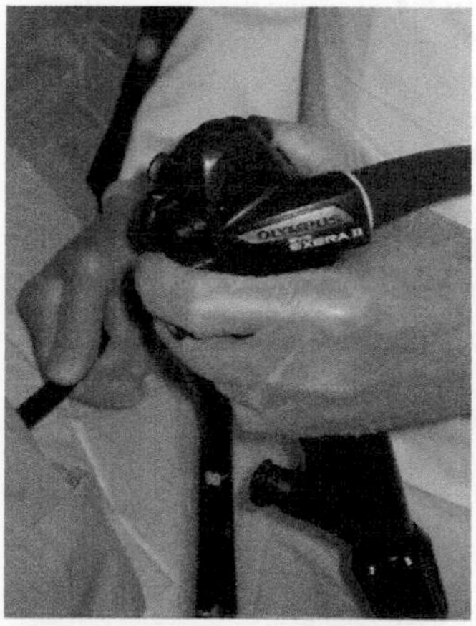

Fig 6.2 Correct scope handle grip.

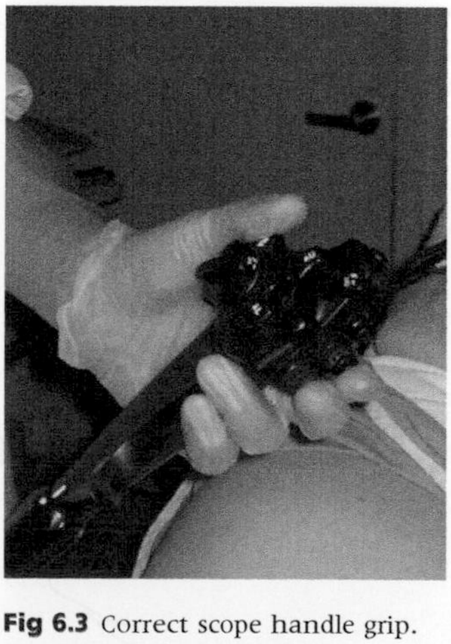

Fig 6.3 Correct scope handle grip. The index and middle fingers depress the trumpet valves.

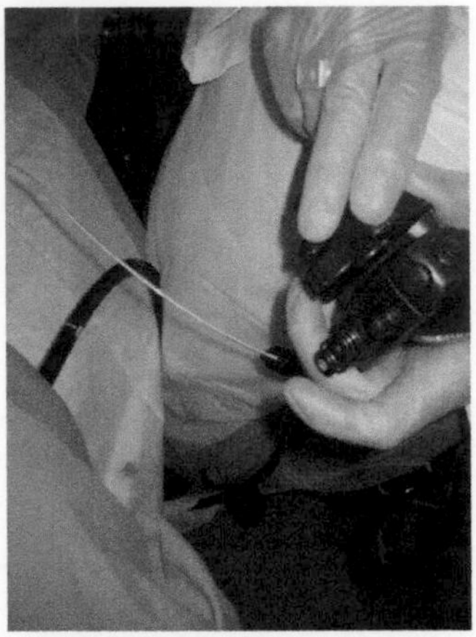

Fig 6.4 Securing the scope shaft. When the right hand moves to the dial control, the right thigh compresses the scope against the stretcher, securing its position.

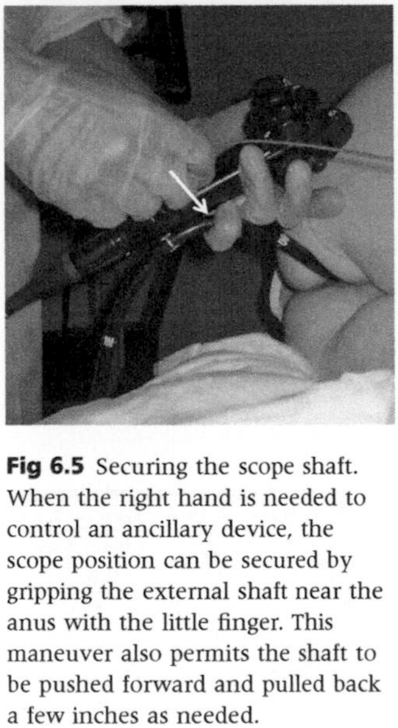

Fig 6.5 Securing the scope shaft. When the right hand is needed to control an ancillary device, the scope position can be secured by gripping the external shaft near the anus with the little finger. This maneuver also permits the shaft to be pushed forward and pulled back a few inches as needed.

edge of the stretcher with the right thigh (Fig 6.4) or holding it with the little finger of the left hand (Fig 6.5).

Optimizing ergonomics when performing colonoscopy

- Position endoscopic video monitor near eye level, approximately 1.8 m away
- Elevate stretcher to a comfortable height
- Wear comfortable, supportive footwear
- Exert all forces (torque, pushing, etc.) gently, in order to minimize strain on elbow
- Maintain relaxed, straight posture
- Ask assistant to note awkward-appearing or stressful actions

Technique of intubation

Every intubation is in some respects similar and unique. Each demands a sequence of tactics. The actions of the right and left hands must be well coordinated, and maneuvers should be delicate, deliberate, and parsimonious, not jerky, rapid-fire, forceful, or unconsidered. Experienced endoscopists achieve cecal intubation efficiently and safely in more than 95% of cases.

Skillful intubation takes time and effort to master. As the experience of colonoscopy is tactile and visual, written descriptions can provide only an initial guide; there is no substitute for practicing, initially under the eye of an experienced mentor.

Keys to efficient intubation

Keep focused on the endoscopic image

The endoscopist must consciously create an environment that fosters mental focus. Infrequent glances away from the monitor are unavoidable, but these should be kept to a minimum. Some practitioners prefer the room to be quiet; others prefer music; some prefer to narrate the sequence of actions and observations of the case; a few find that casual conversation sustains concentration and reduces tension, although to others this can be distracting.

Angulate the tip of the scope

Angulating the tip of the scope allows the colonoscopist to navigate around turns. The tip is angulated either with the dial controls or with torque. With the tip deflected, clockwise torque will shift the tip toward the right, whereas counterclockwise torque will move the tip toward the left (Fig 6.6). Many experienced colonoscopists

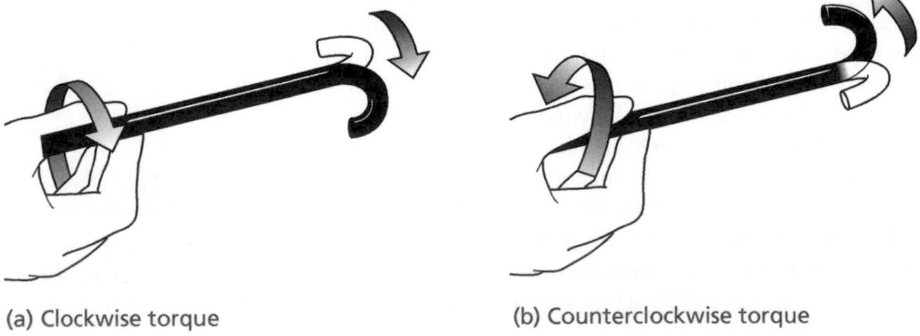

Fig 6.6 Effects of torquing the deflected scope tip.

find it easier to turn using torque than with constant manipulation of the dial controls.

It is easier to use the left thumb to rotate the large dial counterclockwise or downward (deflecting the tip upward) than to push it clockwise or upward. Accordingly, it is easier to rotate the scope shaft so that the colonic lumen is oriented toward the 12 o'clock position so that a downward thumb motion on the dial (upward tip deflection) moves the tip up into the lumen.

When the tip is maximally deflected by the up/down wheel, another 15° of tip deflection can be attained by simultaneously turning the smaller left/right control. This is particularly helpful for traversing a narrowed, tortuous sigmoid colon. However, hyperdeflecting the dial controls can damage the scope's cables.

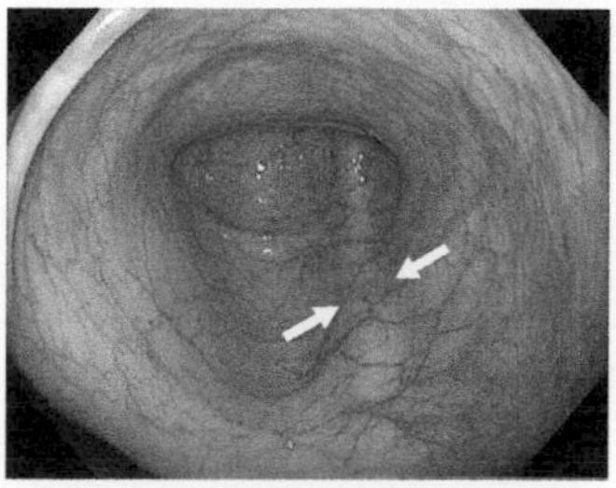

Fig 6.7 The longitudinal teniae coli, as seen here at splenic flexure, indicate the long axis of the colon.

Always know the position of the lumen

The endoscopist should never push blindly. The lumen must be kept in view as constantly as possible. If a "red out" or "white out" is encountered, this means that the lens is pressed against the mucosa. When the tip of the scope is in contact with the colon wall, the dial controls do not deflect the tip of the scope normally. Instead the knuckle (i.e. the tip bending section) of the scope will move, as the position of the tip is fixed. Pulling back the instrument will restore a luminal view and permit tip deflection with the dial control.

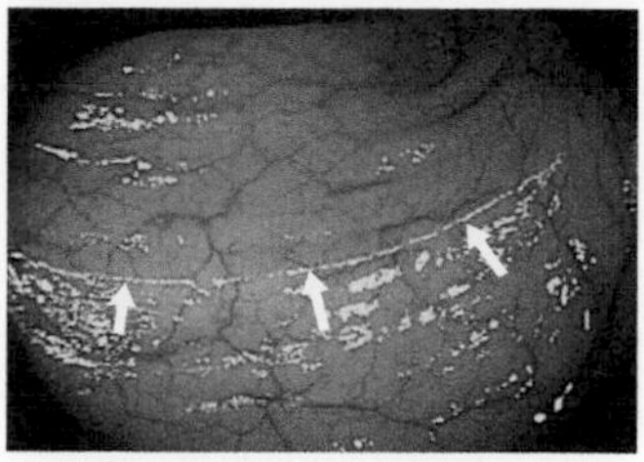

Fig 6.8 Reading the light reflections. Light is reflected in the innominate grooves and the circular muscle. The lumen will be in the direction of the arrows.

Visual clues predict the location of the lumen. In general the lumen is located at the convergence of the folds seen ahead in the distance. The tip is advanced to this area; air (or water) is introduced; and the folds will generally open up, revealing more lumen.

The colonic muscles also provide clues. The three teniae coli course longitudinally along the colon, and are often visible, indicating the colon's long axis (Fig 6.7). The circular muscle fibers in the muscularis propria form subtle circular ridges around the circumference of the colon, reflecting light in an arcuate pattern (Fig 6.8). Reading these 'highlights' allows the endoscopist to identify the direction of the lumen. When an arc of light is seen, even if fragmented in appearance, the endoscopist should make an imaginary circle using the arc as part of its circumference, and the lumen is always in the direction of the center of that circle. The subtle innominate grooves of the mucosa also identify the circumference of the colon.

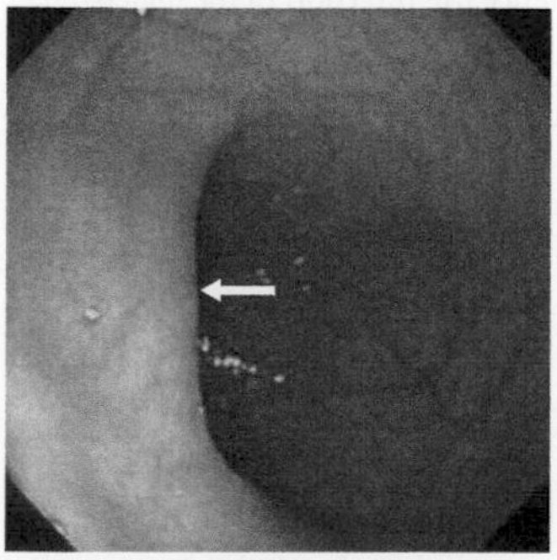

Fig 6.9 Reading the circumferential folds. The lumen is behind the "blind fold."

At a bend in the colon, the colonoscope illuminates the wall that is straight ahead, leaving the lumen darker. This is analogous to the effect of automobile headlights in a bend of a dark tunnel: the wall in front of the headlights is brightly lit, whereas the road ahead is darker.

If a large fold is noted coursing across the image, then the lumen is almost always located behind that fold (the "blind fold"; Fig 6.9) The scope tip should be gently advanced under/over the fold and the lumen can be "teased" open with delicate motions of the tip of the scope.

In some cases of severe sigmoid diverticular disease the diverticular orifices may be larger than the true colonic lumen; but highlights from the hypertrophic circular muscle layer can be used to predict the

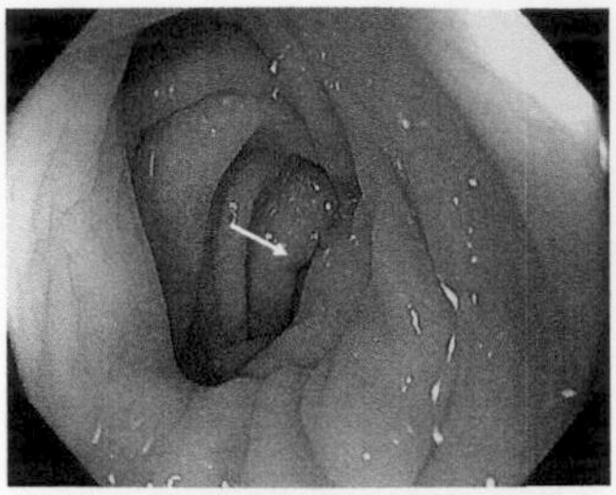

Fig 6.10 Finding the lumen in dense diverticular disease. The thickened, hypertrophied folds and narrowed lumen make identification of the lumen difficult. Care must be taken to distinguish the true lumen (arrow) from a large-mouthed diverticular orifice.

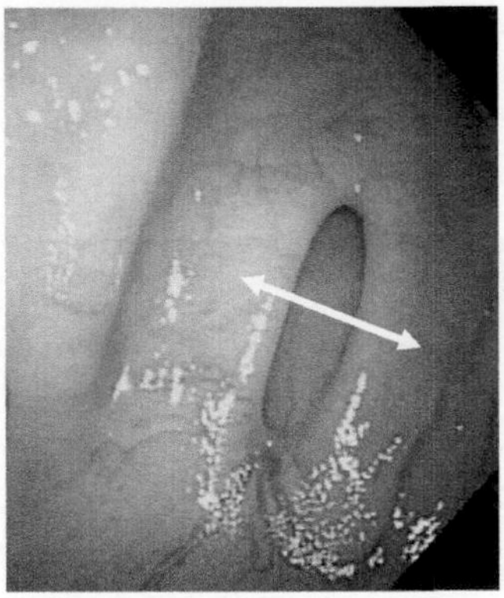

Fig 6.11 Finding the lumen in diverticular disease. Owing to the circular fibers of the muscularis propria, diverticular orifices are typically elliptical. The short axis of the orifice (white arrow) corresponds to the long axis of the colon (and hence the direction of the lumen).

Identifying the Lumen: Landmarks

- Arc-shaped light reflections
- Dark areas in distance
- The "blind fold"
- Convergence of folds

location of the lumen (Fig 6.10). The elliptical diverticular orifices also provide a clue as to the location of the lumen, as the lumen is usually located at a right angle to the long axis of the orifice. The true lumen must be differentiated from the mouths of diverticula, which have a characteristic elliptical, muscular appearance (Fig 6.11). The "bottom" of a diverticulum is generally also readily seen when it is *en face*.

Insufflate and evacuate air strategically

Air insufflation distends the colon and opens up the folds, improving visualization. When air is withdrawn, the colon diameter becomes smaller and its length diminishes, just as a balloon shrinks when air is released. Air aspiration thus may help advance the scope at times when pushing the scope does not—especially in the ascending colon.

In a healthy colon continuous insufflation of air will rarely lead to perforation, because the anus and (in some patients) the ileocecal valve provide escape valves. However, air pressure may create a perforation if these escape valves are closed, e.g. the ileocecal valve is competent and a sigmoid stricture narrows the lumen to the point that the scope creates an air seal. When the scope is within a narrowed segment and air is continuously insufflated in an attempt to keep the lumen open, it is possible to 'blow out' the cecum (Fig 6.12). Therefore when difficulty is encountered in traversing a tight sigmoid segment, air should be introduced cautiously, and navigation performed using fine tip motions, with the assistant gauging the degree of abdominal distention.

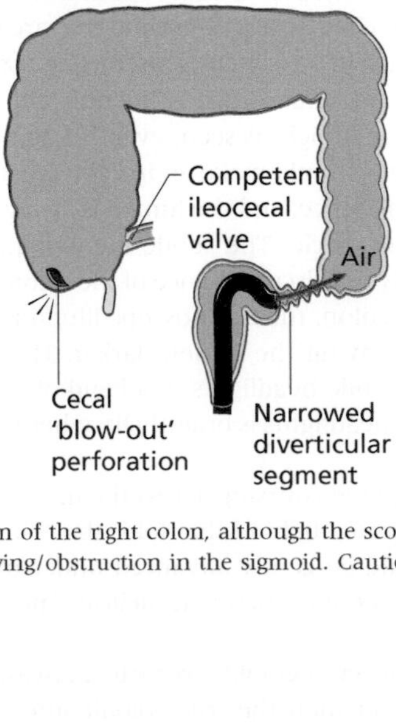

Fig 6.12 Perforation of the right colon, although the scope did not pass through the narrowing/obstruction in the sigmoid. Caution: do not overinflate.

Using water instillation

Some endoscopists instill warm water when they encounter a difficult sigmoid colon. Anecdotally, this may relax the sigmoid musculature, making it easier to traverse the segment. Several groups have reported success distending the entire colon with water instead of air. During intubation, the air pump is turned off, and water is instilled continuously. When the patient lies in the left lateral position, the cecum is usually in a superior position, and the advancing water column pushes air proximally toward the cecum. Therefore, the cecum is usually air-filled when it is reached, and is recognizable by the usual landmarks. This "water method" is reported to decrease sedation requirements and may even permit unsedated colonoscopy.

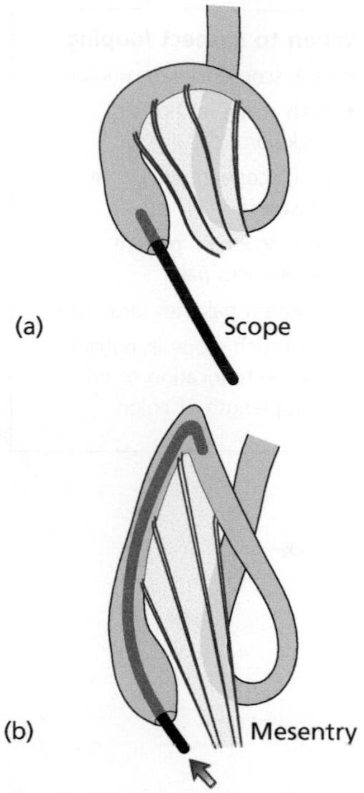

Fig 6.13 Intubating the sigmoid colon. As the scope is advanced from the rectum (a) through the sigmoid (b), the sigmoid mesentery may be stretched, causing pain.

Be alert to looping

During scope insertion, the attachments of the mesocolon to the peritoneal cavity cause the instrument to spiral clockwise on insertion. This occurs repeatedly. When there is a loop in the scope, advancing the shaft may not advance the tip, but may further bow or "loop" the scope. An enlarging loop can pull on the mesenteric attachments, causing pain (Fig 6.13). If the radial strain from an expanding loop is too great, a linear colonic tear may occur.

Looping is suspected when:

• the shaft of the scope is advanced, but the image does not change, implying that the tip is not advancing (i.e. "one-to-one" correlation between shaft and tip movement is absent);

• insertion of the shaft causes the scope tip to move (paradoxically) backwards (Fig 6.14);

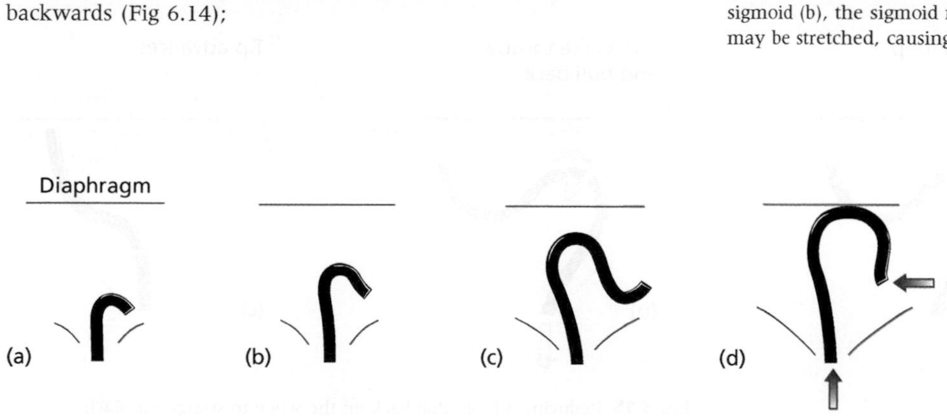

Fig 6.14 Paradoxical tip movement from looping. The scope tip may move backward when the shaft is advanced.

When to suspect looping

- Push scope in: image unchanged
- Push scope in: tip falls backward (distally)
- Push scope in: encounter resistance
- Push scope in: patient experiences pain
- Assistant palpates large loop
- Too much scope in patient relative to location of tip along length of colon

- the patient is experiencing undue pain;
- the endoscopy assistant palpates a large loop;
- the amount of scope within the patient is disproportionate to the location of the tip (e.g. 120 cm of scope have been inserted and the tip is still in the sigmoid);
- inordinate resistance to advancing the scope is felt.

Even after a loop has formed, advancing the shaft may result in forward tip progress. Occasionally, it is necessary to "push through a loop" in order to traverse a recalcitrant segment of colon. To avoid perforation, this must be done tentatively and without undue force.

Reduce the loops

Loops can usually be eliminated ("reduced") by pulling back on the shaft while torquing the scope shaft clockwise. The clockwise motion secures the position of the scope tip, so it does not fall back. During the pullback, the dial controls are rotated to keep the lumen in view. This pullback maneuver straightens the scope, often reducing the length of scope inside the patient by as much as 50%. The scope-straightening maneuver should be performed repeatedly during colonoscopy and often following each advance of the scope (Fig 6.15). Failure to do so may make it impossible to traverse upper colon angulations such as the hepatic flexure. Occasionally loop reduction requires counterclockwise torque.

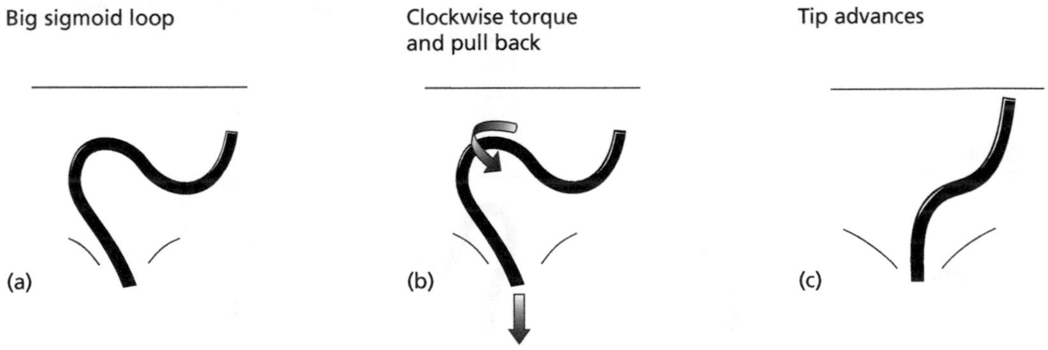

Fig 6.15 Reducing a loop. Pull back on the scope to straighten. Each advance will create another loop.

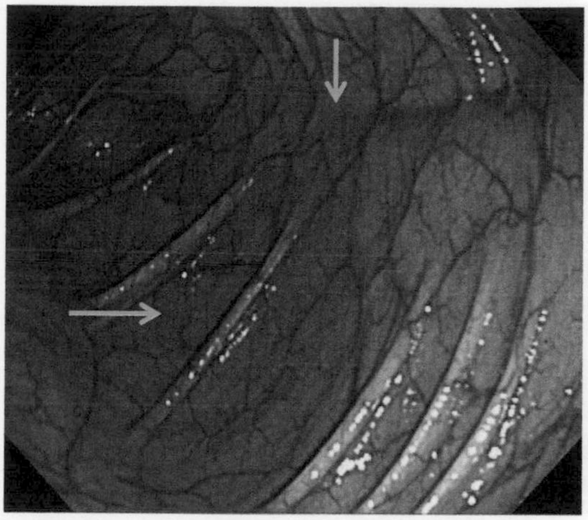

Plate 6.1 Hepatic flexure (normal). In the region of the hepatic flexure, the liver is visible through the thin-walled colon as a triangular, purplish, flat, structure (arrows).

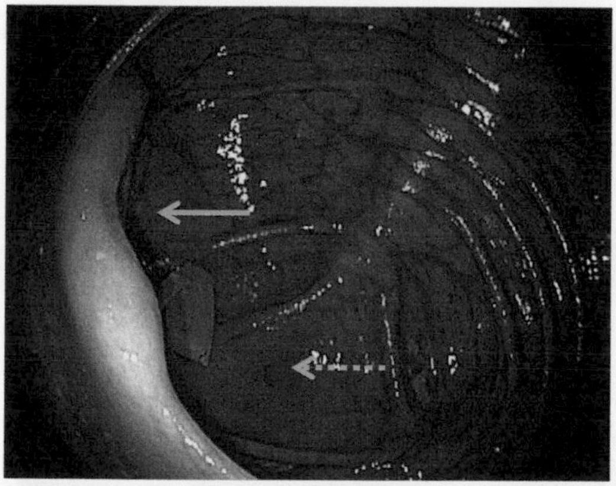

Plate 6.2 Ileocecal valve (normal). Viewed from its side during routine colonoscopy, the ileocecal valve (solid arrow) is identified by its yellowish color, central notch, location within the ileocecal fold, and relationship to the appendiceal orifice (dotted arrow), cecal caput, and converging teniae coli.

Practical Colonoscopy, First Edition. Jerome D. Waye, James Aisenberg, and Peter H. Rubin.
© 2013 John Wiley & Sons, Ltd. Published 2013 by John Wiley & Sons, Ltd.

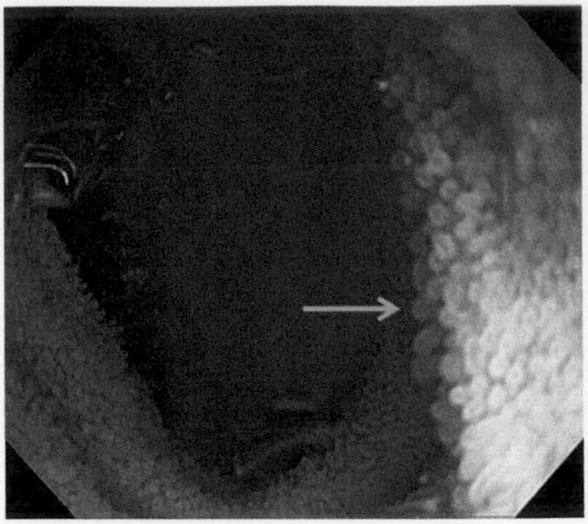

Plate 6.3 Villi of terminal ileum (normal). When water is instilled into the distal ileum, the villi are magnified and more clearly visible.

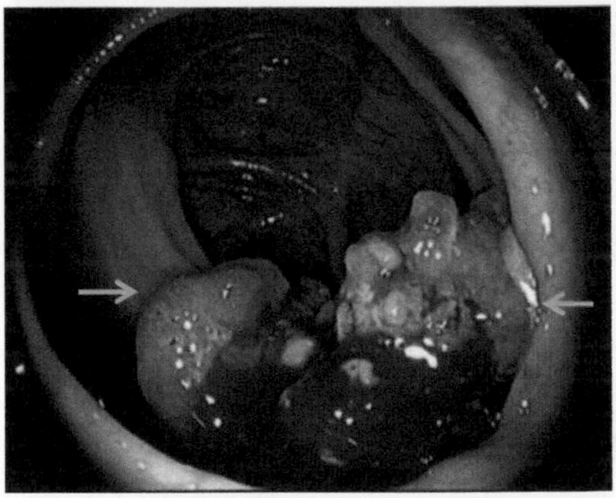

Plate 7.1 Adenocarcinoma of ascending colon. This broad-based exophytic lesion (arrows), detected during the evaluation of occult gastrointestinal bleeding, demonstrates several malignant features: spontaneous bleeding, large size, irregular shape, and surface ulceration/necrosis. The patient underwent right hemicolectomy; the adjacent lymph nodes were negative for cancer. The ileocecal valve and sling folds, seen just beyond it, establish its location.

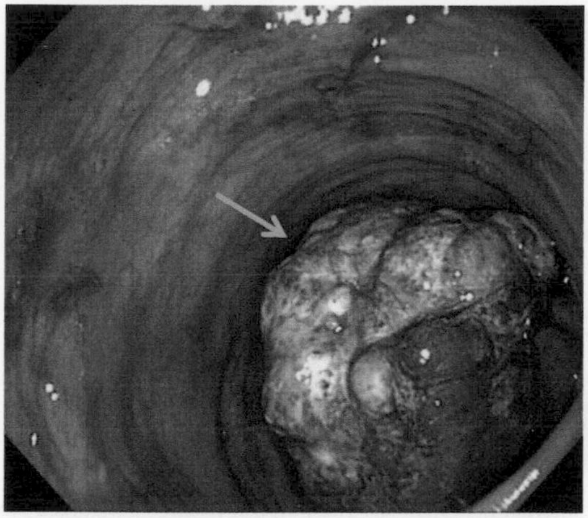

Plate 7.2 Sigmoid carcinoma. This lesion was encountered during the evaluation of unexplained rectal bleeding. The size, necrotic and irregular surface, irregular shape, surface exudate and ulceration, firmness, and varied coloration all suggest carcinoma. The patient underwent left hemicolectomy.

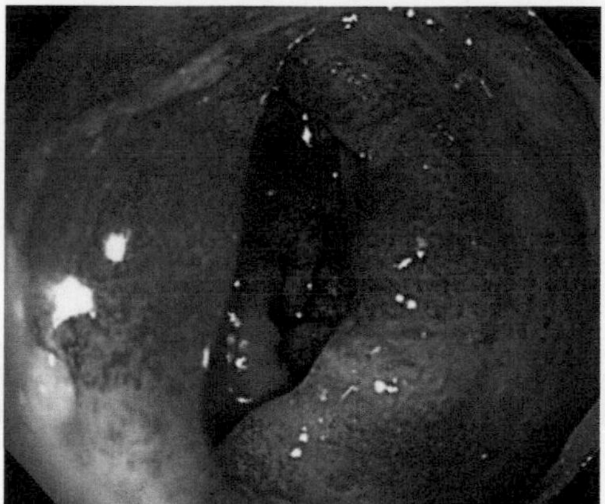

Plate 7.3 Red folds of diverticular disease. Identified in individuals with diverticular disease and haustral hypertrophy, this striking appearance reflects intramucosal hemorrhage and may be asymptomatic or cause bleeding. The abnormality is seen in a short segment of the sigmoid colon. In this case, the characteristic haustral hypertrophy, erythema, edema, and luminal narrowing are seen. Biopsy may confirm the diagnosis.

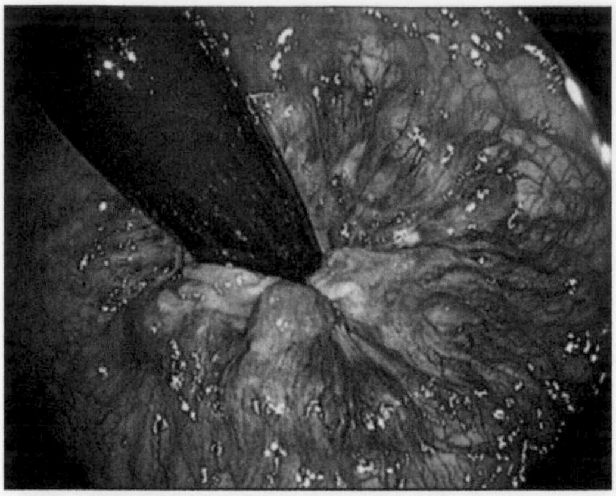

Plate 7.4 Internal hemorrhoids. The purplish rosette of engorged blood vessels, seen best on retroflexion, defines internal hemorrhoids and should be described in the colonoscopy report.

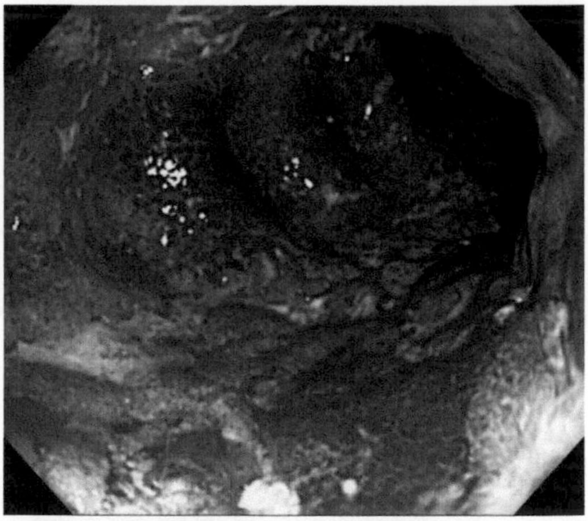

Plate 7.5 Left-sided colonic ischemia. This patient presented with abrupt-onset lower abdominal pain and rectal bleeding. A 20-cm segment of abnormal mucosa was identified in the left colon. The rectum was spared. Endoscopic hallmarks of ischemia include a segmental "watershed" distribution and mucosal edema, erythema, friability, ulceration, and exudate. In more severe cases, the mucosa may appear purplish or cyanotic. Mucosal biopsy may be useful to confirm the diagnosis. In this case, the patient improved with conservative measures.

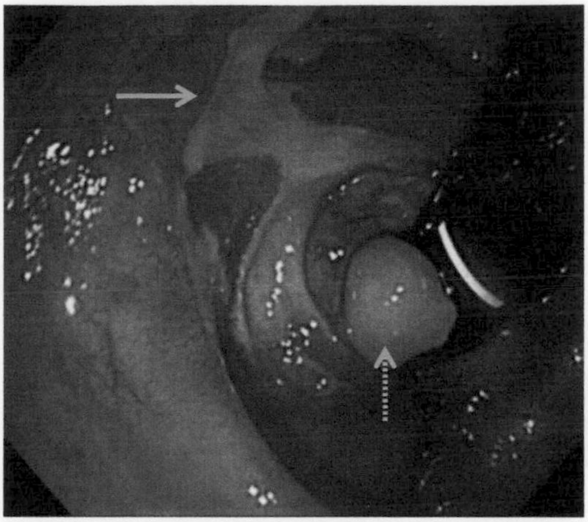

Plate 7.6 Solitary rectal ulcer. Visualized in retroflexion, the lesion is seen as a large pale ulcer (solid arrow) with exudate at the base, and surrounding erythema. These may not be solitary and may have polypoid elements, and are typically associated with constipation and/or rectal prolapse. Mucosal biopsy will confirm the diagnosis. Also seen is a yellowish hypertrophic anal papilla (dotted arrow).

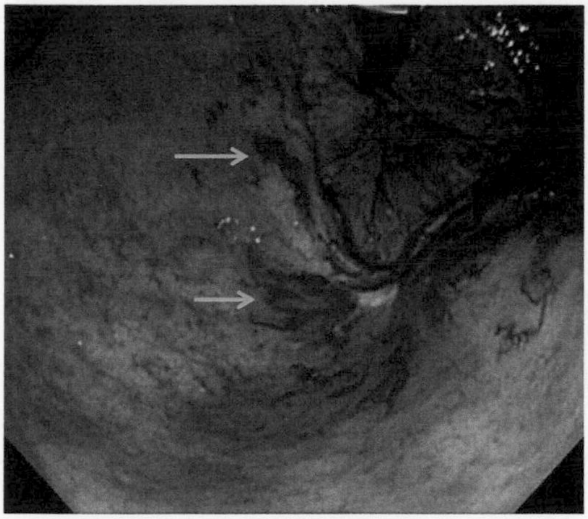

Plate 7.7 Radiation proctopathy. This patient presented with painless hematochezia several years after brachytherapy for prostate carcinoma. Multiple abnormal, prominent, bright red, ectatic, serpiginous, vessels are visible in the distal rectum, seen best with the scope in retroflex orientation. These can be ablated by electrocautery or argon plasma coagulation.

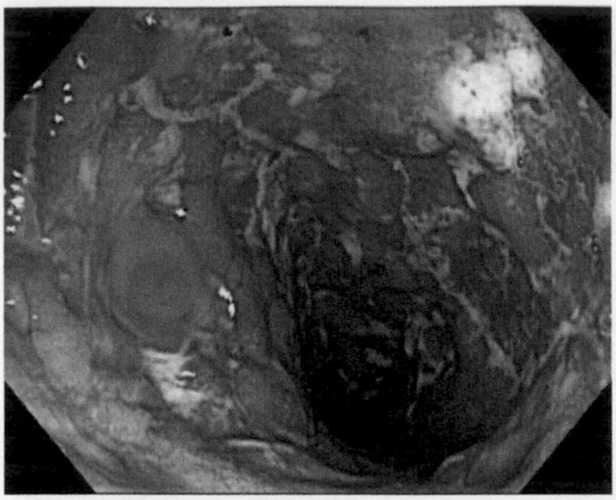

Plate 7.8 Active ulcerative colitis. This narrowed, tubular segment of descending colon is ulcerated, edematous, erythematous, with surface exudates and complete loss of the underlying normal vascular pattern.

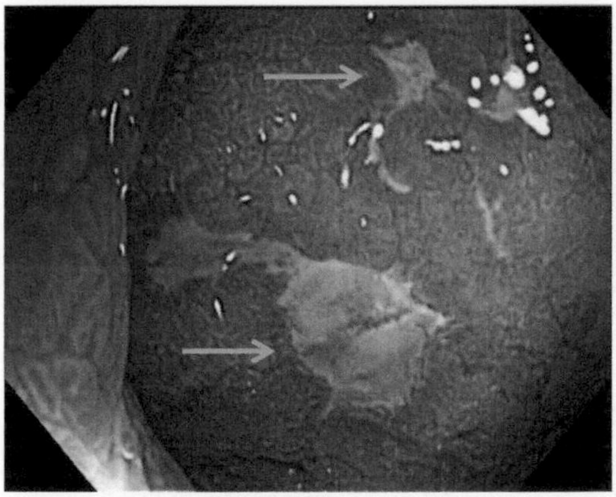

Plate 7.9 Ulcers in Crohn's colitis. Crohn's ulcerations may appear as small aphthoid ulcers or as irregular, stellate ulcers like these. Biopsies seldom reveal granulomas.

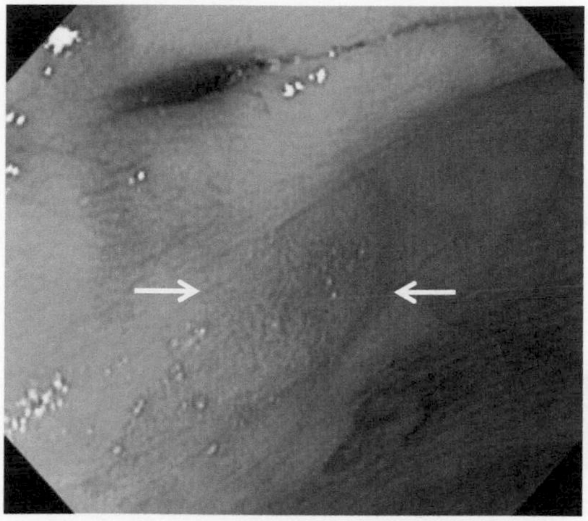

Plate 7.10 Dysplastic polyp seen during colitis surveillance using chromoendoscopy. The mucosa has been sprayed with dilute methylene blue, revealing a small lesion (arrows). This polyp has the appearance of a sporadic adenoma, and was removed by snare polypectomy. The margins of the polypectomy site were biopsied to assure no residual dysplasia. (Paris 0–IIb).

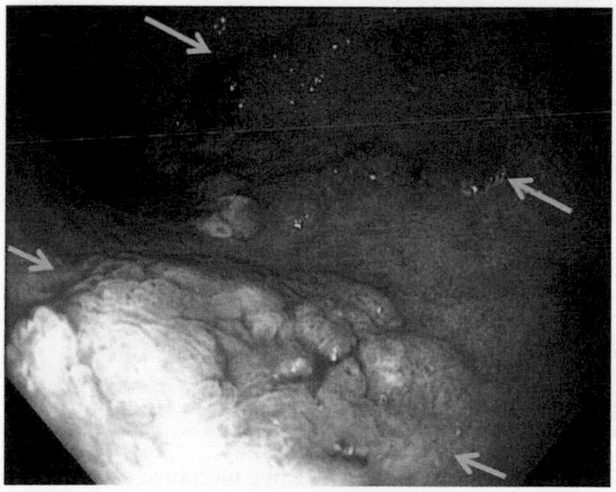

Plate 7.11 Colitis-associated dysplastic polyps. These two lesions (arrows) were identified during surveillance colonoscopy in the distal rectum of a patient with >15 years of chronic ulcerative colitis. Features differentiating these lesions from "pseudopolyps" include: flat and "spreading" shape; irregular, villiform, nodular, surface; and absence of friability and of exudative cap. Biopsy revealed low-grade dysplasia. Because the lesions were multiple, large, atypical, and not amenable to colonoscopic resection, the patient was referred for total proctocolectomy. Multiple sites of dysplasia were found in the surgical specimen, but no carcinoma. (Paris 0–IIb and c).

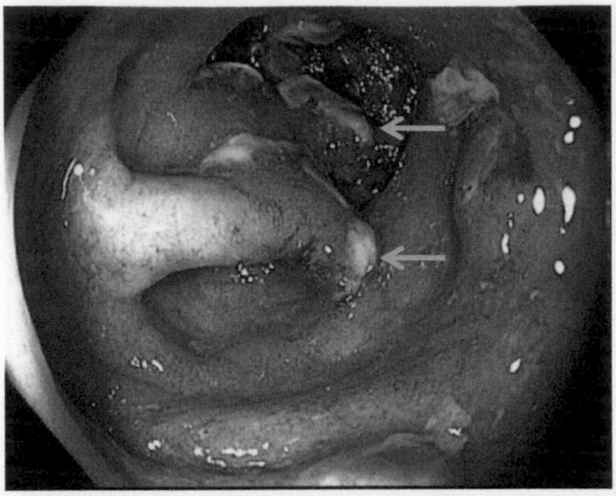

Plate 7.12 Inflammatory polyps in ulcerative colitis. The white exudates on the polyp tips (arrows) are characteristic. These lesions are typically multiple, friable, and have negligible malignant potential.

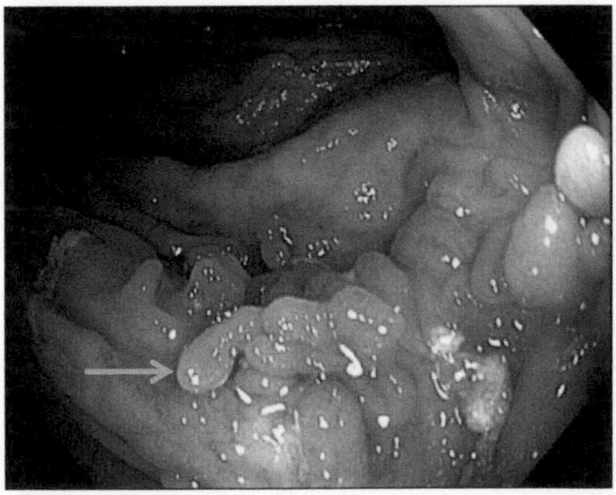

Plate 7.13 Pseudopolyps in chronic, inactive ulcerative colitis. Seen during routine surveillance, the pseudopolyps (arrow) appear as multiple, filiform, uniform, smooth-surfaced protrusions. These polyps have negligible malignant potential and need not be biopsied or removed.

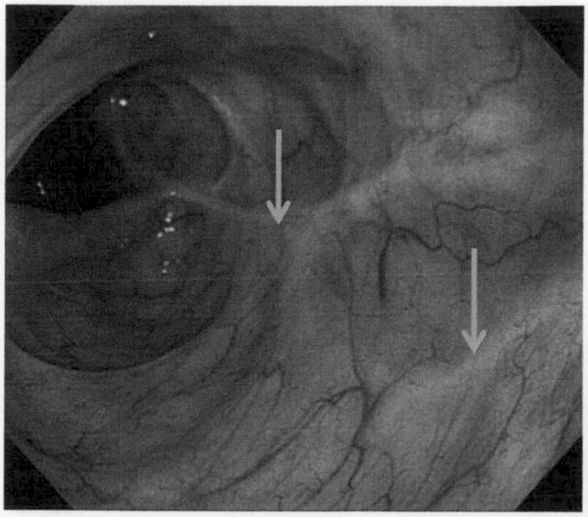

Plate 7.14 Mucosal scarring in healed colitis. During routine surveillance colonoscopy in a patient with healed chronic ulcerative colitis, a lattice of pale scarring is seen, indicative of healing of previous colitis. There is no evidence of active colitis. The mucosa appears hypovascular, and relatively featureless.

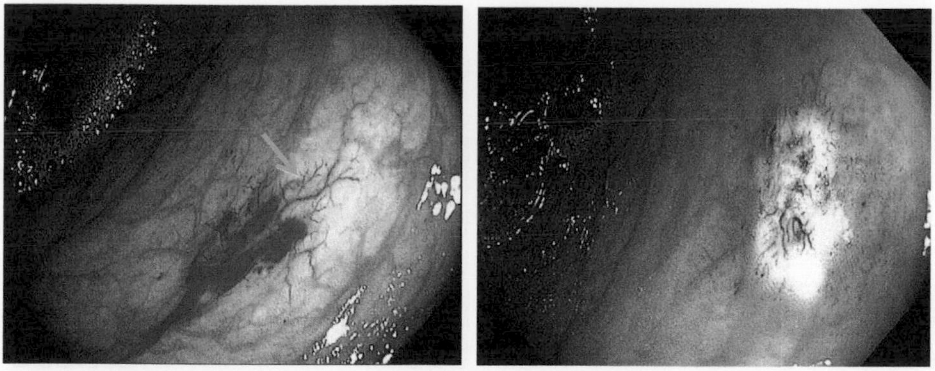

Plate 7.15 Bleeding angioectasia. This spontaneously bleeding lesion was identified in the ascending colon of a patient experiencing occult chronic gastrointestinal blood loss. The lesion displays characteristically distinct, arborizing, deep red, ectatic vessels (arrow). The lesion was ablated with cautery (right panel), stopping the bleeding. Nonbleeding angioectasias may be encountered incidentally during colonoscopy, and in this setting are generally not ablated.

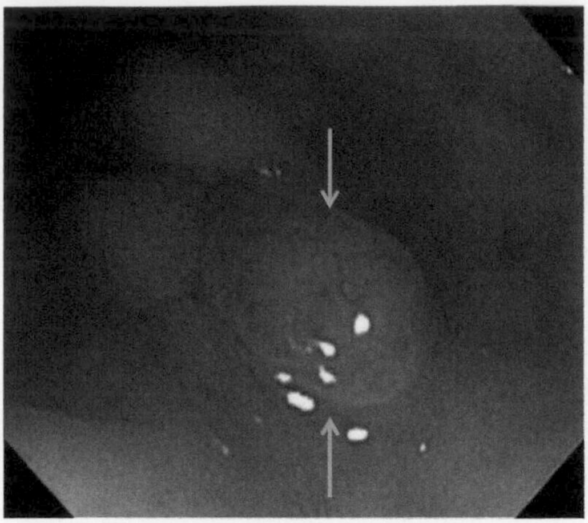

Plate 10.1 Hyperplastic polyp in the rectum. These common lesions are characteristically multiple, small, and (under white light) exhibit a smooth, glistening, pale, hypovascular surface. Under narrow band imaging, hyperplastic polyps will appear pale and bland, with a lacy or absent vascular pattern and homogenous pale pits (Paris 0–IIa).

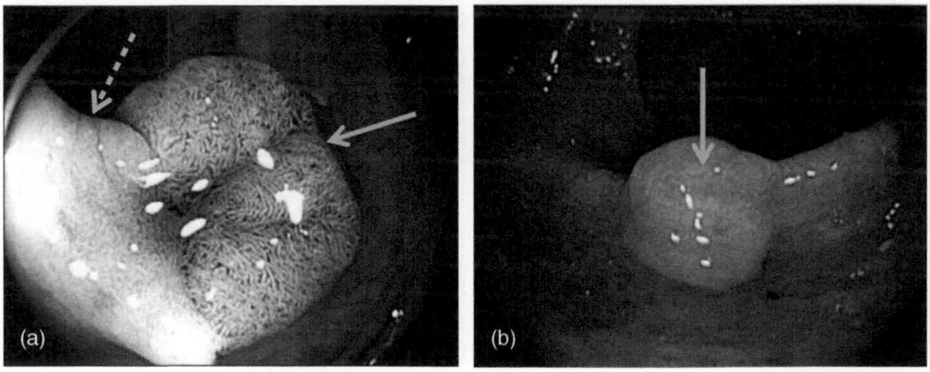

Plate 10.2 Distinguishing a pedunculated adenomatous polyp ((a) Paris 0–Ip) and a sessile serrated polyp ((b) Paris 0–IIa) using NBI (without magnification). The surface vessels in the head of the adenoma (solid arrow, left) are numerous and brown, giving the area a characteristically dark, brownish appearance. Between the vessels are white tubular structures, which create a reticular pattern. This vascular pattern is absent in the polyp stalk (dashed arrow, left) and in sessile serrated polyps (right), which characteristically are pale and lack significant surface vessels.

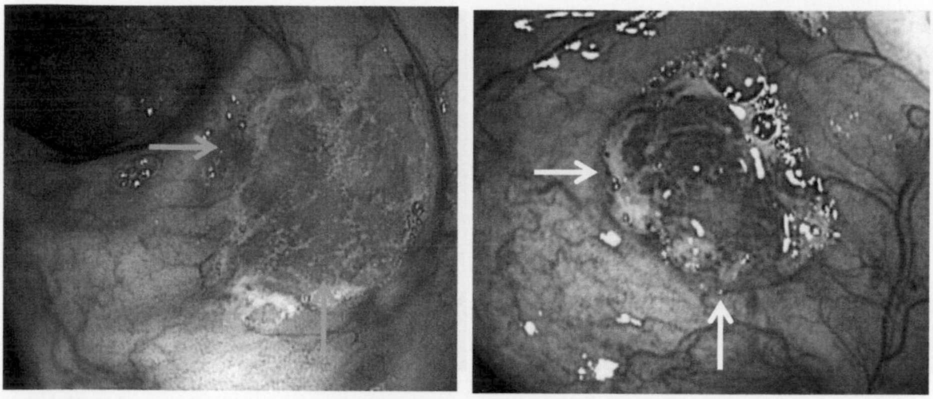

Plate 10.3 Serrated sessile lesion. This 1-cm sessile serrated adenoma/polyp (arrows) is easily overlooked. The lesion is flat and obscures the underlying vascular pattern. It is pale, yellowish, and contains a surface mucous cap. These morphological features are characteristic of sessile serrated adenomas/polyps (SSA/Ps). Narrow band imaging (right panel) highlights interruption of underlying vascular pattern by an SSA/P, and the mucous cap takes on a characteristic reddish appearance (Paris 0–IIb).

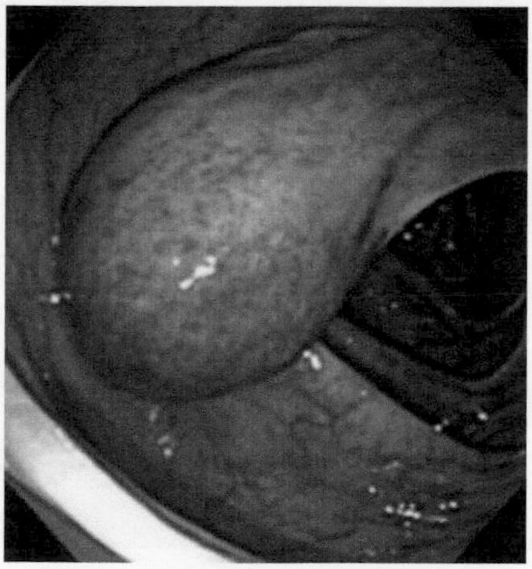

Plate 10.4 Pedunculated lipoma. The polyp appears red at its tip as a result of chronic trauma, with intramucosal hemorrhage and inflammation. The underlying submucosal lipoma creates a yellowish coloration of the body of the lipoma, while the stalk retains the coloration of normal mucosa. When probed with a forceps, the body of the polyp is soft and easily indented. Biopsy of the surface of a lipoma may be normal, or may detect the underlying fat.

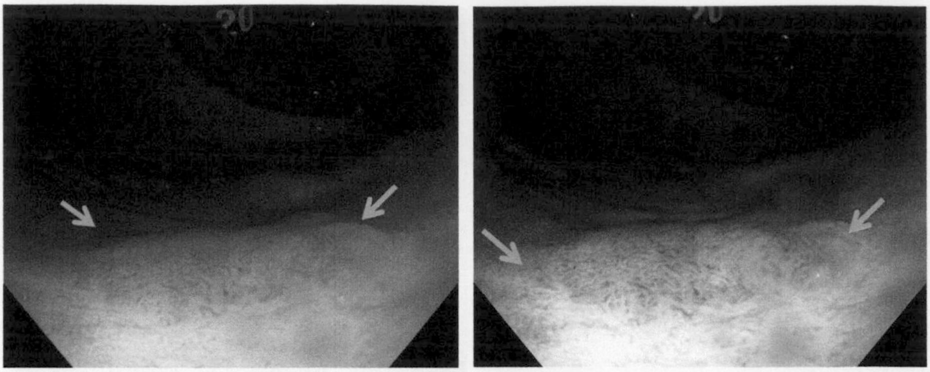

Plate 10.5 Flat adenoma. Seen with the scope in retroflexion, this subtle 1.4 polyp is distinguished from the normal mucosa by slight elevation above the mucosal plane, slight nodularity, cerebriform surface architecture, and slightly increased vascularity. This lesion highlights the importance of meticulous colon cleansing and fastidious and thorough mucosal inspection during scope withdrawal. Narrow band imaging (right panel) highlights the meshed vascular pattern of the adenoma (Paris 0–IIa).

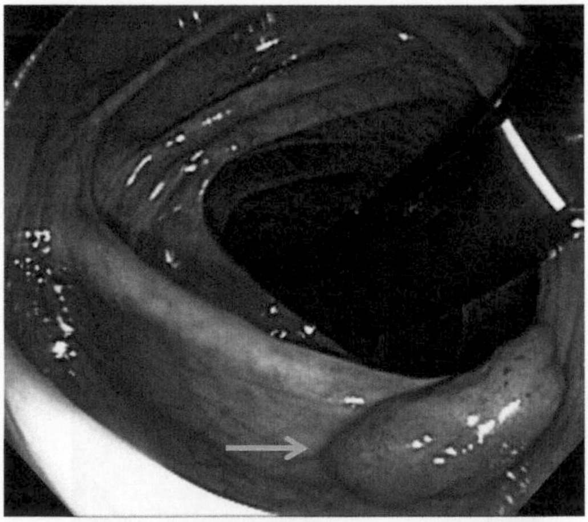

Plate 10.6 Polyp on back of haustral fold. This sessile transverse colon 1.5-cm polyp (arrow) is best visualized with the scope in the retroflexed position. In the antegrade scope position, the proximal margin of the polyp could not be visualized. Submucosal saline injection and snare polypectomy can be performed with the scope in this configuration. During scope withdrawal, the mucosa on the back side of each large fold must be systematically examined (Paris 0–Is).

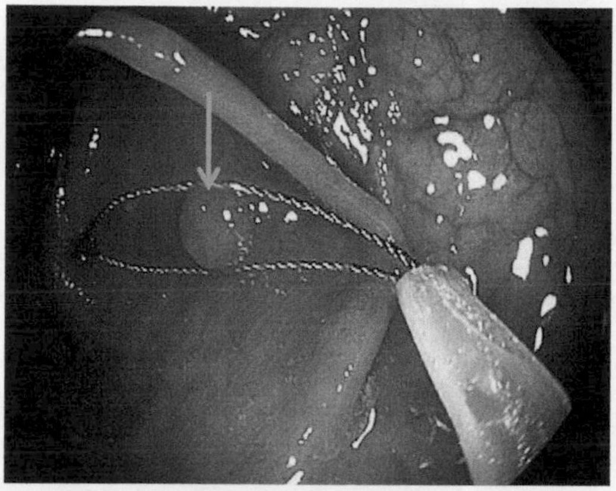

Plate 10.7 "Cold" snare resection of a diminutive polyp. This 3-mm sessile lesion is resected without cautery. Bleeding is minimal and self-limited. Cold resection can be utilized for most serrated and adenomatous polyps that are approximately 6 mm or less in diameter.

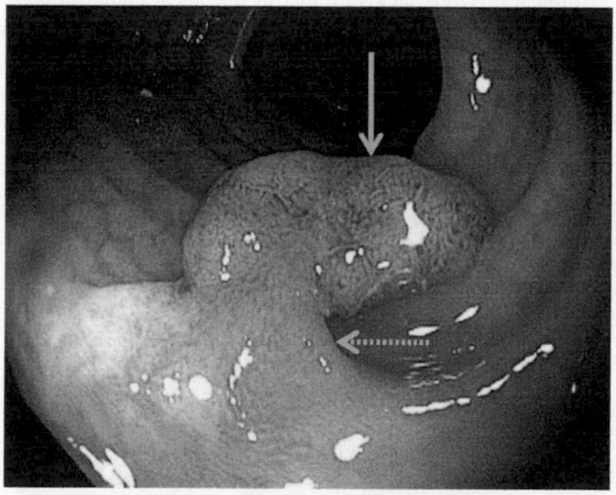

Plate 10.8 Pedunculated polyp. This 1.3 cm descending colon tubulovillous adenoma should be resected with cautery-assisted snare polypectomy. The snare will be closed around the stalk of the polyp at the level of the dotted arrow. The pedicle is created by the chronic traction on the polyp by colonic contractions (Paris 0–Ip).

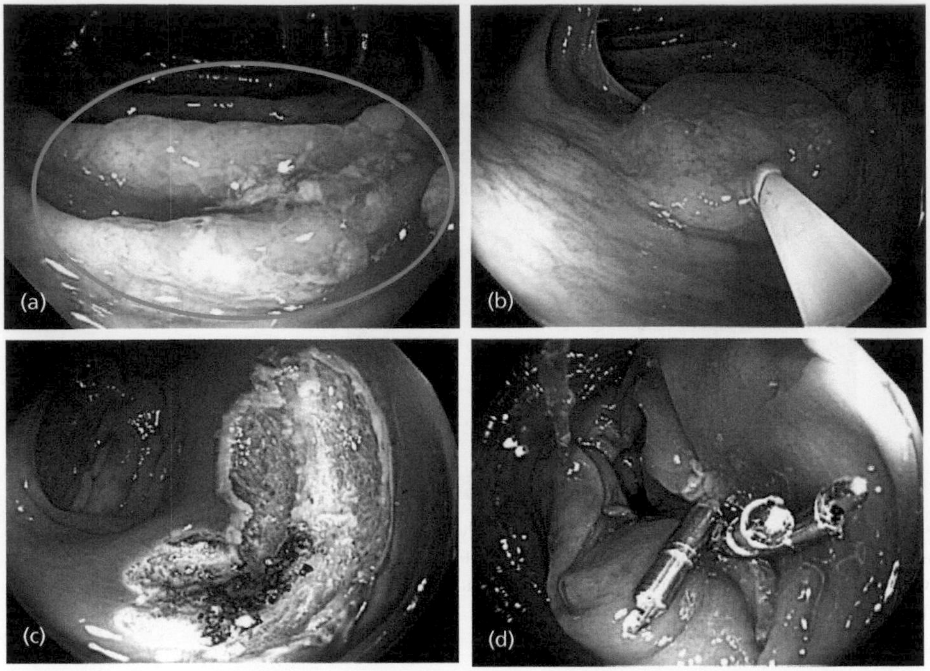

Plate 11.1 Complex resection of flat polyp. This flat, 3-cm, transverse colon polyp (Paris 0–IIb) crosses over two haustral folds (a) has a mucous cap, suggestive of serrated histology. The polyp was elevated with saline (b), using a direct puncture into the body of the polyp. Note that the back of the polyp has been elevated preferentially, making it more accessible to visualization and capture. The polyp was resected piecemeal using snare cautery, revealing the white, lacy submucosa (c). Local bleeding was controlled with direct application of cautery with a probe (brown area in center of defect (c)) and clips were applied to protect against possible bleeding (d). The patient recovered uneventfully. Histology demonstrated a sessile serrated adenoma/polyp with areas of cytological dysplasia.

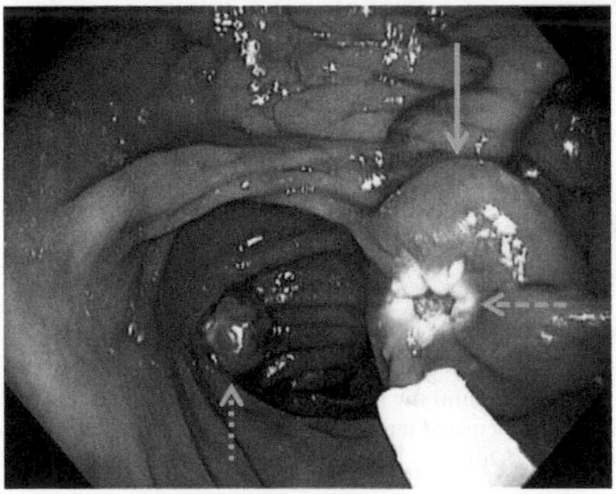

Plate 11.2 Polypectomy site immediately following saline-assisted resection. After snare resection with cautery, the mucosa at the site of this flat, 1.8-cm transverse colon polyp remains elevated by the injected saline (solid arrow). The retracted coagulation zone (dashed arrow), and a small area of submucosa at its center, are visible. The resected polyp (dotted arrow) has fallen to the opposite wall of the colon and awaits retrieval. The white snare catheter is visible in the foreground.

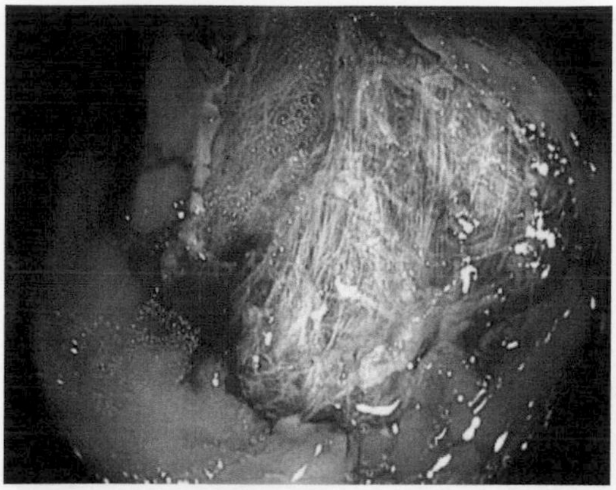

Plate 11.3 The mucosal defect immediately following saline-assisted snare cautery resection of a large sessile polyp. The white, lattice-like submucosa is plainly visible and is an expected observation. There is no disruption of muscularis propria. The minor bleeding from the margins can be treated thermally if desired. There is no visible residual polyp. The mucosal defect should be carefully examined for signs of residual tumor following a complex polypectomy.

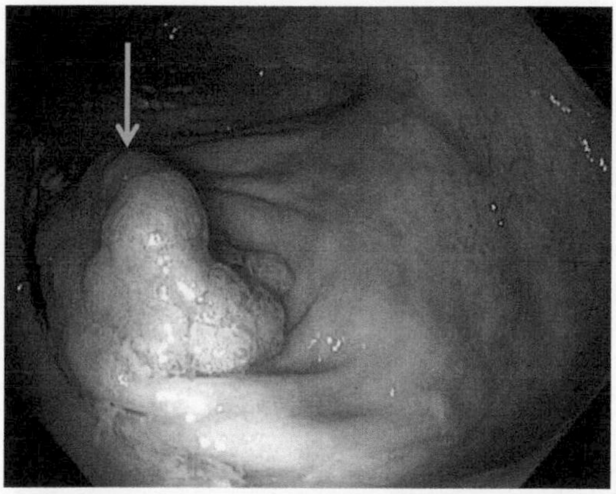

Plate 11.4 Advanced adenoma. This 1- cm sessile tubulovillous adenoma (arrow, Paris 0–Is) arises at the appendiceal orifice. Because the "back" margin of the polyp was located inside the appendix and could not be visualized, the patient was referred for laparoscopic resection.

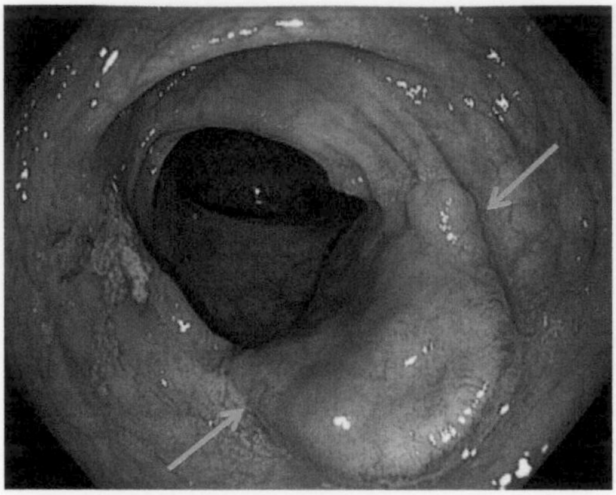

Plate 12.1 Malignant polyp. Worrisome characteristics of this 3-cm sessile descending colon polyp (arrows) include its large size, subtle central depression, and firm texture, and smooth non-granular appearance. The patient underwent curative surgical resection. (Paris 0–IIb and c.)

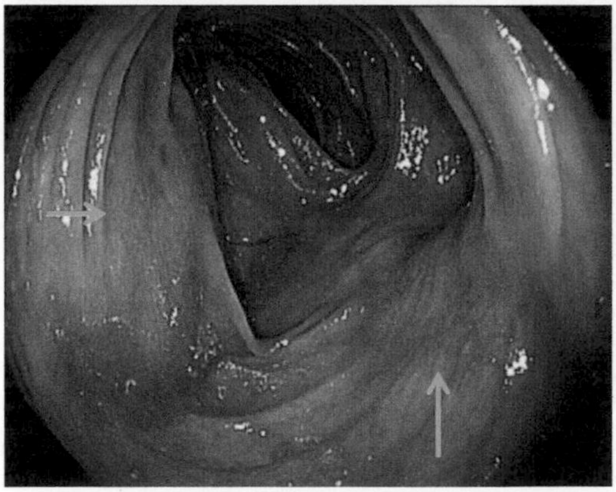

Plate 12.2 Tattoo at polypectomy site visualized at follow-up colonoscopy. Separate markings (arrows) had been placed around the circumference of the colon wall, maximizing their visibility at colonoscopy or surgery.

After several loop reductions, the shaft outside the patient may form a loop because of the repeated unidirectional twists. This external twist is cumbersome, and can be eliminated by twisting the shaft in the opposite direction and manipulating the dial controls to keep the lumen in view (Fig 6.16).

Prevent loop formation

Repeated looping with failure to advance the scope indicates that adjunctive maneuvers are necessary. Carefully positioned pressure by the assistant employing either the palm or the fingertips often helps by altering intra-abdominal anatomy and the resistances encountered by the scope. The assistant should apply the pressure gradually and firmly, with one or two hands. Often suprapubic pressure is helpful when the shaft has been inserted 20 to 30 cm; in other instances mid-abdominal or right or left upper quadrant pressure is helpful. Pressure may help "push" the wall of the colon "toward" the tip of the scope (Fig 6.17). The location is empirical: if one spot doesn't help, a second location is tried. Most of the time, pressure is maintained for only about 30 seconds, as it either helps and the scope is advanced or a different location needs to be tried. Many colonoscopists choose to identify the best spot themselves, reaching over the patient to palpate the abdomen with the right hand.

Another way to prevent the shaft from looping is to pleat (telescope) the colon over the shaft of the scope. This is accomplished by jiggling the shaft back and forth a few centimeters with rapid in and out movements.

Rotating the patient from left lateral decubitus to supine, right lateral or, occasionally, to prone position may also alter the internal anatomy and resistances, allowing intubation to proceed.

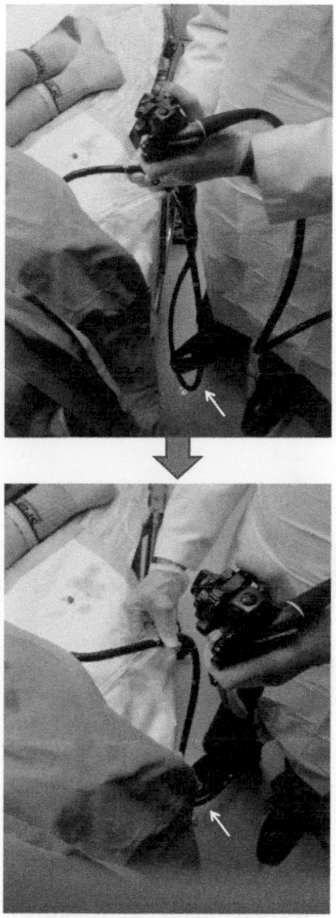

Fig 6.16 Resolve an external loop. The scope is withdrawn and torqued, straightening the external loop. The dial controls are used to keep the lumen in view during this maneuver.

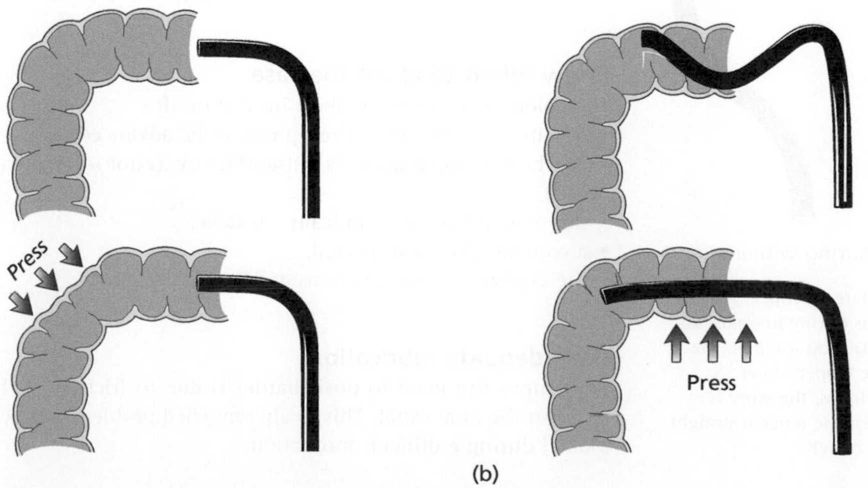

(a) (b)

Fig 6.17 Abdominal pressure may help to advance the scope, either by pushing the colon over the scope (a) or pushing on the scope (b).

If the scope has advanced to the right colon but looping prevents cecal intubation, it is sometimes useful to pull the scope all the way back to the left colon and simply repeat the entire intubation. This lengthy withdrawal—which on the surface appears to "waste" progress and effort—may in fact straighten or pleat the colon, rendering a colon that seemed intractable on the first attempt quite straightforward on the second.

Although fluoroscopy can be helpful, experienced colonoscopists rarely employ it, as it is cumbersome, involves radiation, and is rarely necessary. A device called the "Scope Guide" uses magnetic, nonradiographic impulses to generate an image of the scope as it progresses (or does not progress) through the large bowel. This tool may be useful for the especially difficult colonoscopy and for the novice during training.

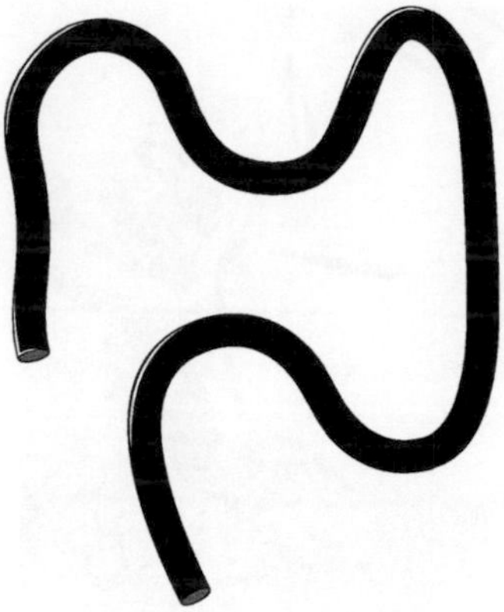

(a) Scope during intubation

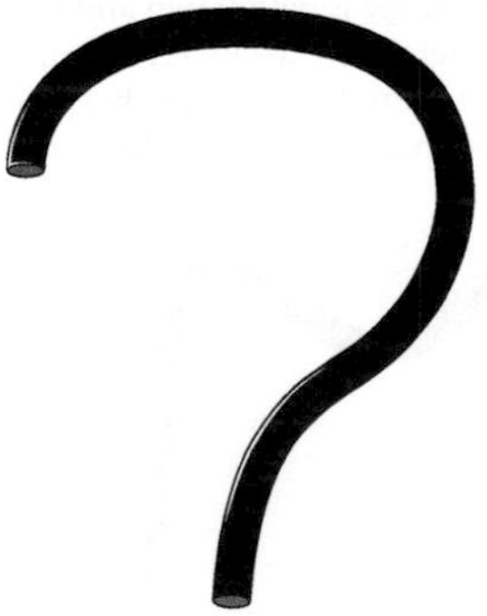

(b) Scope during withdrawal

Fig 6.18 Different scope configurations during insertion and withdrawal. During insertion the scope may be looped. After reduction of loops, the scope is straight. When the scope is straight, tip control is better.

Never push against fixed resistance

Skilled colonoscopists rely on finesse rather than force. At times, moderate, transient axial force is required to advance the scope. However, this force should never exceed a low threshold; if the scope is not advancing there is a reason, and it is time to try a new tactic. Fixed resistance can be caused by scarring (adhesions), extremely large loops (where force is transmitted to the bend rather than the scope tip), and fixation by advanced diverticular disease, tumors, or other abnormalities. If the resistance is fixed, the colonoscopist should never try to "push through" it; this is a potential cause of perforation.

Remove some polyps during intubation

The colon is configured differently during insertion and withdrawal (Fig 6.18). In the latter phase, it may be telescoped over the scope, potentially concealing polyps in the crevices between the folds. If a large polyp is seen during insertion, resection can be deferred until the withdrawal phase; however, a small polyp seen during insertion can be extremely difficult to detect on the way out. The momentum of intubation must be interrupted and the lesion resected.

Know when to abort the case

The colonoscopist should abort intubation if:

- despite all maneuvers, the tip cannot be advanced;
- the bowel preparation is unsatisfactory (photo-document the debris);
- the patient becomes clinically unstable;
- a complication is suspected;
- the equipment malfunctions and cannot be fixed.

Use adequate lubrication

Sometimes the need to push harder is due to friction of the dry scope in the anal canal. This easily remedied problem can be overlooked during a difficult intubation.

Lubricating the insertion tube

- Resistance to insertion tube at anus due to friction occurs commonly
  - Confounds tactile feedback to colonoscopist regarding resistance arising from colon
  - Increases strain on right arm
  - Consider when high resistance to pushing scope in
- Keep lubricant accessible and reapply frequently
- Throughout case, only grip insertion tube with pad/gauze
  - Improves control
  - Decreases likelihood that lubricant will get onto gloved right hand (and from there onto dial controls)
- Avoid getting lubricant on the dial controls
  - Makes them hard to control
  - If lubricant gets on the dial controls, stop case and wipe off

Be aware how much scope you have inserted

The centimeter markings on the insertion tube provide valuable information regarding the configuration of the scope inside the patient. If the scope is straight, the cecum will usually be reached with 75–80 cm of scope inserted. The skilled practitioner fastidiously straightens the instrument throughout intubation, often inserting the scope to approximately the 120-cm mark, before pulling it back. Insertion beyond 120 cm should trigger reassessment of the intubation.

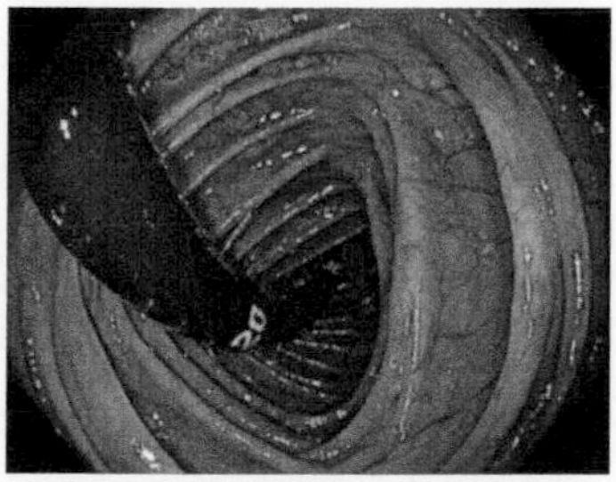

Fig 6.19 The triangular folds of the transverse colon, here seen with the scope in retroversion.

Look for landmarks

During intubation, landmarks predict the approximate location of the tip of the scope. These include the tight muscular folds of the sigmoid colon, the fluid pool at the splenic flexure, the triangular folds of the transverse colon (Fig 6.19), the sharp angulations of the flexures, and the blue hue of the liver (Plate 6.1). Although useful, these landmarks are imprecise, and must not be used to specify the location of a lesion that requires surgery. Precise localization of a lesion is accomplished by submucosal injection of a marker (see Chapter 10). The only unequivocal colonic landmarks are at the rectum and the cecum, provided of course that the cecum is correctly identified.

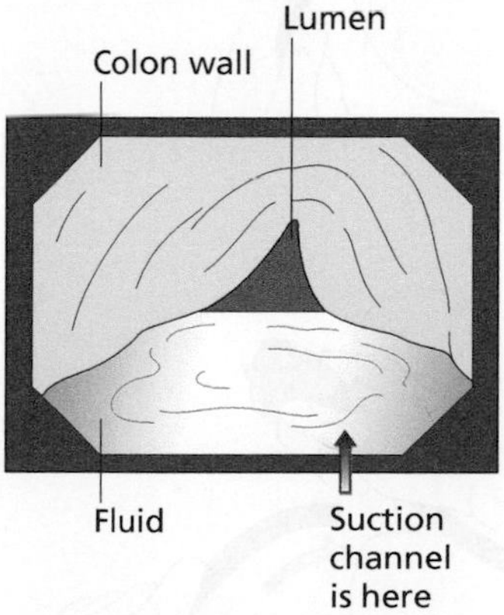

Fig 6.20 Proper orientation of the scope for suctioning intraluminal fluid. The suction channel is at the 5 o'clock position. The scope is positioned so that the channel sits just above the fluid pool and suction is initiated. This orientation prevents suctioning of mucosa or collapse of the air-filled lumen.

Wash and suction

Debris is evacuated during intubation and withdrawal. Thin, aqueous debris can be suctioned easily, but thicker fecal or food debris must be diluted with water before it can be suctioned. Attempting to suction seeds can clog the channel and should be avoided. Proper scope tip positioning avoids inadvertently and repetitively entrapping mucosa in the channel during suctioning. On standard colonoscopes, the suction port is located at the 5 o'clock position. To suction a pool of fluid, the scope should be torqued and turned until the surface of the pool is horizontal and at 6 o'clock or the bottom of the image (Fig 6.20). The lens is positioned just above this surface, so that the orifice of the channel is located at the top of the pool. As the suction button is depressed the fluid is felt streaming through the channel. As the pool surface becomes lower, the suction port can be gradually lowered correspondingly, using the up/down dial control.

Cleaning (washing) the mucosa with water during the case

- Washing enhances visualization during virtually all colonoscopies
- Water reduces mucosal friction
- Water helps to elicit/magnify mucosal detail
- Anti-foaming agents (e.g. simethicone) dissolve bubbles
  - Add simethicone to water at a ratio of approximately 1:50 and inject through the working channel (do not add to water bottle)
- Instruct patients to avoid seeds for 5 days before the procedure
  - Seeds clog scope and interfere with suction
- Built-in irrigation systems, controlled with foot pedal, simplify and enhance mucosal washing
- Avoid suctioning mucosa
  - Always suction intraluminal fluid with scope tip positioned just above surface of the pool (see Fig 6.20)
  - Insufflate air and simultaneously suction (may help keep lumen distended)

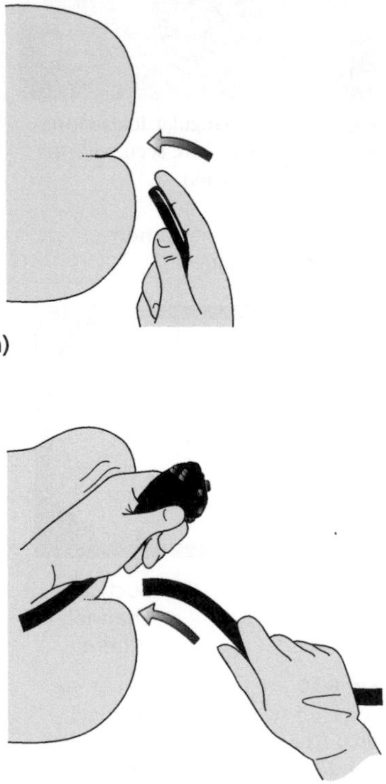
(a)
(b)

Fig 6.21 Insert the scope into the rectum.

Colonic intubation: segment by segment

Inserting the scope into the rectum

The tip of the colonoscope is lubricated and is gently passed through the anal canal. This can be accomplished by several methods (Fig 6.21).

- The scope tip is held in pencil grip position, with the gloved index finger extended slightly beyond the tip. After the fingertip locates the anal orifice, the scope is slid blindly along the finger and advanced into the anus.
- The tip is held in a screwdriver grip, extended about 6 cm beyond the right fist. The left hand holds the head of the scope while the back of this hand elevates the right buttock. The right hand then inserts the scope tip into the anus.
- The head of the scope is rested across the left shoulder, freeing the entire left hand to elevate the buttocks. The right hand inserts the scope tip into the anus as above.

As the tip enters the rectum, the initial view is likely to be a "red out," as the tip is pressed against the mucosa of the nondistended rectal vault. A full view is obtained by slight withdrawal of the shaft, air insufflation, and tip deflection.

The rectum and sigmoid

As the rectum rises out of the pelvis, it moves anteriorly, passing above the bladder before turning toward the left inguinal area. The sigmoid colon varies markedly in length and configuration; some sigmoids are fairly straight and short; others are lengthy and redundant. Because of its tortuosity, the sigmoid is the most common site of scope looping (Fig 6.13), and may be the most difficult segment to traverse. In all passages through the sigmoid (as in the rest of the colon) the scope length should be frequently reduced by pulling back on the shaft (Fig 6.15). Suprapubic pressure may prevent the scope from rising toward the umbilicus and stretching the mesentery (Fig 6.22).

The most difficult part of the examination, especially in slender women, may be traversing the angle at the top of the rectum, where the sigmoid colon begins. The lumen can usually be seen at the 3 o'clock position, but the acuteness of this angle may stymie the colonoscopist. Pushing does not advance the tip, but instead causes the knuckle of the scope to rise toward the diaphragm, stretching the mesentery and causing pain. Delicate coordination of tip deflection, torque, and in-and-out motions are required. For instance, with the tip maximally deflected to the right, moving the scope in and out while torquing clockwise may reorient the lumen from the 3 to the 9 o'clock position; after this occurs, the right/left dial is rotated maximally left, and the scope can be slid through the recalcitrant segment. A change in patient position to supine and/or deep suprapubic pressure may help as well.

In severe sigmoid diverticular disease, delicate, minute, deliberate alterations in tip position are required. Occasionally, a gastroscope, which has more acute tip deflection capability and a shorter bending section, is required. Forceful motions are avoided, and the use of air is minimized. The right hand grips the shaft close to the anus and the left thumb anchors the up/down dial.

Overtubes or stiffening devices maintain a straight scope, but these are cumbersome and in general not necessary.

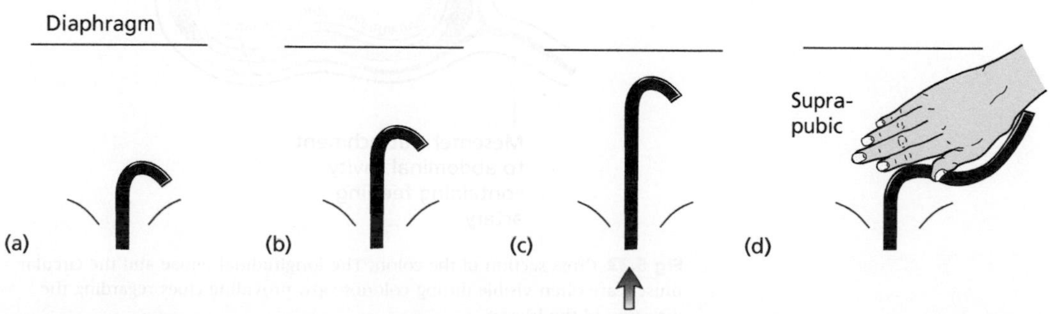

Fig 6.22 Impede sigmoid loop formation during insertion by using suprapubic pressure.

How to maneuver through a narrowed, diverticular sigmoid colon

- Very rarely is a sigmoid truly not traversable due to diverticular disease
- "Read" landmarks carefully before advancing the scope
  - Often hard to determine location of lumen
  - Avoid intubation of diverticular orifice
- Use carefully calculated, slowly executed, "mini-moves" involving fine adjustment of tip deflection, torque, and axial force
- Do not "ride" air button
- Irrigate segment with water
- Eliminate loops whenever possible
- Consider switching to narrower-caliber scope (e.g. pediatric colonoscope or adult gastroscope)
- Repositioning the patient is rarely helpful

The descending colon and splenic flexure

The descending colon is often relatively straight, fixed retroperitoneally, and easily traversed. If the scope is straight, the splenic flexure is typically encountered approximately 50–70 cm from the anal verge. The splenic flexure usually is fixed at the apex by the phrenocolic ligament. With the patient in the left lateral position, a fluid pool often accumulates in the splenic flexure. In many patients, the bulging blue outline of the spleen is visible through the colon wall. When the scope rounds this bend, it passes beyond the pool and into the air-filled transverse colon. When the instrument reaches the splenic flexure, the endoscopist should pause and straighten the scope, removing loops both inside and outside the patient. Further progress may be facilitated by left-sided mid-abdominal pressure, which can help keep the colonoscope shaft straight.

The transverse colon and hepatic flexure

The haustral folds of the transverse colon have a distinctive triangular configuration due to the constraining effect of the three longitudinal teniae coli (Figs 6.23 and 6.19). Once the scope tip has passed the splenic flexure, it is often helpful for the assistant to apply pressure in the mid-abdomen. The scope usually progresses readily through the transverse colon. The hepatic flexure is identified by a sharp bend and by the bluish hue of the liver (Plate 6.1).

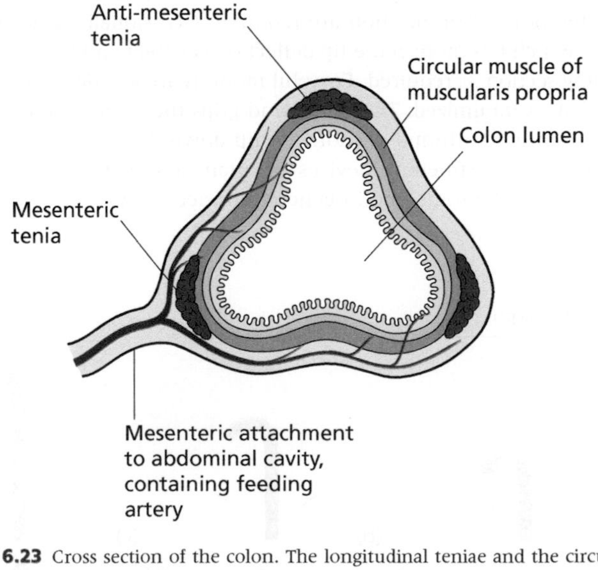

Fig 6.23 Cross section of the colon. The longitudinal teniae and the circular muscle are often visible during colonoscopy, providing clues regarding the direction of the lumen.

The angulation plus the relatively long distance from the anus to the flexure can make intubation difficult. Loops should be reduced, and excess air removed. Applying torque (usually clockwise) and aspirating some air may move the scope tip forward. In some cases the fold at the inner aspect of the flexure can be "hooked" and pulled back with the angulated tip. Often, external abdominal pressure in the left lower abdomen can help prevent new sigmoid loops from forming. The endoscopist may be able to locate a place in the hepatic flexure or mid-epigastrium to apply pressure that will help to advance the scope.

The ascending colon and cecum

The endoscopist must identify the cecum unequivocally. Seeing no further lumen ahead is *not proof* that the cecum has been reached. The hepatic flexure can masquerade as the cecum. The large transverse fold that contains the ileocecal valve can often go into spasm, mimicking the caput coli and concealing the true caput.

The strict criteria for cecal identification include:

• visualization of the appendiceal orifice;
• identification (and preferably intubation) of the ileocecal valve (Figs 6.24 and 6.25);
• identification of the cecal "crow's foot" sign in the caput of the cecum, where the three tenia coli converge (Plate 6.2).

If these criteria are not met, the procedure is reported as an *incomplete examination*. The endoscopist should discuss the limitation with the patient; when appropriate, the patient should undergo either a repeat colonoscopy by a more expert colonoscopist or a computed tomographic colonography (CTC).

When the scope tip is in the cecum, it may transilluminate the abdominal wall in the right quadrant near McBurney's point, producing a visible, localized, orange glow. Likewise, the wall of the colon as viewed on the monitor may be indented when the right lower quadrant of the abdominal wall is pressed with the finger. These two signs are suggestive of cecal intubation but are not reliable, as the transverse colon is also an anterior structure and can mimic these signs.

In the lengthy, redundant colon, the right colon provides the greatest challenge to intubation. Looping and overdistension must be avoided, and abdominal compression is often of benefit. Aspiration of air will often promote forward motion of the scope through the ascending colon. At times, a deep breath by the patient may help, as downward motion of the diaphragm may push the scope tip toward the cecum. When less cumbersome maneuvers fail, the patient should be rotated into the supine or the right lateral decubitus position.

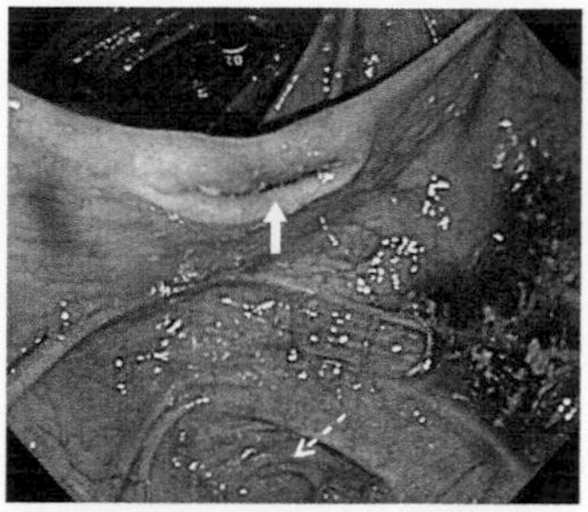

Fig 6.24 Retroflexion in a large caput cecum. The ileocecal valve (arrow) and appendiceal oricifice (dashed arrow) are both seen. The shaft of the scope is seen in the ascending colon at the top of the image.

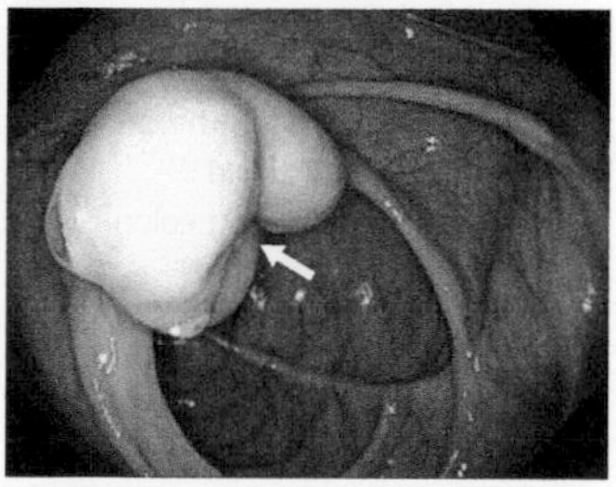

Fig 6.25 Lipomatous ileocecal valve. The arrow indicates the valve orifice.

Confirming cecal intubation

- **Reliable signs**
  - Appendiceal orifice
  - Terminal ileal intubation
  - Ileocecal valve, if identified unequivocally by
    - Intubation/visualization of villi
    - Notch at ileal orifice
    - Lipomatous appearance
  - Convergence of tineae coli at apex of caput ("crow's foot")
- **Unreliable signs**
  - Transillumination of abdomen
  - Visualization of prominent transverse fold that "looks like" the ileocecal valve
  - Indentation of cecum when abdomen is pushed with index finger

Intubating the difficult right colon and cecum

- Reduce loops
- Utilize abdominal pressure, including "sandwich" technique
- Rotate patient from left lateral decubitus position to supine or right lateral decubitus position
- Ask patient to take a deep breath
- Aspirate intraluminal air
- If using pediatric scope, switch to adult scope
- If using variable stiffness scope, set scope on stiffest setting
- If other tricks fail, withdraw scope to sigmoid and reintubate (repleating colon over scope)

The distal (terminal) ileum

Intubation of the ileum confirms that colonoscopy is complete, and occasionally yields important pathology, such as a carcinoid tumor, lymphoma, or Crohn's disease. Although ileal intubation is normally achievable, in some cases of ileitis or if the valve is unusually angulated, it is not possible. In other cases (e.g. chronic ulcerative colitis involving the cecum) the valve may be agape and hard to recognize.

The scope is straightened, loops are removed, excess air is evacuated, and the location of the valve orifice is estimated. The contour of transverse fold containing the valve often has a shallow cleft, representing the site of the valve orifice (Plate 6.2). The fold may also have a central bulge, caused by the musculature of the valve. Some valves are especially lipomatous (Fig 6.25), with the center of the yellowish bulge identifying the position of the valve. Sometimes, sputtering of air or flow of ileal juices reveals the location of the orifice.

With the position of the valve in mind, the colonoscopist passes the scope tip into the caput cecum, a few centimeters from the appendiceal orifice, and angulates the tip of the colonoscope toward the (no longer visible) transverse fold. Some experts prefer positioning the valve at the 6 o'clock position, whereas others rotate the scope so that the valve is at 12 o'clock. The scope is then slowly withdrawn. The intention is to traverse the proximal lip, "pry open" the pliant valve, and "fall" into (engage) the orifice of the ileum. Delicate adjustments in the dial controls are helpful. Often the sequence must be repeated several times or in several orientations in order to succeed. The recognition of granular mucosa and villi are signs of success (Plate 6.3). Air and water are instilled, opening the ileum.

The following are tips for ileal intubation.

- If the valve is angled toward the apex of the caput cecum, it may be necessary to make a U-turn in the cecum and intubate it in this configuration.
- Use the bow and arrow sign. The appendiceal orifice usually appears crescent-shaped. Position the tip of the scope near the appendiceal orifice. Imagine the crescent as the archer's bow, and imagine an arrow positioned across the bow in the ready position; the tip of the arrow will point to the orifice of the ileocecal valve (Fig 6.26).

The bow and arrow sign

- The appendiceal orifice is usually crescent-shaped
- Imagine the orifice as a bow
- Imagine an arrow positioned in the bow
- The arrow head will point in the direction of the ileal orifice

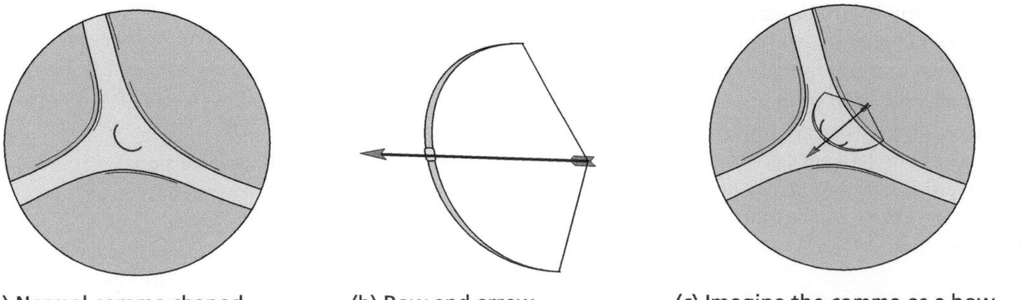

(a) Normal comma-shaped appendiceal orifice

(b) Bow and arrow

(c) Imagine the comma as a bow. An arrow points to the opening of the ileocaecal valve

Fig 6.26 Bow and arrow sign.

• The cecum is asymmetrical; the ileal orifice can be found on the shorter wall (Fig 6.27). That means that when the tip is in the cecum, the valve is located on the wall closest to the scope tip. Angulate the tip toward the closer wall and withdraw the scope as noted above (Fig 6.28).

Finding the ileal orifice after ileocolic anastomosis

- May be challenging to identify
- Anastomosis often not end-to-end
- Insertion may be end-to-side, and may be located 5–10 cm distal to the blind end of the colon
- Localization may require scope tip retroflection

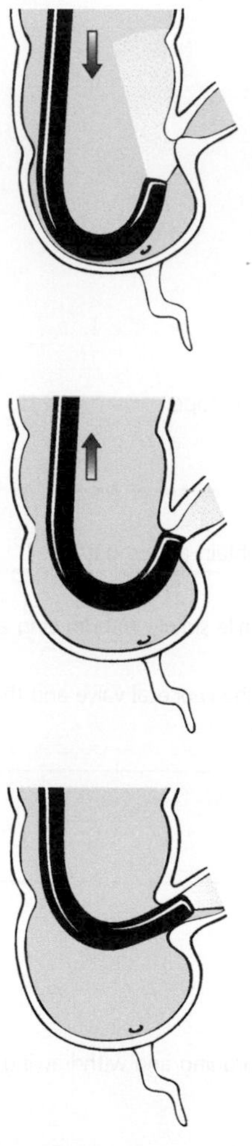

(a) (b) (c)

Fig 6.27 IC valve intubation. The scope is retroflexed in the caput (view as in Fig 6.24) and gently withdrawn, teasing open the valve.

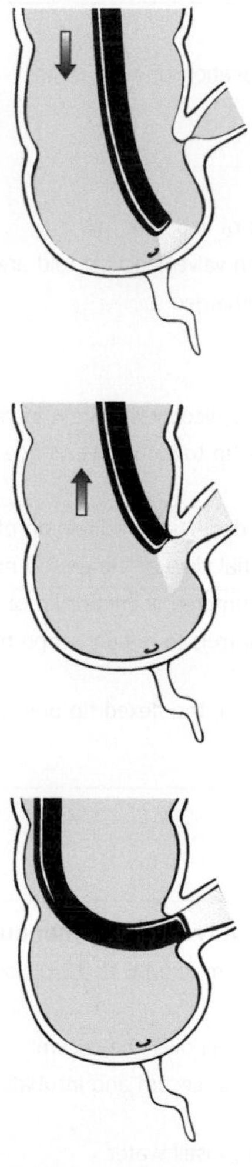

(a) (b) (c)

Fig 6.28 IC valve intubation. The scope is advanced into the caput and the tip is "dragged" back along the medial wall of the cecum until the proximal lip of the valve is encountered. Small adjustments in the tip position are then made with the right hand until the tip "pops" into the ileum.

The terminal ileum mucosa is recognized by the granular appearance produced by the villi. Deep ileal intubation may be achieved in many cases with persistent and skillful technique. Instillation of water magnifies the villi and causes them to "float up," allowing for clear photo-documentation (Plate 6.3).

Entering the terminal ileum

- Before attempting intubation, identify location of valve orifice
- Landmarks for valve orifice
  - Notch in ileocecal fold
  - Midway point in ileocecal fold
  - Midway point in lipomatous segment of ileocecal fold
  - Direct visualization of orifice/villi (when valve/ileocecal fold are angled "up")
  - Site where ileal effluent/gases are discharged
  - Bow and arrow sign
  - Cecum is asymmetric
    - With scope tip at appendiceal orifice, ileocecal valve is in colon wall nearer to the scope
- Using dial controls, gently deflect scope tip toward valve orifice
- Slowly withdraw scope
- Use right hand (torque) to maintain tip deflection in direction of orifice
- While withdrawing scope, maintain partial view of lumen (do not hyperflex tip and obtain a "red out")
- During withdrawal, first large fold encountered is inferior lip of valve
- After first fold encountered, use dial controls to deflect scope tip toward that fold while slowly withdrawing and torquing scope
- When favorable tip orientation is achieved, the flexed tip pries open the two lips of the ileocecal valve and the ileum is entered

Intubating the recalcitrant ileocecal valve: Useful maneuvers

- Rotate the scope so valve orifice shifts from (e.g.) 6 to 12 o'clock position
- Rotate the patient
- Have assistant compress the abdominal wall over the cecum
- If cecum is capacious, retroflex scope tip in cecum and intubate orifice by carefully torquing and withdrawing the scope
- If scope hesitates at the lips of the valve, instill water
- Consider possibility of scarring or ileitis as cause for difficulty
- Wait for valve to spontaneously open and spill ileal fluid and then try again to intubate

Intubating the "impossible" colon

Sometimes the angulations of the sigmoid are so acute or the lumen is so narrowed that a colonoscope cannot traverse it. The common settings are postoperatively (e.g. due to pelvic adhesions) or severe diverticular disease and in slender women. Switching to a nimbler gastroscope may permit successful passage. Although shorter and less rigid than the colonoscope and therefore more prone to looping, the gastroscope may achieve total colonoscopy in this setting, in part because the sigmoid pathology that caused the difficulty in the first place acts as a stent (splint), keeping subsequent sigmoid loops from forming.

In some patients, it may appear impossible despite all maneuvers to pass the scope beyond the hepatic flexure or ascending colon. If looping is not the cause, this problem occurs because the colon is inordinately long or flaccid, most often in obese or tall persons. Because the pediatric colonoscope is less rigid than the adult scope (even if the variable stiffness function is utilized), changing to an adult instrument may be of benefit. Pulling the scope all the way back to the sigmoid and repeating the intubation may help. Very rarely, an especially long scope, such as a long 220-cm push enteroscope, may be required. Lastly, it may be prudent to refer the patient to an expert colonoscopist or for CTC, instructing the radiologist to focus on the ascending colon or cecum.

Withdrawal phase of colonoscopy

The withdrawal phase of a colonoscopy may be the only opportunity for a decade of the patient's life to detect malignant or premalignant lesions of the colon. The colon lining is enfolded, convoluted, and expansive, and polyps can be hidden. Under the best of circumstances, polyp detection is imperfect: "tandem" colonoscopy studies, in which two colonoscopies are performed during a single patient visit, reveal a "miss rate" of 10–20%. Thus, scrupulous technique, adequate time, and intense focus are required.

Cleaning the mucosa

After an appropriate bowel preparation, most colons are fairly clean, containing only small pools of clear or bile-stained fluid, some bubbles, and perhaps a little debris that can readily be removed by aspiration. If there is a modest amount of debris or turbid fluid, the endoscopist must strive to remove it, repetitively washing and suctioning. If debris cannot be removed, roll the patient from the left lateral decubitus to the supine or right lateral decubitus position: because of gravity, the fluid/debris will shift, unveiling the obscured tract of mucosa.

If despite all efforts the colon cannot be adequately cleaned, abort and reschedule the examination. Make this decision early in the exam, to avoid wasting time or risking complication. Often, additional laxatives given the same day will finish the cleansing, and (if scheduling permits) the procedure can be successfully completed.

The colonoscope must be withdrawn slowly, centimeter by centimeter, while each segment of the colon is meticulously inspected (Fig 6.29). The process is tedious, but is rewarded when a polyp concealed in a crevice is detected. Repetitive examination of

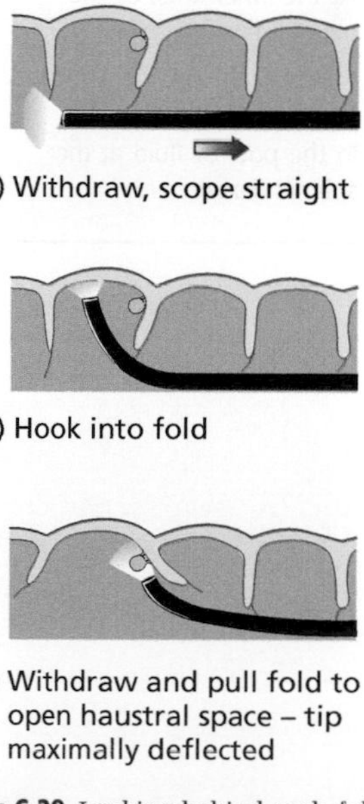

(a) Withdraw, scope straight
(b) Hook into fold
(c) Withdraw and pull fold to open haustral space – tip maximally deflected

Fig 6.29 Looking behind each fold. During careful withdrawal, examining the "valley" behind each fold in sequence. Polyps can easily be missed behind large haustral folds.

Withdrawal technique: Guiding principles

- Do not rush (in general should be >6 minutes)
- Appropriate withdrawal time/case varies, depending on anatomy (i.e. longer for convoluted, lengthy colon)
- Perform repetitive examination of difficult colon segments and notorious blind spots
- Wash colon thoroughly
- Inspect systematically behind all folds (Fig 6.31)
- Pry apart apposed folds
- If "fly-by" occurs, reintubate and examine the area that was suboptimally inspected

Where polyps are missed: Five blind spots

1. Behind the ileocecal valve
2. Behind the rectal valves of Houston
3. At the inner knee of the hepatic flexure
4. Between thickened diverticular folds
5. In the pool of fluid at the splenic flexure

difficult segments is essential. At times, the scope tip is kept still while the colonoscopist inspects the segment in view. In general, very little right/left dial control is needed during the withdrawal phase of the examination, as the combination of torque and up/down dial movement allows fine tip control.

It has been suggested that an average of 6 minutes be spent in the withdrawal phase of the procedure, but the appropriate withdrawal time varies, depending on the colonic anatomy: a long, convoluted colon that has prominent folds requires more time than a relatively short, straight one.

In order to achieve thorough inspection, it is often useful to examine each segment of colon circumferentially. This is accomplished by deflecting the tip about 45° with the dial controls, and then torquing the colonoscope shaft. As the torque is transmitted, the tip will then sweep the 360° circumference of each section, much like the second hand on a clock.

Know the trouble spots

Some colonic segments are straight and fold-free and, as such, relatively easy to examine; others may easily conceal lesions.

The cecum is the most capacious segment of colon and the most difficult to reach. The scope tip must be passed beyond the transverse fold that contains the ileocecal valve, into the caput of the cecum, and any fluid or debris in the caput must be removed. Otherwise, subtle flat polyps in the caput coli or polyps concealed behind the ileocecal valve will be missed.

The back (proximal) sides of the ascending colon folds are not seen during standard straight-on viewing. The scope tip can be deflected so as to "flatten out" the folds, and then the scope can be torqued to examine the valley behind the fold. Retroflexion of the scope in the cecum is also helpful (see below).

During intubation the colon is pleated over the shaft of the scope like an accordion. During withdrawal, a colonic segment may suddenly "unpleat" and re-elongate, causing an entire segment of colon to fly by. When this occurs the segment must be reintubated and reexamined. The endoscopist can advance and withdraw the tip slowly and use torque and tip deflection to stabilize the tip position. It may be necessary to examine such segments repeatedly. Pleating also creates blind areas ("potential spaces") between the infolded mucosa. To look into these areas, the tip is deflected into the crevice between two folds and the folds teased apart. Irrigation also helps separate adherent folds.

In sigmoid diverticulosis, the folds are hypertrophied so the crevices are especially inaccessible. Muscular spasm is common, and the distending effect of air insufflation is decreased. Scope tip mobility is restricted and the folds are often red or edematous, resembling polyps. Inverted diverticula also may mimic polyps. Fecaliths, washed by the laxatives out of the diverticular orifices, may obscure the mucosa. To overcome these obstacles, the scope should be withdrawn slowly and patiently. Repetitive intubation and examination of folded and hypertrophied segments is valuable.

An effort should be made to examine all the crevices, teasing them open with the tip of the scope.

The splenic and hepatic flexures are potential blind spots (Fig 6.30). A conscientious effort must be made to examine and reexamine the dome and inner aspect of these flexures. Often several passes are needed to be confident that the segment has been cleared. The tip is used to flatten the folds in these regions and fluid debris is removed, so that the entire surface can be seen. The dome of the hepatic flexure is seen well in the retroflex position.

Because of their prominence, the large rectal folds (valves of Houston) can conceal polyps. Therefore, this area must be examined intensively.

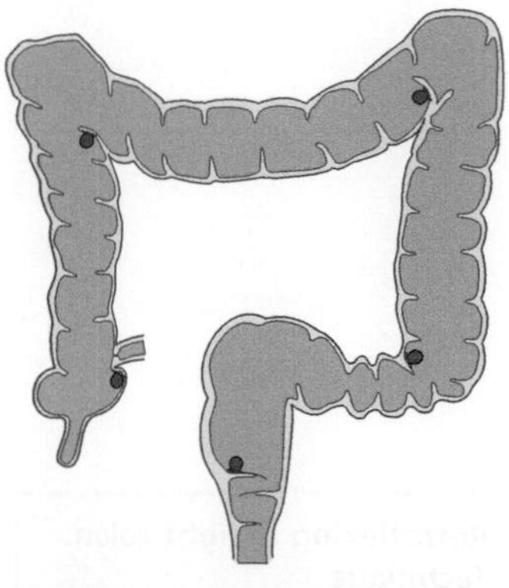

Fig 6.30 Five blind spots where polyps are missed. Careful attention to these locations is essential to a thorough examination.

Special techniques to increase visualization

Retroflexion

Maximally flexing the tip of the colonoscope and then gently advancing the shaft can achieve a retro-view. This maneuver is commonly used in the rectum (Fig 6.31). The capacious rectal vault accommodates the maneuver, and it enhances inspection for low rectal and anal pathology. Caution must be taken (or the maneuver avoided entirely) in patients with active proctitis or a narrowed, scarred rectum—as may occur following radiation treatment for prostate cancer, or resolution of severe colitis. In this setting, the nondistensible rectum may be vulnerable to perforation.

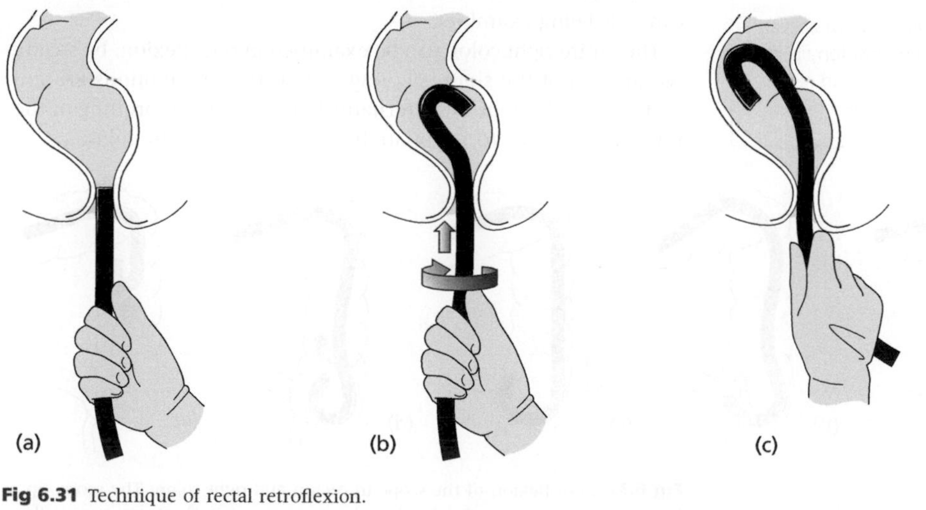

Fig 6.31 Technique of rectal retroflexion.

Right colon polyps: Techniques to increase detection

- Use split-dose bowel preparation
- Look specifically for "sentinel signs" of sessile serrated adenomas
- Wash away residual debris
- Retroflex scope in cecum and withdraw in this configuration through ascending colon
- Push down large folds with probe (e.g. closed biopsy forceps)in order to examine the back side
- Systematically examine the "valleys" between all the folds

Retroflexing in right colon: Technique

- Straighten the scope (take out loops)
- Confirm that pushing in scope results in forward (not paradoxical) tip motion
- Position tip in caput or capacious segment of ascending colon
- Maximally up-deflect tip (using dial control)
- Gently push scope in several cm and torque
- Lumen with shaft of scope will usually appear
- If not, maximally right-deflect tip wheel and withdraw while turning clockwise
- If lumen still does not appear, straighten tip, position tip in different location, and repeat series of maneuvers

To perform a U-turn in the right colon, position the tip of the scope in the cecum or in a capacious segment of ascending colon (Fig 6.32). The insertion tube must be relatively straight, so that the scope tip advances in response to pushing with the right hand. Deflect the tip up and right, and then gently advance approximately 5 to 10 cm while torquing clockwise. If the anatomy is favorable, the tip will "flip" into the retroflexed position, with the distal 20 cm of scope in view. If this view does not appear promptly, the scope position or orientation should be altered, and the maneuver attempted again. The maneuver should be made with minimal force, in order to avoid the possibility of perforation. If advancing the shaft does not result in retroflexion, then move the right/left dial maximally right and withdraw the scope while torquing the shaft clockwise (this may require more than 180° of twist).

Once retroflexion is achieved, the visual image will respond paradoxically to inward and outward movements on the insertion tube. This paradoxical effect is familiar to the endoscopist, as it occurs when the gastroscope is in U-turn in the stomach and the cardia is being examined.

The entire right colon can be examined in retroflexion, by steady withdrawal of the shaft, steering it with twisting motions around folds. Often this requires alternatively right and left torquing of the retroflexed scope, to negotiate backward through the folds.

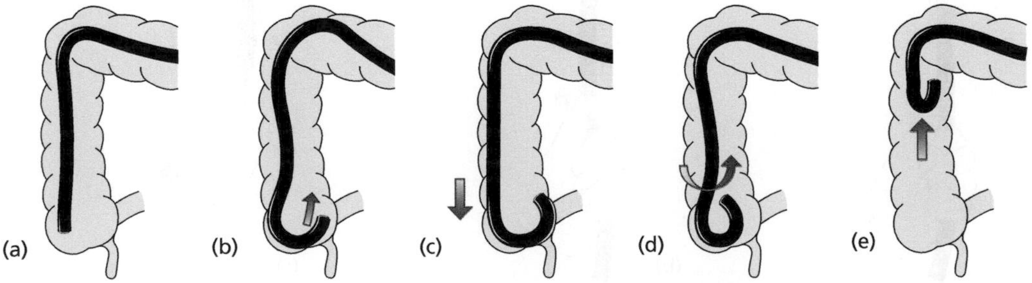

Fig 6.32 Retroflexion of the scope in cecum and right colon. The scope tip is positioned in the proximal right colon or cecum (a). The tip is maximally deflected using the up/down control (b). The scope is gently advanced (c) and torque and right/left tip deflection (d) are added as needed. Once the retroflexed view has been obtained, the scope can be withdrawn, permitting examination of the backs of the ascending colon folds and the underside of the hepatic flexure.

Even in expert hands, right colon retroflexion is not always possible, particularly if the colon is long and redundant, or if the ascending colon is relatively narrow or nondistensible, as is the case with right-sided diverticular disease.

To enhance polyp detection, the "third eye retroscope" was developed. This is a miniature endoscope with its own light source. It is passed through the biopsy channel of the scope and its tip flexes 180° as the mini-scope emerges from the biopsy channel. Its integral light source illuminates the proximal side of the colon folds. The third eye image is displayed on the endoscopy monitor side by side with the conventional forward viewing image. Studies show that this device increases polyp detection, but utilization has been scanty, in part due to cost.

A clear plastic hood, attached to the tip of the colonoscope, may also be used to afford an enhanced view by pushing folds aside. It is uncertain whether this technique increases polyp detection. Likewise, a forceps or snare pushed out through the working channel may function as a probe and be used to push on the colonic folds to flatten them.

Retroflexion in the right colon

- Achievable in most colons
- Difficult to achieve if:
  - tip does not respond reliably to right-hand actions, as in elongated/tortuous colon;
  - ascending colon spastic or hypertrophied (e.g. due to right colon diverticular disease).
- Always use minimal force
- Remove loops first to ensure that the tip is responsive
- Test "one-to-one" scope responsiveness before initiating
- Can perform in cecum or proximal ascending colon
- Can perform with pediatric-type instruments or adult scopes
- Torque while withdrawing scope to see entire right colon
- Increases polyp detection rate
- Provides excellent visualization of dome of hepatic flexure (often hard to see otherwise)
- Can perform polypectomy/fluid injection/biopsy in retroflexion

Decompress the colon during withdrawal

After the examination, the residual air in the large bowel may cause discomfort. The insufflation of CO_2 gas, which is rapidly absorbed and excreted through the lungs, rather than room air, mitigates this problem, but is not in widespread use. Remove as much air as possible during scope withdrawal. At the end of the case, palpate the abdomen to assess the degree of abdominal distention; occasionally, a quick run up the colon to remove air is worthwhile. Decompression is usually rapidly accomplished by changing the patient position from left lateral (with the cecum superior) to the right lateral, permitting air to rise to the sigmoid and be expelled.

When to consider rolling the patient

- To assist with colon intubation
  - Roll supine or to right lateral to advance through the ascending colon to cecum
- To move a pool of fluid
- To assist the patient in expelling gas after the procedure (roll prone or right lateral)
- To move a polyp into more favorable position for polypectomy
- To uncover a lost polyp
- To enable thorough examination of a segment
- Some experts reposition patients by protocol during every case, in the belief that this increases polyp detection rate

Summary

Skilled insertion and withdrawal technique are at the core of successful colonoscopy practice. Every colonoscopist develops a personal style, but certain basic principles and methods favor good results. The exam may be difficult, but this can be overcome by close examination, persistence, and a repertoire of technique.

Further reading

1. Hazewinkel Y, Dekker E. Colonoscopy: basic principles and novel techniques. *Nat Rev Gastroenterol Hepatol* 2011;8:554–64.
2. Huh KC, Rex DK. Advances in colonoscope technique and technology. *Rev Gastroenterol Disord* 2008;8:223–32.
3. Korman LY, Egorov V, Tsuryupa S, *et al.* Characterization of forces applied by endoscopists during colonoscopy by using a wireless colonoscopy force monitor. *Gastrointest Endosc* 2010;71:327–34. Epub 2009 Nov 17.

4. Lee RH, Tang RS, Muthusamy VR, *et al.* Quality of colonoscopy withdrawal technique and variability in adenoma detection rates (with videos). *Gastrointest Endosc* 2011;74:128–34. Epub 2011 Apr 30.
5. Leung FW, Mann SK, Salera R, *et al.* Options for screening colonoscopy without sedation: sequel to a pilot study in U.S. veterans. *Gastrointest Endosc* 2008;67:712–7. Epub 2008 Feb 14.
6. Rex DK. Maximizing detection of adenomas and cancers during colonoscopy. *Am J Gastroenterol* 2006;101:2866–77.
7. Rex DK, Chen SC, Overhiser AJ. Colonoscopy technique in consecutive patients referred for prior incomplete colonoscopy. *Clin Gastroenterol Hepatol* 2007;5:879–83. Epub 2007 Jun 4.
8. Simmons DT, Harewood GC, Baron TH, *et al.* Impact of endoscopist withdrawal speed on polyp yield: implications for optimal colonoscopy withdrawal time. *Aliment Pharmacol Ther* 2006;24:965–71.
9. Van Rijn, JC Reitsma JB, Stoker J, Bossuyt PM, van Deventer SJ, Dekker E. Polyp miss rate determined by tandem colonoscopy: a systematic review. *Am J Gastroenterol* 2010;101:343–350.
10. Waye JD, Yessayan SA, Lewis BS, Fabry TL. The technique of abdominal pressure in total colonoscopy. *Gastrointest Endosc* 1991;37:147–51.
11. Waye JD, Rex DK, Williams CB, editors. *Colonoscopy: Principles and Practice*. 2nd ed. Blackwell Publishing Ltd, Oxford; 2009, pages 537–559.

CHAPTER 7
Colonoscopic Findings

Colorectal cancer

The diagnosis of adenocarcinoma of the colon is obvious when a large, circumferential, friable mass is encountered (Plate 7.1, Plate 7.2). Some carcinomas appear hard, scirrhous, and pale, whereas others are exophytic, friable, and soft. Because only the surface is sampled, forceps biopsies may reveal only adenomatous change. In order to minimize sampling error, multiple biopsies should be taken from different parts of the tumor, and some experts snare a sizable lobule of tumor.

If a large colorectal carcinoma obstructs the lumen, bowel preparation may require retrograde cleansing with enemas, and it may be impossible to traverse the obstruction. In this setting, the colonoscopist should be careful not to overinsufflate because the lesion may function as a one-way valve, increasing the risk of pneumatic cecal perforation. If the obstruction is partial, it may be possible to traverse the tumor with a pediatric colonoscope or a gastroscope. It is important to visualize the colon proximal to the lesion in order to exclude a synchronous carcinoma; if this is not possible colonoscopically, computed tomographic colonography (CTC) should be considered.

Unless the lesion is unequivocally located within 10 cm of the anal verge or the cecal caput, or unless it is extremely large, it is best to mark permanently ("tattoo") the site for the surgeon (see Chapter 11, Figure 11.2). The size and length of the lesion should be estimated, and its approximate location noted (Video Clip 7.1). In general, synchronous polyps should be removed, unless they are adjacent to the cancer and will be resected in the subsequent surgical specimen. If polyps are left *in situ*, their location should be described to the surgeon. The lesion should be photographed and, if appropriate, video recorded.

The diagnosis of cancer is less obvious when the lesion is more localized and/or resembles a benign polyp (see "Malignant polyps", Chapter 12). The size of the polyp *per se* may not be a reliable indicator of malignant transformation, as small polyps may be cancerous, and enormous polyps may be benign. Likewise, the elevation (height) of the polyp is not a reliable indicator, as flat or minimally elevated lesions may be malignant. Flat lesions with a central depression have a particularly high risk of being malignant.

Is the polyp cancerous?: Worrisome characteristics

- Surface ulceration
- Central depression in a minimally elevated polyp
- Large size
- Visible villous components
- Spontaneous bleeding or friability
- "Feels" hard when pushed by forceps
- Snare cuts through with unusual difficulty
- Does not elevate with submucosal injection
- Appears to tether the adjacent mucosa

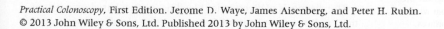

Practical Colonoscopy, First Edition. Jerome D. Waye, James Aisenberg, and Peter H. Rubin.
© 2013 John Wiley & Sons, Ltd. Published 2013 by John Wiley & Sons, Ltd.

Rectal carcinoids

- Characteristics
  - Yellowish
  - Firm
  - Submucosal
  - Usually <1 cm diameter
- If small (<1 cm), risk of spread is low and snare excision ("shelling out" lesion) may be adequate
- Cautery may be used to obliterate the base
- As submucosal, may be difficult to achieve a clear resection margin
- If lesion is larger or no adequate margin, consider full-thickness excision by colorectal surgeon
- India ink tattoo site if surgery is considered
- Second most common location of carcinoids found during colonoscopy = terminal ileum

Colonoscopic findings

- Colorectal carcinoma
- Colon polyps
  - Mucosal
  - Submucosal
- Diverticulosis, -itis
- Hemorrhoids
- Ischemic colitis
- Solitary rectal ulcer syndrome
- Radiation proctopathy, colitis
- Diversion colitis
- Inflammatory bowel disease
- Ileal pouch abnormalities
- Graft-versus-host disease
- Vascular lesions
- Infectious colitis
- Dieulafoy lesions
- Microscopic colitis
- Cathartic-induced lesions

Colorectal polyps

Colorectal polyps are discussed in Chapter 10.

Anal carcinoma

Most palpable anal abnormalities are benign, but occasionally a cancer will be felt and identified during the colonoscopic examination.

The anus is examined with the scope in retroflexion. The lens is pulled distally to within a few inches of the dentate line, to permit close inspection. The retroflexed scope is then rotated 360° in order to visualize the circumference of the anus (Video Clip 7.2). Rigid anoscopy with a beveled anoscope offers a complementary view. Malignant and premalignant anal changes can be subtle and difficult to distinguish from inflammatory or fibrotic changes. Papillomas and small anal carcinomas are firm, nonfriable, frondlike, and pale. They arise from the squamous lining at the dentate line. Care must be taken to avoid pain during anal biopsy, as sensory receptors innervate portions of the anal canal.

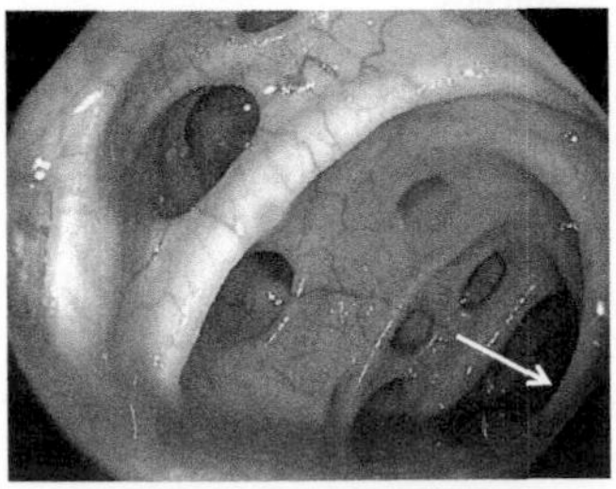

Fig 7.1 Diverticulosis coli. Care must be taken to distinguish the true lumen (arrow) from wide-mouthed diverticular orifices.

Diverticulosis

Diverticular orifices are found during most colonoscopies in middle-aged and older patients, most commonly in the sigmoid (Fig 7.1). Often they are associated with muscular hypertrophy and spasm. Diverticular orifices are at times larger than the adjacent, true lumen. Diverticulosis is usually an incidental finding, but the extent and location should be reported.

The diagnosis of diverticular bleeding is often based on presumption, as it may not be possible to see active bleeding from an individual orifice, or an adherent clot or a visible vessel within one. Recent studies suggest that prompt colonoscopy after a rapid bowel purge pinpoints a site of diverticular bleeding in approximately 40% of patients presenting with severe hematochezia. The lesion is typically a localized ulceration that penetrates into an arteriole in the neck or base of the diverticulum. Hemostasis can be achieved in up to 90% of these cases.

Acute diverticulitis poses a contraindication to colonoscopy, as the infection can compromise the integrity of the wall of the involved colonic segment. Occasionally during colonoscopy pus can be seen draining from a diverticular orifice in an edematous and erythematous segment of sigmoid colon, suggesting subclinical or recent diverticulitis.

Commonly, the colonoscopist will observe red mucosa in a segment of diverticular disease (Plate 7.3). This represents microhemorrhage and hemosiderin deposition due to mucosal blood vessel injury from the high intra-colonic pressures. "Diverticular colitis," a form of segmental colitis, is of uncertain etiology, but may be ischemic (Video Clip 7.3).

Diverticula can invert, creating a small luminal protuberance that can be mistaken for a polyp. Careful inspection usually differentiates the two entities: the inverted diverticulum is more symmetrical, is surrounded by concentric rings of innominate mucosal grooves, has extremely regular, smooth mucosa on its surface, and can be dimpled (and sometimes "de-inverted") with the biopsy forceps. A biopsy of the tip of the protuberance will confirm normal mucosa; snare transection of a large inverted diverticulum should be avoided.

Rectal hemorrhage: Etiologies

- Hemorrhoids
- Diverticular disease
- Ischemic
- Colitis
  - Idiopathic
  - Infectious
- Vascular lesions
  - Angioectasia
  - Dieulafoy lesions
- Ulcer
  - Infectious
  - Drug-induced (e.g. nonsteroidal anti-inflammatory drugs, or NSAIDs)
  - Solitary rectal ulcer

Hemorrhoids

Internal hemorrhoids (Plate 7.4) are usually found incidentally, and should be described in the colonoscopy report. Hemorrhoids may be responsible for severe hematochezia, pain, and itching. For large volume, chronic, or refractory bleeding, hemorrhoidal ablation by surgical or endoscopic means may be required.

Ischemic colitis

The colonoscopic hallmarks of ischemia are segmental edema, erythema, friability, exudates, mucosal hemorrhage, and ulcerations (Plate 7.5). Occasionally, hemorrhagic blebs, the endoscopic equivalent of radiographic "thumbprinting," may be seen. In more severe cases, the colon lining may appear bluish and cyanotic. Mucosal biopsies help differentiate ischemia from infectious or inflammatory bowel disease, revealing "ghosts" of colonic crypts, and a characteristic pattern of inflammation and hemorrhage. Most commonly, ischemia affects the sigmoid colon or the splenic flexure, the "watershed" areas that have the poorest collateral blood flow. The diseased segment may range in length from several centimeters to half a meter or more. In milder cases, the inflammation appears as a "strip" of inflammation along the antimesenteric wall of the colon, but usually it is circumferential (Video Clip 7.4).

Colonoscopy should be performed with minimal force and air insufflation, and the scope advanced far enough to make the diagnosis. If the disease is mild or the segment is short, the scope can be gently advanced through the segment, in order to determine the proximal extent and severity.

Solitary rectal ulcer

In patients with rectal bleeding and chronic defecatory dysfunction, colonoscopy may reveal a conspicuous distal ulcer (Plate 7.6), often with a heaped-up border. The term "solitary rectal ulcer syndrome" (SRUS) is misleading: the lesions may be multiple, and may develop exuberant granulation tissue and appear polypoid (Video Clip 7.5). The lesions are usually located in the anterior rectum. Biopsy shows pathognomonic changes of ischemia, hyperplastic mucosa, and fibrosis of lamina propria with interspersed muscle fibers. Uncommonly, solitary rectal ulcers can result in significant hematochezia, and treatment with a thermal modality may be required.

Radiation colopathy and proctopathy

This entity is most commonly encountered in the rectum of men who have received external beam radiation or brachytherapy for prostate cancer or in women who have had radiation for cervical cancer, where the effect may be in the distal sigmoid. The characteristic colonoscopic finding is a myriad of ectatic blood vessels, often within a background of atrophic mucosa (Plate 7.7). Bleeding is the most common symptom. Rarely radiation injury can cause chronic inflammation, ulceration, and stricture, and result in pain, tenesmus, and incontinence. Radiation injury may be discovered as an incidental finding during colonoscopy, but in patients who have rectal bleeding, the abnormal vessels are friable and may ooze.

When symptomatic, the bleeding of radiation proctopathy can be treated with a superficial thermal modality such as the argon plasma coagulation (APC), often in several sessions (Video Clip 7.6). Alternatively, heater-probe or bipolar-probe coagulation can be utilized, but caution is necessary to avoid deep thermal injury, which could result in a nonhealing ulcer in radiation-damaged tissue or a fistula to the urethra. The visual end point of treatment should be a shallow white coagulum at the site of the visible mucosal lesion. Many experts consider APC to be the first-line treatment modality.

Diversion colitis

After diverting colostomy, the bypassed colonic mucosa can become inflamed, presumably as a result of deprivation from the nutrients contained in the fecal stream. Colonoscopically, the mucosa appears diffusely friable and edematous, with decreased vascular pattern and surface exudates, similar to the appearance of mild-to-moderate idiopathic colitis. The abnormality typically resolves with restoration of gastrointestinal continuity.

Inflammatory bowel disease

Colonoscopy in ulcerative colitis (UC) reveals mucosal edema, friability, exudates, granularity, loss of vascular pattern, and ulceration (Plate 7.8; Video Clip 7.7). These findings characteristically involve the entire circumference of bowel, and begin in the rectum and extend cephalad continuously. UC may involve the rectum, a portion of the colon, or the entire colon. Occasionally, the ileocecal valve will be scarred open, and the distal ileum will be mildly inflamed, presumably owing to the reflux of colonic contents ("backwash ileitis"). Patients with distal colonic inflammation may demonstrate inflammation around the appendiceal orifice ("cecal patch"). Biopsies in UC reveal nonspecific acute and chronic inflammation.

Crohn's disease (CD) is often segmental (i.e. discontinuous). In some cases, the colitis displays the same characteristics as UC: erythema, ulceration, friability, edema, and loss of the normal vascular pattern. More commonly, the features are large, irregular, serpiginous, coalescing ulcerations (Plate 7.9). The normal or edematous mucosa between ulcers may appear elevated, giving the appearance of "cobble-stoning." In a given colonic segment, CD is not necessarily circumferential. The distal ileum is frequently involved. The aphthous lesion that may be seen in CD is a small, canker sore-like ulceration. It may be solitary or in clusters and is not pathognomonic. Biopsies of involved mucosa in CD may appear identical to UC; noncaseating granulomas are seldom detected but when present, establish the diagnosis.

In a small subset (5–10%) of patients, it is not possible to differentiate between UC and CD on endoscopic and histological grounds. These patients may have features of both diseases. They are classified as having "indeterminate colitis."

In a colitic patient, the colonoscopist should inspect the distal ileum. Deep ileal intubation may be impossible in CD if the valve and distal ileum are strictured. In such cases there is usually telltale ulceration of the lips of the ileocecal valve, and the biopsy forceps can be inserted through the stenotic valve to sample distal ileum (Fig 7.2).

Colonoscopy is utilized to establish diagnosis, to judge anatomic extent, mucosal activity, and response to therapy. Thus, in UC colonoscopy will differentiate among proctitis, proctosigmoiditis, left sided, or universal (pan-) colitis, which in turn can lead to more effective and targeted therapy. In CD, colonoscopy is helpful preoperatively in defining the extent of colitis and, in cases of ileosigmoid fistulas, determining whether the colon is intrinsically diseased, requiring segmental resection or simply resection of the end point

Four settings in which CD and UC may look similar

1. Severely active colitis
2. After topical treatment of mild-to-moderate UC (owing to drug-induced "rectal sparing")
3. After systemic therapy of UC, if healing has been patchy (segmental residual inflammation may resemble CD)
4. Quiescent disease (colon may be foreshortened, ahaustral, tubular; mucosa normal, or have diminished vascular pattern, granularity, lattice-like fibrosis, and/or scarring)

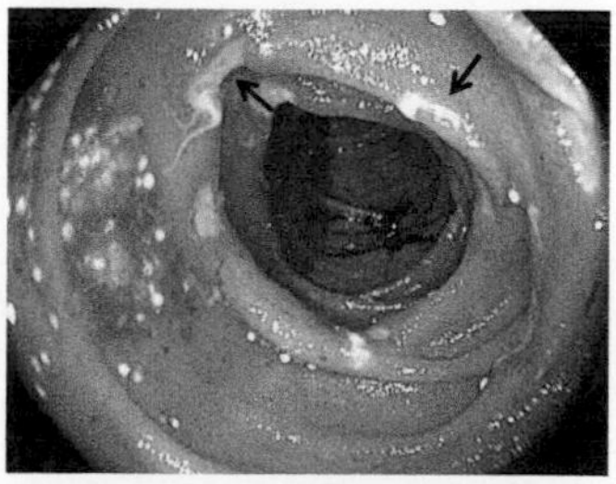

Fig 7.2 Neo-terminal ileal Crohn's disease. Three months previously, the patient underwent ileocolic resection. The appearance of small erosions with surface exudates is characteristic of early recurrence, and may suggest the need to intensify treatment. Granules from the 5-ASA preparation have pooled in the dependent portion of the bowel (lower left).

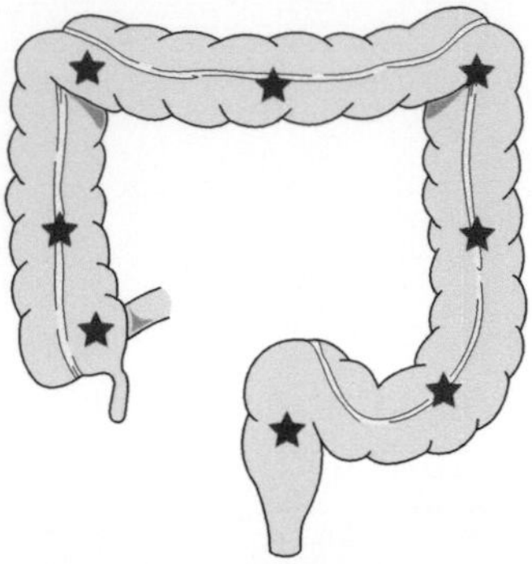

Fig 7.3 Surveillance biopsies for dysplasia in chronic inflammatory bowel disease are taken from at least eight stations throughout the large bowel: in the cecum, ascending colon, hepatic flexure, transverse colon, splenic flexure, descending colon, sigmoid colon, and rectum. Four biopsies are taken at each station and all biopsies from each station are placed in one container, so that eight specimen jars are sent to the laboratory. Targeted biopsies of any abnormality are sent in separate containers.

of fistulization from diseased small bowel. Colonoscopy is also useful to detect post-resection CD recurrence. Also, when there is inadequate response to therapy, colonoscopy can determine the extent, location and severity of inflammation, and thus drive therapeutic decision-making.

The severely colitic colon is prone to perforation and toxic dilation even in the absence of instrumentation and air insufflation. If strongly indicated (e.g. to rule out cytomegalovirus) in a toxic and immunosuppressed patient, a limited inspection of the rectosigmoid with minimal air insufflation is generally safe.

Patients with colitis affecting at least one-third of the length of colon and disease duration of greater than 8 to 10 years are at increased risk for colon cancer (Video Clips 7.8 and 7.9). It is standard practice to survey this population for dysplasia with colonoscopy (Video Clip 7.10). Surveillance entails careful mucosal inspection; random four-quadrant mucosal biopsies obtained every 10 cm (or every segment of large bowel; Fig 7.3); and targeted sampling of any suspicious abnormality (Video Clip 7.11). Chromoendoscopy (Plate 7.10) with targeted biopsy may detect dysplasia more accurately than the conventional random-biopsy method, but is not widely accepted (Video Clip 7.12). The colonoscopist should be vigilant in looking for subtle, villiform, flat, or minimally elevated polyps, which may represent dysplastic precursors to colorectal cancer (Plate 7.11; Video Clip 7.13).

Colitis-associated polyp: Inflammatory or dysplastic?*

Lesion characteristic	Favors inflammatory polyp	Favors colitis-associated dysplasia
Location	In colitic segment	In colitic segment, more likely in distal colorectum
Number	Multiple (may be tens–hundreds)	Solitary or few
Shape	Usually pedunculated/filamentous or semipedunculated, lobulated	Usually sessile or flat
White exudate on tip?	Yes	No
Very friable/ erythematous?	Yes	No
Surface texture	Glistening, smooth	Cerebriform, villous

*In some cases it is impossible to distinguish between dysplastic and nondysplastic polyps by gross morphology

Detecting colitis-associated dysplasia

- Adhere to recommended surveillance intervals
  - Implement electronic recall system
  - Educate patients and staff regarding importance of surveillance
- Adhere to recommended biopsy protocols
- Perform surveillance when patient in remission (if practical)
- Inspect and sample all colitic segments
  - If impassable stricture, develop appropriate strategy
- Maintain high index of suspicion in:
  - high-risk patients:
    - primary sclerosing cholangitis;
    - family history of colorectal cancer;
    - long-standing, active, pan colitis;
    - history of previous dysplasia.
  - high-risk colon segments:
    - strictures (especially in UC);
    - rectosigmoid > proximal colon.
- Achieve high-quality bowel cleansing
- Consider chromoendoscopy
- Use high-resolution, high-definition scopes
- Look for atypical polyp appearance

Is the dysplasia colitis-associated or sporadic?*

Lesion characteristic	Favors colitis-associated	Favors sporadic
Location	Always in colitic segment	May be in uninvolved segment
Patient risk factors	Long-standing colitis, primary sclerosing cholangitis, active disease, etc.	Advanced age, previous sporadic adenomas
Shape	Often atypical for sporadic adenoma (sessile, highly villous, cerebriform surface, lateral spreading)	Usually typical for sporadic adenoma
Dysplasia in surrounding mucosa	Sometimes	No
Histology of polyp	Adenomatous, very rarely serrated	Adenomatous or serrated

*In some cases it is impossible to distinguish between dysplastic and nondysplastic polyps by gross morphology and histology

Polypectomy in colitis

- Always photograph lesion before and after resection
- In general, adhere to same techniques and principles as if normal mucosa
- Saline lift rarely works well in colitic segment owing to fibrosis/inflammation
- Consider tattooing site: tattooing in involved segment may be technically difficult because of fibrosis/ inflammation; puncture with injector needle in nearby uninvolved site if possible
- Biopsy adjacent mucosa to rule out adjacent dysplasia

Colonoscopy in colitis: What to describe in the report

- Colitis extent
- Appearance of terminal ileum
- Colitis activity
- Inflammatory-type polyps, if present
- Unusual features (e.g. bridging, foreshortening, etc.)
- Areas of sparing
- Specific characteristics of any suspicious polyps
  - Location
  - Morphology (photograph also)
  - Appearance of adjacent mucosa (colitic?)
  - Endoscopic intervention

The endoscopic report must describe the tissue-sampling technique and all pertinent observations.

Nondysplastic, inflammatory polyps commonly referred to as "pseudopolyps," arise as a result of an overly exuberant mucosal healing response (Video Clip 7.14). They are typically multiple, friable, and may exhibit a white exudate at their tips (Plates 7.12 and 7.13). These gross characteristics usually distinguish them from dysplastic polyps. Pseudopolyps possess negligible malignant potential, so there is no need to resect them, unless they are causing bleeding or the diagnosis is uncertain. They may be small and distributed sparsely throughout the colon, or they may be large and innumerable. This second distribution pattern makes surveillance colonoscopy more challenging with respect to detecting an "important" dysplastic polyp. But close inspection and perhaps chromoscopy may be useful in identifying dysplastic polyps.

Dysplastic polyps in colitic patients may be colitis-associated or sporadic. If the polyp is in a segment of the colon unaffected by the colitis (e.g. if the patient has proctosigmoiditis and the polyp is in the transverse colon) then the distinction is easy. If it is in a colitic area, it may be impossible to differentiate the two. Certain factors suggest a sporadic polyp: a "typical" appearance of an adenoma, unifocality, shorter duration of colitis, and older patient age. Close communication between pathologist and gastroenterologist is important. The management of colitis-associated dysplasia is controversial and should be tailored to the individual situation. Several studies suggest that in the well-selected patients, polypectomy and close surveillance is a reasonable alternative to colectomy, and this lower-morbidity alternative has gained favor in recent years in many centers. The choice between a surgical and nonsurgical approach will depend on numerous considerations, including dysplasia grade, disease duration, patient age, colonoscopist expertise, patient risk tolerance, clinical symptoms, and number of sites of dysplasia. From a technical standpoint, dysplastic polyps in colitis patients can be removed by most of the same polypectomy techniques used in noncolitic patients (Video Clip 7.15). It is helpful to biopsy the margins of the polypectomy site separately to assure eradication of all dysplasia.

Mucosal "bridges," segmental strictures, and scarring (Plate 7.14) also signify healed colitis. Mucosal bridges and scarring are of little consequence. Stricturing is more common and less concerning in CD than in UC; many experts suggest that a stricture in UC should be considered a cancer until proven to be benign. In CD, anastomotic strictures may result from scarring, ischemia, or recurrent CD, and can be dilated endoscopically.

Endoscopy of ileal pouches

The Kock pouch (KP) procedure entails closure of the perineum and creation of a continent ileal pouch that is brought out to the anterior abdominal wall as a flat stoma; it is emptied with a catheter. The ileal pouch-anal anastomosis (IPAA) colectomy is achieved by creating a J-shaped pouch of distal ileum that is anastomosed to rectum or anus with anal sphincters having been preserved. Defecation is transanal, and therefore this has become the preferred continent ileal pouch procedure today.

Patients who have undergone IPAA and KP are susceptible to several postoperative complications. Common indications for "pouchoscopy" are diarrhea, incontinence, and (for IPAA) dysplasia, surveillance of residual rectum. With KP, a common complication is inability to intubate the valve. Pouchoscopy is generally performed with a gastroscope after a mild oral cathartic. Often lavage through the scope channel will be necessary to complete cleansing. The mucosa of the pouch is carefully inspected. The pre-pouch ileum is identified and examined. Complete inspection of the pouch requires retroflexion of the scope.

Difficult intubation in KP may occur in two ways: a stricture at the skin exit of the valve or within the valve lumen; or by slippage or "de-intussusception" of the valve. These findings can be identified endoscopically. KP valve slippage results in angulation of the valve lumen, so that the emptying catheter cannot traverse it. Slippage usually requires surgical revision, whereas a stricture can in some cases be dilated endoscopically or with minor surgery. At endoscopy of a slipped KP valve, the lumen may be elusive and the scope tip may enter a cul-de-sac. If the lumen is not evident or resistance is encountered, the scope tip should be carefully redirected using angulation and torque. KP incontinence may occur if the valve has become patulous or if a fistula has developed. A patulous valve is suggested by absence of resistance to the scope, but a fistula, usually at the base of the nipple valve, may be difficult to identify at endoscopy.

"Pouchitis" is a form of ileitis, and may result in diarrhea, bleeding, incontinence, and extraintestinal symptoms. Endoscopically, pouchitis is characterized by mucosal ulcerations, exudates, erythema, and friability, which can range widely in severity and may resemble CD, although the two entities are different. Mild inflammation is seen in most ileal reservoirs, and in the absence of clinical symptoms is not significant.

IPAA patients may develop stricture at the ileo-anal anastomosis, pre-pouch ileitis, or anastomotic breakdown with fecal leakage and pelvic abscess. Anastomotic strictures are appreciated at digital examination, and can be dilated under anesthesia with a bougie, a balloon, or a gloved finger. A small caliber scope may help traverse the stricture. Although pre-pouch ileitis may suggest CD, it usually is not. In IPAA patients, anastomotic breakdown is often difficult to appreciate endoscopically, and may require an imaging study with contrast.

Some IPAA patients with symptoms suggestive of pouchitis actually have retained rectal mucosa with active colitis ("cuffitis"). This can be confirmed by mucosal biopsy. If there is residual rectal mucosa and the colitis is of long-standing, then dysplasia surveillance (with biopsy of the mucosa adjacent to the anal sphincter) should be considered.

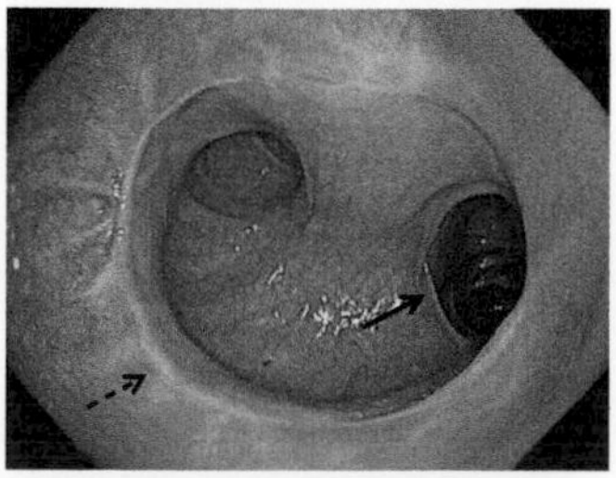

Fig 7.4 Colocolonic anastomosis (unremarkable). Scarring is visible in the forefront (dashed arrow). The functional limb of the anastomosis is at right (solid arrow) while a blind end is seen at upper left.

Vascular ectasias

These small mucosal vascular lesions can be discovered incidentally during colonoscopy, or can be the cause of either frank or occult rectal bleeding. Typically located in right colon and cecum, they are less than 2 cm in diameter, blanch on compression, and may be multiple. The colonic lesions display an unmistakable cherry-red coloration and "sunburst" pattern, with ectatic vessels radiating out from a central hub.

Because they are small, they are easily overlooked. Detection requires meticulous purging of the colon, a high index of suspicion, and careful examination on both sides of haustral folds, aided if necessary by retroflexion in right colon. When encountered incidentally during colonoscopy, vascular ectasias do not require treatment. If they are responsible for gross bleeding, iron deficiency, and/or anemia, then they should be ablated with bipolar coagulation, heater probe, or APC (Plate 7.15; Video Clip 7.16). The endoscopic end point is visible whitening of the entire lesion and cessation of bleeding. Ablation stops clinical bleeding in approximately 70% of cases. Bleeding may recur, necessitating repeat endoscopy, and perhaps evaluation of the small bowel for vascular lesions.

Graft-versus-host disease

Gastrointestinal involvement by graft versus host disease (GVHD) is common, and should be considered in any patient who develops diarrhea after bone marrow transplant. The diagnosis can be established by colonoscopy with mucosal biopsy and often requires only flexible sigmoidoscopy. Macroscopically, the mucosa may appear normal, or display nonspecific colitic features, such as erythema, ulceration, edema, and exudate.

Infectious colitis

Infectious colitis may involve the entire colon, or may be localized. Ileal involvement may accompany colonic involvement (e.g. in *Salmonella*, *Campylobacter*, *Yersinia*, or tuberculosis infections), but this distribution is not pathognomic of infection, as it is seen in Crohn's ileocolitis, *Shigella*, *Entamoeba histolytica*, and cytomegalovirus infections. *Entamoeba* may produce colonic friability, and "flask-shaped" ulcerations that have red borders and central exudates, often preferentially afflicting the proximal colon. Enteroinvasive *E. coli* can produce friable, ulcerated mucosa, more commonly in right colon. Viral colitis (e.g. cytomegalovirus or herpes virus) can visually mimic UC, but may also cause multiple deep localized ulcers. Cytomegalovirus colitis should be considered in all immunosuppressed patients and may complicate idiopathic colitis. Biopsies (particularly of the rims of ulcers) may reveal characteristic cytoplasmic inclusion bodies.

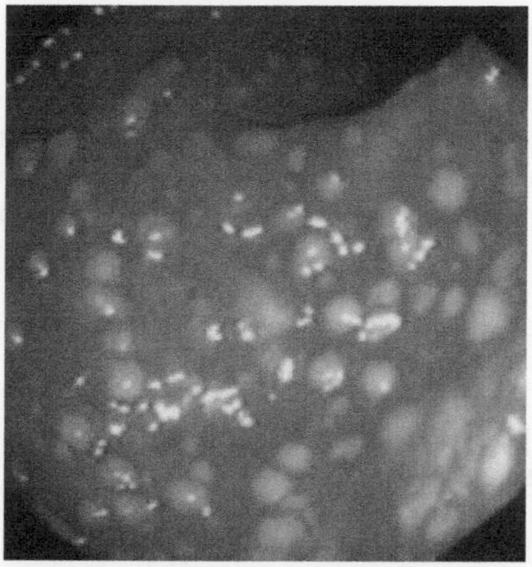

Fig 7.5 Pseudomembranous colitis. The pattern of multiple punctate exudates is highly characteristic of *Clostridium difficile* infection.

The diagnosis of *Clostridium difficile* colitis can be established by detection of toxin in the stool, but is at times made by colonoscopy. Classically, colonoscopy reveals "pseudomembranes"—yellow-white plaques of exudate studding the mucosal surface (Fig 7.5). Pseudomembranes are usually found throughout the colon and rectum, but can on rare occasion be only right-sided. The ileum is uninvolved. Pseudomembranes are not pathognomic for *C. difficile* infection, and *C. difficile* infection may exist in the absence of pseudomembranes. Biopsy reveals a characteristic inflammatory exudate. If the colitis is severe, colonoscopy should be limited to the rectosigmoid and air insufflation should be minimal.

Intestinal tuberculosis may appear identical to CD. Tuberculosis may involve right colon, ileocecal valve, and ileum and, like CD, it may be segmental, ulcerate, and lead to stricturing. Diagnosis is established with biopsy.

The most common organisms responsible for sexually transmitted proctitis are *Neisseria gonorrhoeae*, *Herpes* virus, *Chlamydia trachomatis*, and syphilis. Colonoscopically, the rectum may be nodular, erythematous, and coated with pus. The more proximal colon is spared. The diagnosis is established by culture and response to antibiotics.

Occasionally, whitish, small, filamentous wiggling structures are seen on the mucosal surface. These are usually pinworms but if fixed to the wall may be whipworms. Either can be captured with the forceps for analysis (Video Clips 7.17 and 7.18).

Colonoscopic aspiration of stool is a convenient means of obtaining a sample for microbiological analysis. Biopsy may be helpful as well. In amebiasis, colonic biopsy may reveal diagnostic trophozoites. Characteristic organisms can be seen also on colonoscopic biopsies in *Strongyloides* infestation. In order to increase diagnostic sensitivity, multiple biopsies should be obtained from affected mucosa.

Microscopic colitis

- Exclude in patient with unexplained diarrhea
- Increased incidence in women >60 years old
- Mucosa usually appears normal
- In a minority of cases, mucosa is subtly, diffusely nodular, with mosaic-like appearance
- Colonoscopic perforations related to "fracturing" have been reported
- Obtain random biopsies from right and left colon
- Alert the pathologist that microscopic colitis is in the differential diagnosis
- May require special stain to see collagen band

Dieulafoy lesions

Rarely, sudden-onset hemorrhage results from disruption of an anomalous "persistent-caliber" vessel in the colonic submucosa (a "Dieulafoy" lesion). Careful mucosal inspection after rapid bowel purgation may disclose the lesion—a small ulcer, containing a red spot or pigmented protuberance. The lesion can be ablated colonoscopically with cautery and/or clipping. However, the site should also be marked, as segmental colectomy may be required.

Microscopic, lymphocytic, and collageneous colitis

In microscopic colitis, the mucosa typically appears normal, although subtle edema and/or erythema may be noted, particularly in the proximal colon (Video Clip 7.19). Thus, random biopsy must be taken from left and right colon, and even if the gross appearance is normal. Microscopic evaluation reveals increased lamina propria lymphocytes and/or a thickened subepithelial collagen band.

Colonoscopic abnormalities due to medications

Drug	Lesion
Phosphate-based preparations	Aphthous erosions, distal > proximal colon
All cathartics/purgatives	Mild acute colitis Erosions, ulcer on ileocecal valve
Hydrogen peroxide or glutaraldehyde after incomplete scope rinsing	Acute colitis, with white patchy appearance, usually seen during scope withdrawal
Nonsteroidal anti-inflammatory drugs (NSAIDs)	Focal ulcers, diaphragm-like membranes
NSAIDS, gold, isoretinoin, potassium, and cytotoxic chemotherapy	Acute colitis
Anthraquinone laxatives	"Melanosis coli" (Video Clip 7.2) • Brown, "alligator-hide" appearance to colon mucosa due to pigment in macrophages • Polyps appear pale against dark coloration • Terminal ileum unaffected

Abnormalities of terminal ileum and ileocecal valve	
A few scattered erosions in terminal ileum	• Common • May be related to prep or nonsteroidal anti-inflammatory drugs • Do not necessarily imply Crohn's disease
Multiple diminutive subepithelial polyps/ nodules in terminal ileum	• Common • Usually nodular lymphoid hyperplasia is common, particularly in young patients • Insignificant clinically
Firm, isolated, pale submucosal nodules	• Usually carcinoid tumor (Video Clip 7.1) • Diagnosis rarely made on standard biopsy (unless lesion ulcerated) • Confirmation usually requires further imaging (CT, octreotide scan, etc.)
Terminal ileum diseases that "masquerade" as Crohn's ileitis	• Ileal tuberculosis • Unusual bacterial infections (e.g. *Yersinia*) • Lymphoma
Strictured ileocecal valve that cannot be intubated	• Crohn's ileitis • Forceps can generally be passed into the ileum for biopsy
Widely and persistently patulous ileocecal valve	• Chronic ulcerative colitis

Further reading

1. Abreu MT, Harpaz N. Diagnosis of colitis: making the initial diagnosis. *Clin Gastroenterol Hepatol* 2007;5:295–301.
2. Baxter NN, Goldwasser MA, Paszat LF, Saskin R, Urbach DR, Rabeneck L. Association of colonoscopy and death from colorectal cancer. *Ann Intern Med* 2009;150:1–8. Epub 2008 Dec 15.
3. Chetty R, Govender D. Lymphocytic and collagenous colitis. an overview of so-called microscopic colitis. *Nat Rev Gastroenterol Hepatol* 2012;9:209–18.
4. Itzkowitz SH, Present DH, Crohn's and Colitis Foundation of America Colon Cancer in IBD Study Group. Consensus conference: colorectal cancer screening and surveillance in inflammatory bowel disease. *Inflamm Bowel Dis* 2005;11:314–21.
5. Jensen DM, Machicado GA, Jutabha R, Kovacs TO. Urgent colonoscopy for the diagnosis and treatment of severe diverticular hemorrhage. *N Engl J Med* 2000;342:78–82.
6. Lakoff J, Paszat LF, Saskin R, Rabeneck L. Risk of developing proximal versus distal colorectal cancer after a negative colonoscopy: a population-based study. *Clin Gastroenterol Hepatol* 2008;6:1117–21; quiz 1064. Epub 2008 Aug 8.
7. Nagar AB. Isolated colonic ulcers: diagnosis and management. *Curr Gastroenterol Rep* 2007;9:422–8.
8. Sheibani S, Gerson LB. Chemical colitis. *J Clin Gastroenterol* 2008;42: 115–21.
9. Shen B. Acute and chronic pouchitis-pathogenesis, diagnosis and treatment. *Nat Rev Gastroenterol Hepatol* 2012;9:323–33.
10. Zuccaro G. Epidemiology of lower gastrointestinal bleeding. *Best Pract Res Clin Gastroenterol* 2008;22:225–32.

Chapter video clips

Video Clip 7.1 Melanosis coli with polyp
An adenoma is hidden behind the ileocecal valve in the setting of melanosis coli.

Video Clip 7.2 Squamous papillomas in the rectum
Multiple diminutive papules are seen near the dentate line during careful retroflex examination.

Video Clip 7.3 Diverticular colitis
Prominent polypoid red folds seen in a patient with sigmoid colon diverticular disease.

Video Clip 7.4 Segmental colonic ischemia
A segment of sigmoid colon is involved with moderate to severe ischemia.

Video Clip 7.5 Solitary rectal ulcer syndrome
Endoscopic findings of solitary rectal ulcer syndrome include ulceration, erythema, edema, and exudate.

Video Clip 7.6 Radiation proctopathy
Angioectasias in the rectum treated with argon plasma coagulation therapy.

Video Clip 7.7 Cobble-stoning in chronic ulcerative colitis
Severe edema, erythema, and ulceration in a patient with active ulcerative colitis.

Video Clip 7.8 Small carcinoma in chronic ulcerative colitis
Small carcinoma detected during surveillance in chronic ulcerative colitis. Extensive mucosal scarring is also seen.

Video Clip 7.9 Large carcinoma in chronic colitis
Large carcinoma in colitis, mucosal bridging is seen and snare biopsy technique is used.

Video Clip 7.10 Dysplasia in ulcerative colitis
The spray catheter is used for chromoendoscopy, which reveals a dysplastic plaque.

Video Clip 7.11 Nodular carcinoma arising in ulcerative colitis
Small, nodular carcinoma detected during surveillance in patient with chronic ulcerative colitis.

Video Clip 7.12 Chromoendoscopy in colitis surveillance
Areas of flat dysplasia are detected during chromoendoscopy in colitis surveillance.

Video Clip 7.13 Sessile dysplasia in chronic ulcerative colitis
Large area of villiform, sessile dysplasia is seen in chronic ulcerative colitis.

Video Clip 7.14 Giant inflammatory polyp
Giant inflammatory polyp identified in chronic colitis.

Video Clip 7.15 Dysplastic polyp in ulcerative colitis
Identification and snare resection of flat, dysplastic polyp in chronic ulcerative colitis.

Video Clip 7.16 Bleeding angioectasia
Detection and cauterization of ascending colon, bleeding angioectasia.

Video Clip 7.17 Pinworms
Live pinworms seen during colonoscopy.

Video Clip 7.18 *Ascaris*
Live *Ascaris* worm seen during colonoscopy.

Video Clip 7.19 Flat adenoma in microscopic colitis
Large flat adenoma seen in ascending colon in a patient with microscopic colitis. The colitis has caused edema and a mosaic pattern, which is atypical for this disease.

CHAPTER 8
Diagnostic Biopsy

Introduction

Biopsy extends the diagnostic capability of colonoscopy to the microscopic level, allowing the pathologist to view cellular detail and to apply histochemical, immunochemical, and immunogenetic testing. Endoscopic biopsies are superficial, usually sampling mucosa (not often submucosa), and therefore limited but extremely safe. Tissue acquisition is one of the chief advantages of optical colonoscopy over capsule colonoscopy and computerized tomography or magnetic resonance colonography. Although newer technologies such as confocal imaging offer the potential to provide real-time cellular detail during colonoscopy, histological interpretation of biopsy specimens remains the standard of care.

Equipment for biopsy

The forceps consist of two apposing cups, controlled by a wire attached to the handle. A variety of forceps designs are available (Fig 8.1). The cups may be hemispherical, elliptical, or fenestrated, and some contain a central spike. The standard cup is about 2 mm in diameter, which will provide a tissue sample of about 4 cubic mm or 6 mg. Pediatric forceps can collect a specimen of about 3 mg, whereas that from a "jumbo" forceps can be up to 15 mg. Jumbo forceps require a larger (3.6 mm) accessory channel such as that within the adult-model (not pediatric-model) scopes. Larger samples can also be taken with a polypectomy snare. The spike forceps is designed to impale and secure the sample so that two

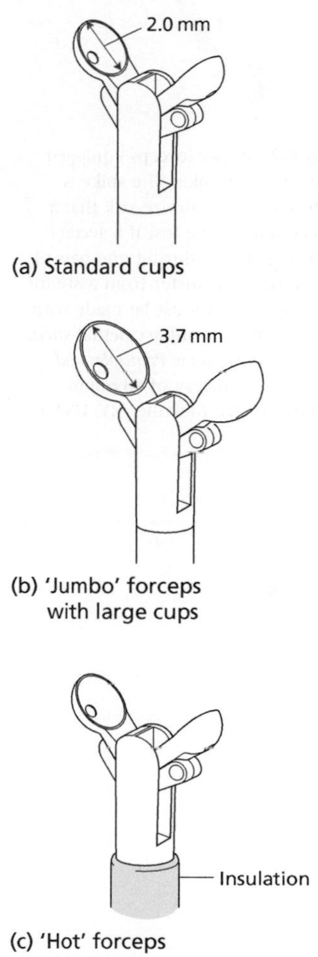

Fig 8.1 Three types of biopsy forceps. The larger ("jumbo") cup is often used for cold forceps polypectomy. The hot forceps are used for hot forceps polypectomy or for cauterization of a bleeding site.

Practical Colonoscopy, First Edition. Jerome D. Waye, James Aisenberg, and Peter H. Rubin.
© 2013 John Wiley & Sons, Ltd. Published 2013 by John Wiley & Sons, Ltd.

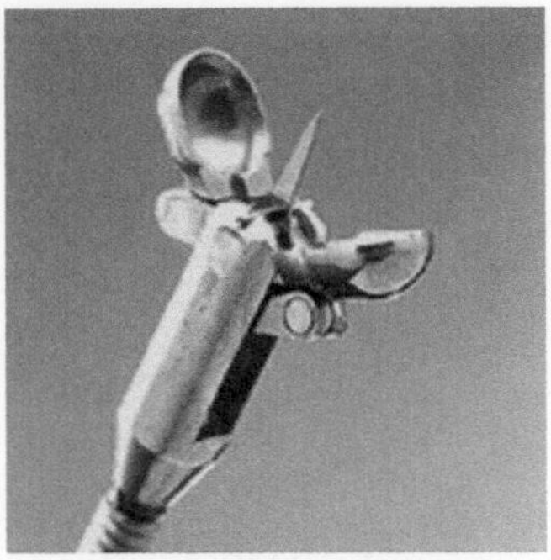

Fig 8.2 Biopsy forceps equipped with needle spike. The spike is intended to minimize risk that a specimen will be lost if a second biopsy is taken during one pass of the forceps. Transfer from assistant to endoscopist must be made with cups shut to avoid accidental stick. (From *Colonoscopy: Principles and Practice*—Courtesy of Olympus America Inc., Melville, NY, USA.)

pieces can be obtained during one pass (Fig 8.2). It is reasonable for the standard forceps to serve as the "default forceps," with other designs serving special situations.

Reusable or single-use (disposable) biopsy forceps are available, and both types are widely acceptable. The single-use varieties offer efficiency, sterility, and prevention of inadvertent tissue carry-over from case to case, but the costs are considerable. Reusable forceps should be tested before each use, and sterilization–reprocessing protocols must be followed assiduously.

"Hot biopsy" forceps are monopolar devices, can be connected to an electrosurgical unit, and require a remote return electrode. The sheath is insulated. This device permits cauterization of the target tissue plus biopsy of tissue that is sequestered in the forceps' cups, out of the electrical conduction pathway. This device can be useful for simultaneous biopsy and eradication of small polyps (less than 5 mm). Specialty forceps, such as rotatable and angulated models, are available but are not essential to daily practice.

How to use biopsy forceps

The endoscopist should specify which forceps variety (large cup, small cup, etc.) to use. The assistant should test the forceps function. During passage of the forceps, the scope tip should be pointed toward the lumen to avoid hitting and inadvertently puncturing the colon wall.

Because the view of the mucosa/lesion after biopsy may be changed, deformed, or obscured by bleeding, the endoscopist should inspect carefully the suspected abnormal area *before* biopsy. The closed forceps can be used to probe the lesion, assessing its firmness, compressibility, friability, and margins. This is particularly helpful for submucosal lesions: for example, if the lesion can be indented it is probably a lipoma (the "pillow sign").

The biopsy should be performed under direct vision with the colonoscope lens a few centimeters above the target. The open forceps is gently advanced into the colon wall onto the target, causing a slight indentation. It may be useful to aspirate intraluminal air to decrease luminal diameter and raise the target into the jaws of the forceps. During tangential biopsy, protrude the forceps tip only a few centimeters from the tip of the colonoscope in order to maximize stiffness of the forceps shaft. To obtain the biopsy the forceps are closed and withdrawn into the channel, avulsing the sample against the faceplate of the scope. If desired, a second bite can be taken, although occasionally this results in losing the first piece.

What to do with the biopsy

The endoscopic assistant should delicately and completely remove the specimen from the forceps, using a needle, blunt dental probe, or toothpick. Rapid rotation of the open forceps in the formalin to shake the specimen loose may separate the layers of the colon wall and hinder accurate microscopic interpretation. The assistant must inform the colonoscopist if the specimen is too small or mostly comprised of blood or exudate. The specimen may be placed directly into the fixative jar, or placed onto Styrofoam or cellulose filter paper. Specimens from one site are usually combined in one formalin bottle. However, all biopsies from one fixative bottle are embedded into one paraffin block, and therefore it has been suggested that no more than four specimens be placed in one bottle. The assistant labels each bottle with the patient's identification and the site of biopsy.

The pathology requisition form must be completed during or immediately after the procedure. If the form is filled out by the assistant, the colonoscopist should review it to verify accuracy.

In complex cases, dialogue between the colonoscopist and pathologist is invaluable. It is often useful to provide the pathologist with a copy of colonoscopic photographs, to permit correlation of gross and microscopic observation.

The pathology requisition: What to provide

- Clinical history (e.g. radiation therapy, organ transplant, immunosuppression, laxative use, nonsteroidal anti-inflammatory drugs)
- Anatomic location that specimen came from
- What lesion looked like *in situ*
- How the biopsy was obtained (i.e. forceps, cold snare, snare+cautery)
- The endoscopist's differential diagnosis
- The question (e.g. rule out amyloidosis, cytomegalovirus, graft versus host disease, etc.)

When to take a biopsy

If the lesion appears vascular (e.g. a colonic Dieulafoy lesion) or if the wall appears dangerously thin (e.g. in toxic colitis), biopsy is contraindicated. Otherwise, biopsy is appropriate whenever the endoscopist determines that histology would aid diagnosis of the observed abnormality. Biopsy is useful for both focal lesions (e.g. ulcerations or erosions, polyps, or tumors) and diffuse abnormalities (e.g. areas of erythema, friability, exudate, or diminished vascular pattern).

In certain settings, such as those below, biopsy of macroscopically normal mucosa is indicated.

• Unexplained, persistent diarrhea (with prior negative stool microbiologic studies), in order to diagnose lymphocytic or collagenous colitis and amyloidosis. Distal ileal mucosa biopsy should also be considered.

• Ulcerative colitis or Crohn's colitis, to determine the extent of disease, or the extent of mucosal healing following treatment.

• Ulcerative colitis or Crohn's colitis, to survey for cancer or precancerous changes.

• Follow-up evaluation of the site of a complex or advanced polypectomy, in order to confirm complete eradication.

• Flat mucosa adjacent to a raised/suspicious lesion in a patient with inflammatory bowel disease.

Indications for diagnostic mucosal biopsy

- Nonvascular mucosal abnormality
  - Ulceration/erosion
  - Polyp/tumor
  - Cystic lesion
  - Erythema/friability/exudate
  - Altered vascular pattern
- Unexplained persistent diarrhea
- Evaluation of ulcerative colitis and Crohn's disease
- Prior polypectomy of advanced polyp

Biopsy in special settings

• When biopsying a suspected malignancy obtain samples from several locations on the lesion (carcinomatous change may be focal).

• For submucosal lesions, (e.g. lipomas, leiomyomas, and carcinoids) "well biopsy" (also known as "bite-on-bite") technique may

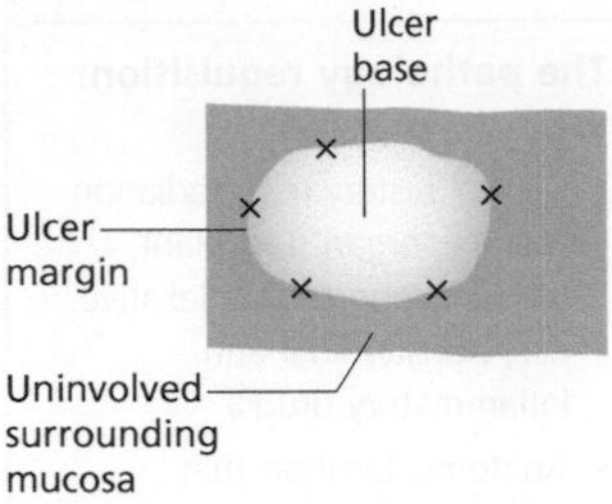

Fig 8.3 Ulcer biopsy sites. Isolated colonic ulcers are unusual and often reflect viral infection. In refractory idiopathic colitis in the immunocompromised host, it is important to exclude a superimposed viral infection. Biopsy of the ulcer rim is especially useful, since the base may be necrotic.

Performing mucosal biopsy: Recommendations

- Test forceps function before passing through scope
- Orient scope into lumen before passing forceps out of tip
- Photograph lesions before biopsy
- In severe colitis, use small-cup forceps and biopsy with caution
- Where appropriate, use closed forceps to probe lesion before biopsy
- Assistant must immediately tell endoscopist whether specimens are adequate/inadequate
- If inadequate, repeat biopsy procedure
- Obtain multiple biopsies of presumed cancer
- Provide pathologist with history, findings, and concerns; include photographs if possible
- Assistant must label specimen bottles and requisition immediately and double-check accuracy

be useful. In this method, the biopsy is repeated several times in one specific site, obtaining sequentially deeper biopsies into the lesion. For lipomas the "well biopsy" technique can demonstrate the yellow submucosal fat.

• Mucosal biopsy may be diagnostic when seemingly polypoid lesions are actually cystic, as in pneumatosis cystoides intestinalis. In this situation, when the endoscopist takes the biopsy the cyst may collapse.

• When biopsying a mucosal ulcer, sample both the ulcer base and the ulcer margin, as the ulcer base may contain only necrotic tissue (Fig 8.3).

• Biopsy protocols for dysplasia surveillance in patients with idiopathic chronic inflammatory bowel disease are discussed elsewhere (see Figure 7.3).

• To test for amyloidosis or Hirschprung's disease, submucosa must be obtained. "Well biopsy" technique with a large cup forceps may be helpful, and the requisition must specify that these diseases are being sought.

• To test for microscopic (collagenous or lymphocytic) colitis, take biopsies throughout the colon, as the recto-sigmoid may be uninvolved.

• After removing a polyp in a patient with chronic colitis (i.e. a potential colitis-associated dysplastic polyp), biopsy the surrounding mucosa. This may determine whether the polyp is colitis-associated or sporadic, and if there is a "field defect" (surrounding dysplasia).

• If more complex analysis of the specimen such as viral culture or flow cytometry is planned, specialized media (e.g. Hank's or RPMI) must be available.

Summary

Biopsy is an important adjunct to colonoscopy. There are nuances to colonoscopic biopsy, which promote safety and accurate diagnosis. An effective working relationship with an expert pathologist is invaluable.

Further reading

1. Barkun AN, Liu J, Carpenter S, *et al.* Update on endoscopic tissue sampling. *Gastrointest Endosc* 2006;66:743–7.
2. Bronwicki J-P, Venard V, Botte C, *et al.* Patient-to-patient transmission of hepatitis C virus during colonoscopy. *N Engl J Med* 1997;337:237–40.
3. Deprez PH, Horsmans Y, Van Hassel M, *et al.* Disposable versus reusable biopsy forceps: a prospective cost evaluation. *Gastrointest Endosc* 2000;51:262–5.
4. Eisen G, Baron TH, Dominitz J, *et al.* Guideline on the management of anticoagulation and antiplatelet therapy for endoscopic procedures. *Gastrointest Endosc* 2002;55:775–9.

5. Fantin AC, Neuweiler J, Binek, *et al.* Diagnostic quality of biopsy forceps specimens: comparison between a conventional biopsy forceps and multibite forceps. *Gastrointest Endosc* 2001;54:600–4.
6. Harpaz N. Pathology of colorectal polyps. In: Waye JD, Rex DK, Williams CB, editors. *Colonoscopy. Principles and Practice*. 2nd ed. Chichester: Wiley-Blackwell; 2009.
7. Jafri S-M, Arora A. Silent perforation: an iatrogenic complication of colonoscopy. *Surg Laparoscop Endosc Percut Tech* 2007;17:45–4.
8. Kozarek RA, Attia FM, Sumida SE, *et al.* Reusable biopsy forceps; a prospective evaluation of cleaning, function, adequacy of tissue specimen, and durability. *Gastrointest Endosc* 2001;53:747–50.
9. Weinstein WM. Colonoscopic biopsy. In: Waye JD, Rex DK, Williams CB, editors. *Colonoscopy: Principles and Practice*. 2nd ed. Chichester: Wiley-Blackwell; 2009.
10. Yang R, Ng S, Nichol M, Laine L. A cost and performance evaluation of disposable and reusable biopsy forceps in GI endoscopy. *Gastrointest Endosc* 2000;51:266–70.
11. Waye JD, Rex DK, Williams CB, editors. *Colonoscopy: Principles and Practice*. 2nd ed. Chichester: Wiley-Blackwell; 2009.

SECTION 3

Operative Procedures

CHAPTER 9

Thermal Techniques: Electrosurgery, Argon Plasma Coagulation, and Laser

Introduction

Thermal techniques are used to remove polyps, ablate tissue, and achieve hemostasis. The colonoscopist should be familiar with the principles and practice of electrosurgical interventions.

Electrosurgery

In electrosurgery, an electrosurgical unit (ESU) converts electrical wall current, which flows at 60 cycles per second (cps), into high-frequency current, flowing at greater than 100,000 cps. Unlike standard low-frequency wall current, high-frequency current does not cause muscular polarization and depolarization, so muscle spasm (electrical shock) does not occur.

Electrical current requires a complete circuit, from source to target and back to source (Fig 9.1). Most therapeutic devices used in colonoscopy are monopolar: the "active" electrode is applied to the target tissue, and electrical current is collected at a remote site by a second electrode, which returns it to the ESU, completing the circuit. Because the active electrode (e.g. a snare closed around a polyp) is small, it achieves a high local current density, which generates intense heat and tissue destruction at the target site. Because the return electrode (the patient return plate or "grounding pad") is relatively large, the electrons are dispersed over a wide surface area and negligible heat is generated, so a burn of the skin will not occur.

The colonoscopist can regulate many characteristics of the energy delivery. The foot pedal controls the amount of time that energy is delivered. The ESU settings regulate the electrical properties of the current: a continuous electrical waveform with low peak voltages ("cutting" current) generates intense local heating, which disrupts cells and results in rapid tissue destruction; whereas an interrupted

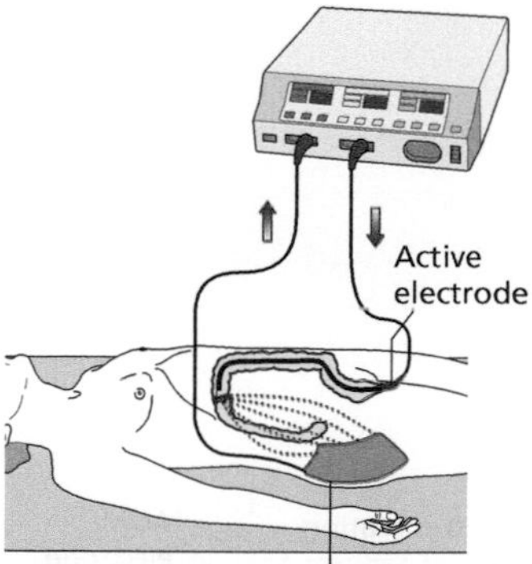

Fig 9.1 Monopolar electrocautery. Current travels from the ESU through the tissue and returns to the ESU via a neutral electrode. Because the neutral electrode is large, intense local heating is not caused.

Practical Colonoscopy, First Edition. Jerome D. Waye, James Aisenberg, and Peter H. Rubin.
© 2013 John Wiley & Sons, Ltd. Published 2013 by John Wiley & Sons, Ltd.

waveform with higher peak voltages ("coagulation" current) generates more moderate heating and favors tissue desiccation and coagulation. Some ESUs automatically adjust current delivery in response to second-by-second changes in tissue impedance in order to keep the power delivery constant. Thinner snare wires create more intense local electrical currents that promote cutting, whereas thicker wires promote coagulation.

Specific colonoscopic interventions call for specific electrosurgical settings. Specific power recommendations are available from the ESU manufacturers. In general, cutting current lowers the risk of injuring the adjacent tissue, promotes rapid, clean transection, and preserves an unaltered specimen for pathologic analysis but has little hemostatic effect. Coagulation current is better for achieving hemostasis and can be useful for obliterating residual adenoma around the margin of a polypectomy. Most ESUs offer cutting current, coagulation current, or blended current. In fact, "cut" settings also result in some coagulation, and "coagulation" settings (unless a very low peak voltage is used) also cause some tissue destruction.

Because it is thin, the colon wall is not ideal for thermal surgery. A perforation or "post-polypectomy coagulation syndrome" may occur if thermal injury extends beyond the submucosa. The distended colonic wall (mucosa, submucosa, and muscularis propria)

Principal thermal effects occurring during electrosurgery

Devitalization

- Irreversible destruction of tissue and its cellular structure
- Occurs when cells reach >41.5°C
- Not visible and hard to control
- Extends beyond the coagulation zone
- May lead to perforation of the colon wall

Coagulation

- Conversion of colloidal cellular systems from solution to a gel state (like boiling an egg)
- Occurs if cells reach >60.0°C
- Creates a visible white color change on mucosal surface, which can be used for visual control during electrosurgery
- Does not indicate extent of devitalization but roughly correlates with it
- Results in a "glue" effect, which may seal the endoscopic accessory to the target tissue

Desiccation

- Heat-induced cellular dehydration and shrinkage due to boiling of cells
- Occurs at temperature >100°C
- Results in glue effect
- Creates insulator effect, which may interfere with electrosurgical cutting during polypectomy
- During APC application, surface desiccation and insulator effect limit the depth of injury

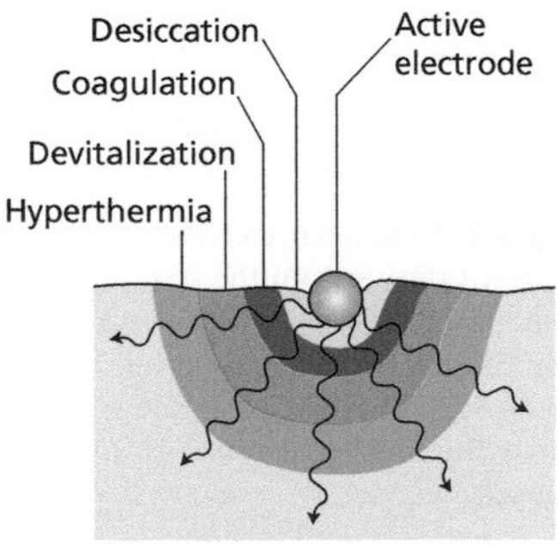

Fig 9.2 Tissue injury during electrocautery. Current density is greatest adjacent to the active electrode. The white area seen during polypectomy corresponds to the coagulation zone.

varies in thickness, from approximately 1.5 to 3.0 mm. It is thickest in the rectum and sigmoid and thinnest in the ascending colon and cecum. The burn should not extend deeper than about half the thickness of the wall—at times less than a millimeter. During polypectomy, perforation is more likely to be due to thermal injury than to mechanical injury related to cutting. Thermal techniques increase the risk of delayed bleeding after polypectomy, because tissue devitalization extends beyond the visible tissue reaction and over time devitalized tissue may slough, occasionally eroding into a blood vessel. Despite these caveats, electrosurgery during colonoscopy is safe and effective when utilized appropriately.

Instruments used for electrosurgery

Heater probes

Contact-based "heater" probes are useful for achieving hemostasis. The heater probe has the same outside diameter as a snare, and a bullet-shaped Teflon-coated nonstick tip that heats to 100°C when activated. This device converts electrical energy into intense heat within its metal tip. When the activated heater probe is touched to biological tissue, heat travels directly from the tip of the instrument into the target tissue. This probe does not require transfer of electrical energy (and thus requires no grounding pad). These probes contain an irrigation channel so that blood or debris can be washed away. The tip is specially coated in order to decrease sticking to desiccated tissue. This device is used to cauterize bleeding sites through compression (coaptation) of medium-sized blood vessels while heat-sealing them. Vessel compression minimizes the dissipation of heat ("heat-sink" effect) into flowing blood.

Multipolar electrode (BiCap)

The multipolar electrocautery (MPEC) probes contain a series of closely spaced electrodes, arranged in a linear or spiral configuration. When the tip is touched to the mucosa and is activated, a circuit is created between the electrodes. Bipolar instruments possess both the active and neutral electrodes in close proximity at the accessory's tip, and electric current flows from one closely spaced electrode to the other, generating intense local heating (Fig 9.3). The electrical thermal energy and pressure on the probe can seal bleeding vessels. These probes do not require a patient return plate, as the electrical circuit is completed locally. MPEC probes provide water irrigation capability, control of duration of energy delivery, and can be applied to the target tangentially or *en face*.

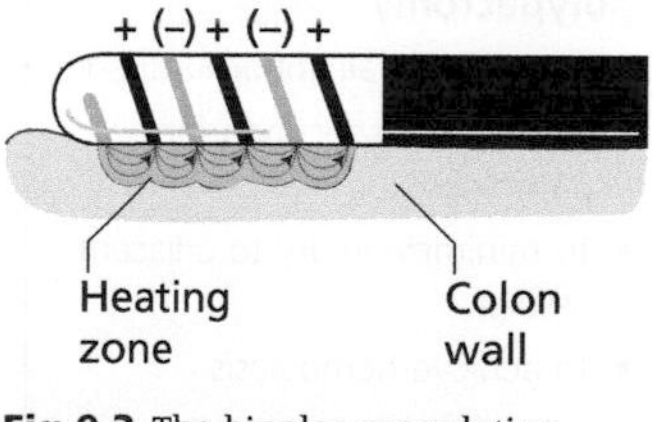

Fig 9.3 The bipolar coagulation probe. This instrument does not require a return plate, as the current flows from one positive electrode into its immediately adjacent negative electrode.

Monopolar accessories

Instead of direct heat transfer, these devices deliver high-density electrical current, which generates heat when it encounters resistance in the target tissue. Monopolar devices include snares, forceps, and probes. Monopolar systems utilize a wide-area return electrode (grounding pad) that receives the current at a distant site—typically the patient's lower back, thigh, or buttock. The return of electrons often follows a circuitous route to the grounding pad.

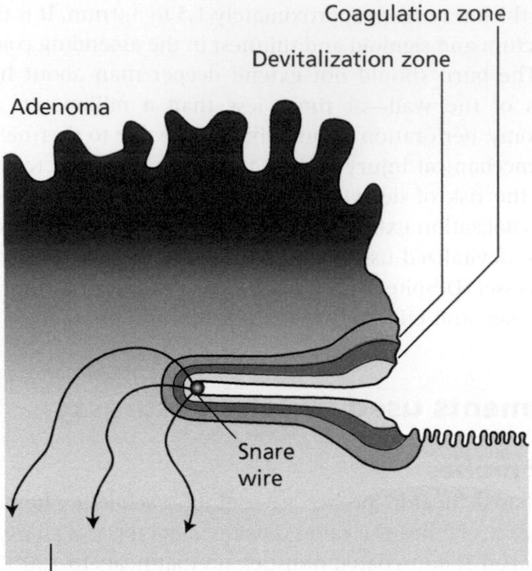

Fig 9.4 Tissue injury during snare polypectomy. Current density is greatest adjacent to the active electrode. Delayed perforation may occur if the devitalization zone involves the entire colon wall.

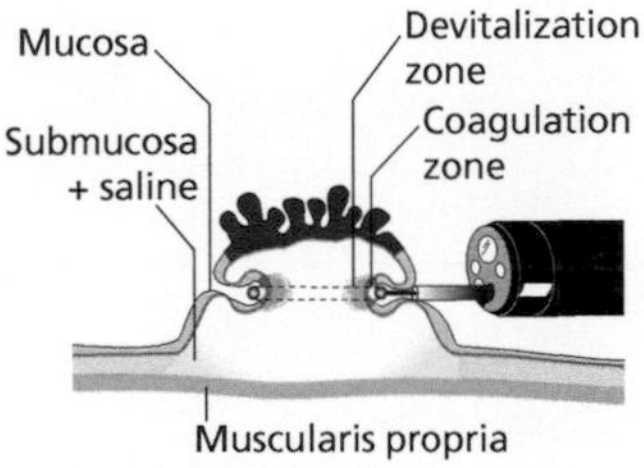

Fig 9.5 Injection of submucosal saline increases the distance from the tissue target of the thermal injury (polyp) and the muscularis propria, thus reducing the risk of perforation.

The four goals of "hot" polypectomy

- To eradicate all abnormal tissue
- To obtain a specimen for pathology
- To minimize injury to adjacent tissues
- To achieve hemostasis

Common uses of electrocautery

Polypectomy

For polyps >5–8 mm in diameter, monopolar electrocautery is usually utilized for simultaneous hemostasis and tissue obliteration (Figs 9.4 and 9.5). Electrocautery is essential for heat-sealing the larger blood vessels contained within the stalks of pedunculated polyps or within the submucosa underlying broad-based flat or sessile polyps. The techniques of polypectomy are described in detail elsewhere.

Coagulation of bleeding vessels

Electrocautery techniques can be used to stop the bleeding from vascular ectasias, polypectomy sites, radiation proctopathy, Dieulafoy lesions, bleeding diverticula, and virtually any other bleeding lesion in the colon. To coagulate superficial, smaller vessels, the monopolar snare, a hot biopsy forceps, or a heater probe can be used. For large vessels, coaptation is generally also required in order to prevent dissipation of heat by flowing blood ("heat-sink" effect).

During polypectomy the snare is often handy and used for controlling immediate post-polypectomy bleeding. The tip of the wire is advanced approximately 5 mm out of the catheter tip, creating a pinpoint tool that can be targeted precisely to the bleeding site. The wire tip is gently touched to the bleeding site and activated and the bubbling and blanching effects of the cautery are directly observed. Because the wire tip is relatively sharp, hard pressure into the colon wall is avoided. This technique may be used in the treatment of angioectasia and radiation proctopathy. If the blunter heater probe or biopsy forceps are used, the tool may be pressed more firmly onto the colon wall. The bipolar probe, which can be applied either axially or laterally, can coapt a vessel while applying current. Unlike argon plasma coagulation (to be discussed below), the thermal injury related to the snare loop, forceps, or probe have uncontrolled depth, so caution must be used; the current is generally activated in short bursts (5–10 seconds in duration).

Thermal devices commonly used in colonoscopy

- Monopolar argon plasma coagulator
- "Heater" probe
- Bipolar probe
- Monopolar polypectomy snare
- Monopolar "hot" biopsy forceps
- Laser

General precautions for electrosurgery

• The ESU service manual explains the indicators and settings, service instructions, and safety precautions. The document should be readily accessible. The therapeutic colonoscopist and the support staff should be comfortable with the operation of the equipment.
• Electrocautery in a poorly prepared colon is ill advised, as retained fecal material raises the danger of combustible gas, which could lead to explosion and perforation. For the same reason, only non-sugar-based bowel cleansing preparations should be utilized.
• High-frequency electrocautery can interfere with electronic devices such as defibrillators or pacemakers. Pacemakers are usually unaffected by colonoscopic electrosurgery, because the cautery electrodes are remote from the pacemaker. Implanted defibrillators can be activated by stray electrosurgical currents and should be turned off before the application of monopolar electrocautery but require monitoring when the defibrillator is shut down.
• The ESU should be stored in an easily accessible location, and when it is in use the displays should be easily visible to the operators.
• Before delivering current, the colonoscopist should personally check that the ESU settings are correct.
• To prevent thermal damage to the patient's skin the neutral electrode must be fixed firmly using appropriate electrode pads.

Electrosurgery: General precautions

- Check ESU settings before use
- Watch the site during application of energy
- Both endoscopist and assistants must be familiar with equipment settings and functions
- Test function before passing ancillary through scope channel
- The ESU displays should be easily visible
- Prevent an aberrant current pathway
  - Ensure proper placement of return electrode
  - Patient and any wires should not touch any metal object
  - Observe that no excess tissue is entrapped in the closed snare
- Application of current in a poorly prepared colon may cause an explosion
  - Do not use enema as only preparation when using electrocautery
  - Exchange gas throughout entire colon during intubation
  - CO_2 insufflation throughout entire colon eliminates explosion
- Cardiac pacemakers are usually unaffected by colonoscopic electrosurgery
- Implanted defibrillators can be activated by electrosurgical currents and should be turned off

Most ESUs issue a warning beep if a connection is loose or the return plate is not in proper contact with the skin.

- If the device fails to test properly, run through a correction algorithm. The problem is often corrected simply by tightening one of the cable/wire connections.
- During electrosurgery, neither the patient nor the wires attached to the patient should touch a metal surface (such as the stretcher bars or examining table) to avoid an aberrant current pathway bypassing the return plate and causing unintended thermal injury.
- The colonoscopist should apply short (e.g. 5–15 second) bursts of energy and respond to the visual effects on the target tissue (e.g. tissue blanching, progression of the snare through the polyp, etc.)
- The energy should be delivered only to the desired target. For example, during polypectomy care must be taken not to entrap an adjacent fold or excessive normal adjacent tissue (see Chapter 10).

Argon plasma coagulation

Principles

In argon plasma coagulation (APC), argon gas is infused into the colon lumen through a dedicated probe and is ionized by high-density electrical current. Electrons flow through the ionized argon gas (termed "plasma") to the nearest electrically conductive tissue, creating visible arcs of light (sparks) between the tip of the catheter and mucosal surface. Direct contact between probe and tissue is not required (Fig 9.6). Thermal injury is limited to the colon wall closest to the probe tip, and is similar to that caused by direct contact during other thermal modalities. When the coagulated tissue becomes desiccated and loses its electrical conductivity, the plasma arc jumps to adjacent non-desiccated tissue, thus decreasing the depth of penetration and risk of transmural burn. As there is no contact, there is no "glue effect" to seal the catheter to the tissue and cause bleeding when the catheter is withdrawn. The APC is monopolar and requires a return electrode, a tank of argon gas, a flow regulator, a dedicated ESU and probes, and a foot control pedal (Fig 9.7). It is not a laser

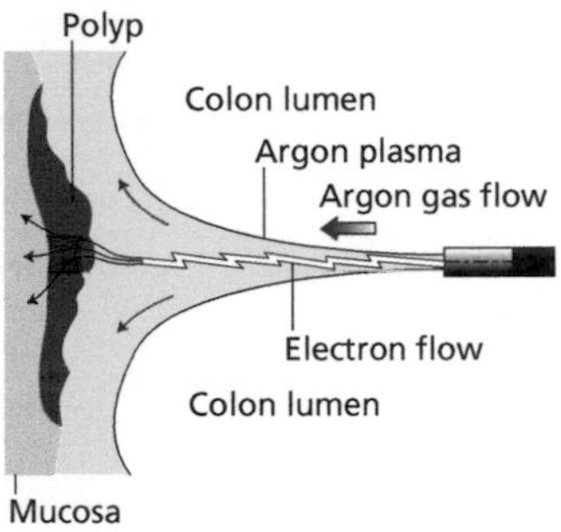

Fig 9.6 Argon plasma coagulator. The probe tip does not touch the mucosal surface. The tissue damage is superficial.

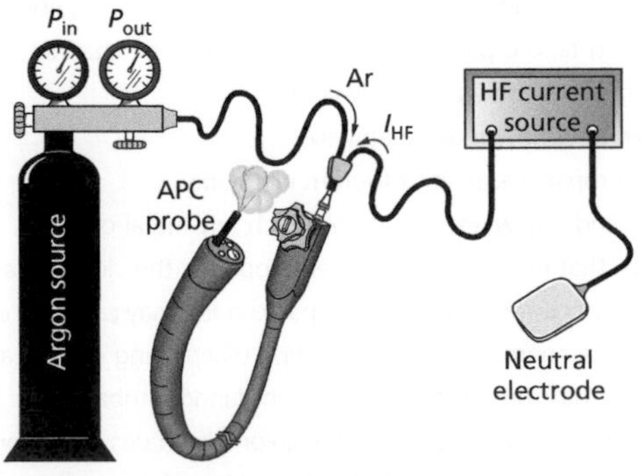

Fig 9.7 Argon plasma coagulator. The argon gas and the electrode pass through the endoscope in a catheter. An argon source and dedicated probe are required.

(see discussion below), although confusion often arises because lasers may also have the term "argon" in their name.

Technique

If the distance between the probe and tissue is too great, electron transfer will not occur and no effect will ensue. The probe tip needs to be placed close to (<1 cm) but not directly on the targeted tissue. The foot pedal activates the flow of argon gas and ionizing electric current. The arc of electrons travels to the tissue closest to the probe tip, be it en face or tangential. The depth of coagulation is controlled by the power settings and the duration of power delivery. If the probe tip is moved during coagulation ("painting" the mucosa), a more shallow thermal effect is created.

Applications

APC can be employed after polypectomy for hemostasis and to destroy residual polyp at the margins of resection. The tissue treated with APC is thermally destroyed and not available for pathology analysis. If there is concern about completeness of polypectomy, biopsies can be obtained before APC ablation or during a follow-up surveillance exam.

APC is also useful for achieving hemostasis from vascular ectasias and for treating radiation proctopathy. The ectatic blood vessels are obliterated with minimal adjacent or deep tissue injury. APC is not ideal for larger vessels, as it does not permit coaptation.

Cautions

Similar to other cautery techniques, APC can ignite combustible gas and should not be employed in a poorly prepared colon.

Laser

Principles

When applied to biological tissues, this extremely high-density energy achieves temperatures of >500°C, causing thermal vaporization (combustion) of desiccated tissue. The only laser employed for endoscopy is the neodymium-YAG.

Technique

The end of the laser light guide is positioned close to the target. Unlike the APC arc, the laser beam is invisible. The thermal effect is proportional to power settings, beam angle, duration of energy application, and the proximity of the source to the target. Care must be taken to avoid thermal damage to normal tissue and to the operator. Eye protection for all participants in the room is mandatory.

Applications

Laser may be useful to debulk tumors that are obstructing or bleeding. As it is not coaptive, it may not be useful if bleeding is coming

Electrosurgery in the colon

- Use approximately 50% of energy used in the upper gastrointestinal tract
  - Heater probe: set at 15 joules
  - "BiCap": set at 10 joules
  - APC (second generation): set at 25 joules

Troubleshooting electrosurgery in the colon

- Make sure ESU is turned on/ plugged in
- Check all connections
- Make sure grounding pad is attached to patient
- Check power setting
- Check for error light/code
- Switch to different endoscopic accessory
- Reboot the system

from larger vessels and may in fact intensify the hemorrhage by vaporizing the blood vessel wall.

Summary

Electrosurgery is useful in therapeutic colonoscopy for polypectomy, control of bleeding, and tissue ablation. Successful utilization of electrosurgery requires balancing its therapeutic benefits with risks of tissue damage, such as bleeding and perforation.

Further reading

1. Ginsberg GG, Barkun AN, Bosco JJ, *et al.* The argon plasma coagulator: February 2002. *Gastrointest Endosc* 2002;55:807–10.
2. Ischise Y, Horiuchi A, Nakayana Y. Prospective randomized comparison of cold snare polypectomy and conventional polypectomy for small colorectal polyps. *Digestion* 2011;84:78–81.
3. Laine L, Long GL, Bakos GJ, Vakharia OJ, Cunningham C. Optimizing bipolar electrocoagulation for endoscopic hemostasis: assessment of factors influencing energy delivery and coagulation. *Gastrointest Endosc* 2008;67:502–8.
4. Lee CK, Lee SH, Park SY, *et al.* Prophylactic argon plasma coagulation ablation does not decrease delayed post polypectomy bleeding. *Gastrointest Endosc* 2009;70:353–61.
5. Nelson DB, Barkun AN, Block KP, *et al.* Technology status evaluation report. Endoscopic hemostatic devices. May 2001. *Gastrointest Endosc* 2001;54:833–40.
6. Nesbakken A, Kristinsson J, Svinland A, Lunde OC. Endoscopic snare resection followed by laser ablation in the treatment of large sessile rectal adenomas. *Scand J Surg* 2011;100:99–104.
7. Parra-Blanco A, Kaminaga N, Kofima T, Endo Y, Tajiri A, Fujita R. Colonoscopic polypectomy with cutting current: is it safe? *Gastrointest Endosc* 2000;51:676–81.
8. Sawhey MS, Salfiti N, Nelson DB, Lederle FA, Bond JH, *et al.* Risk factors for severe delayed postpolypectomy bleeding. *Endoscopy* 2008;40:115–9.
9. Tanigawa K, Yamashita S, Maeda Y, *et al.* Endoscopic polypectomy for pacemaker patients. *Clin Med J* 1995;108:579–81.
10. Van Gossum A, Cozzoli A, Adler M, Taton G, Cremer M. Colonoscopic snare polypectomy: analysis of 1485 resections comparing two types of current. *Gastrointest Endosc* 1992;38:472–5.
11. Waye JD, Rex DK, Williams CB, editors. *Colonoscopy: Principles and Practice.* 2nd ed. Chichester: Wiley-Blackwell; 2009.

CHAPTER 10

Basic Principles and Techniques of Polypectomy

Introduction

A polyp is a localized abnormal growth arising on the colon wall. Polyps vary in size, shape, attachment to the colon wall, location, and histopathology. Polyps may be non-neoplastic or neoplastic, and benign or malignant. Tubular or villous adenomas exhibit epithelial cell dysplasia, whereas sessile serrated polyps do not. Some polyps are clinically inconsequential. About 5% of colon adenomas may progress to cancer, but it is impossible to tell a polyp's destiny from its gross morphology. Therefore, in practice most polyps should be resected. The purpose of polypectomy is to interrupt progression to carcinoma.

Polyps: Useful terms

- "Flat" : elevated <2.5 mm from mucosal surface
- "Sessile": elevated >2.5 mm, without stalk
- "Pedunculated": elevated >2.5 mm, with stalk
- "Diminutive": <0.5 cm diameter
- "Advanced adenoma": >1 cm diameter, villous components, high-grade dysplasia

Polyp appearance, location, and prevalence

Polyp size can be approximated by comparing the polyp to a tool of known dimensions, such as biopsy forceps. Colon polyps are described as flat, sessile, or pedunculated. The "Paris criteria" provide widely accepted nomenclature for describing the colonoscopic appearance of superficial neoplasms (Fig 10.1). Flat polyps

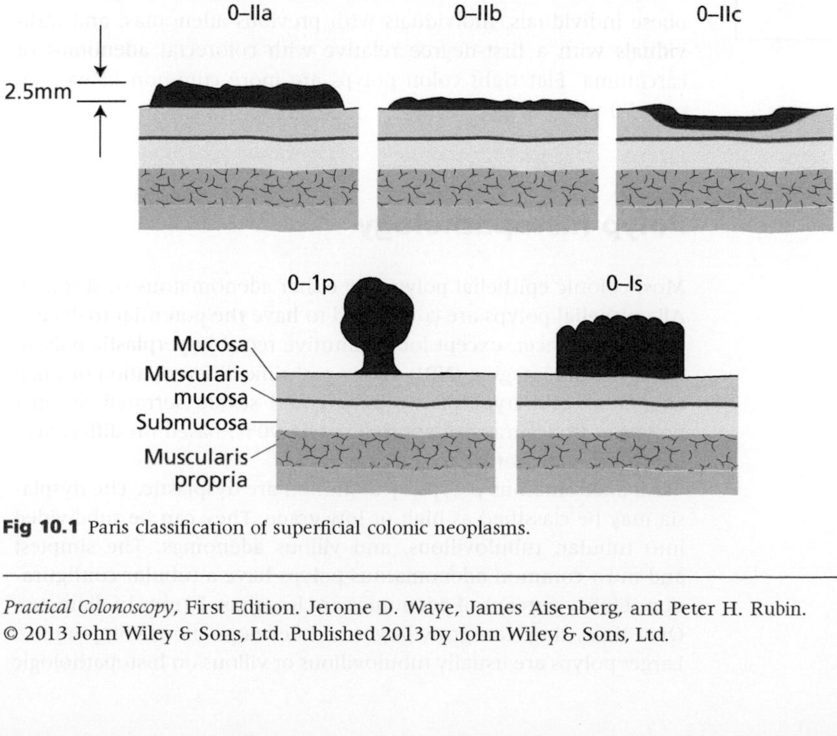

Fig 10.1 Paris classification of superficial colonic neoplasms.

Practical Colonoscopy, First Edition. Jerome D. Waye, James Aisenberg, and Peter H. Rubin.
© 2013 John Wiley & Sons, Ltd. Published 2013 by John Wiley & Sons, Ltd.

Hyperplastic rectosigmoid polyps: Endoscopic features (white light)

- Diminutive or small
- Round
- Multiple
- Surface pale, smooth, glistening
- Normal, homogeneous pit pattern

Polyps: Microscopic classification

- Serrated
  - Hyperplastic
  - Sessile serrated adenomas/ polyps
  - Traditional serrated adenoma
- Adenomatous
  - Tubular adenoma
  - Tubulovillous adenoma
  - Villous adenoma
- "Mixed"
  - Contains serrated and adenomatous
  - Rare

according to the Paris criteria are elevated <2.5 mm above the mucosal surface. Sessile polyps are elevated >2.5 mm above the mucosa, have no stalk, and generally are wider than they are elevated. As polyps grow, peristalsis may pull on the polyp, creating a pedunculated polyp, which has a stalk. This phenomenon is more common in the sigmoid colon, where muscular contraction is most vigorous. Polyps may become quite large in the right colon and rectum without becoming pedunculated.

Most colon polyps are less than 5 mm in diameter and are sessile; these are generally termed diminutive. Diminutive and medium-sized polyps (6–9 mm in diameter) comprise approximately 80% of all colon polyps.

In the general population, 60% of polyps are located between the rectum and the splenic flexure. However, in patients over 70 years of age, there is a shift in the location of polyps toward the right side of the colon. Flat serrated polyps occur predominantly proximal to the splenic flexure. Adenomas are least common in the transverse colon. Polyps are multiple in about 40% of cases. Diminutive hyperplastic polyps of the rectum and distal sigmoid colon are common and are believed to possess no malignant potential. These are recognized by their multiplicity, pale, smooth, glistening appearance, and need not be removed (Plate 10.1).

Adenoma prevalence varies according to genetic risk, age, gender, and nongenetic factors such as obesity or smoking. During careful colonoscopy using modern instrumentation in a Western screening/surveillance population, the prevalence of adenomas reaches approximately 50%. Adenomas are uncommon in individuals <50 years old who have no risk factors and are asymptomatic. Prevalence is increased in older patients, males, African Americans, smokers, obese individuals, individuals with previous adenomas, and individuals with a first-degree relative with colorectal adenomas or carcinoma. Flat right colon polyps are more common in women over 70 years of age.

Polyp histopathology

Most colonic epithelial polyps are either adenomatous or serrated. All epithelial polyps are considered to have the potential to degenerate into cancer, except for diminutive rectal hyperplastic polyps. Narrow band imaging (NBI) allows real-time differentiation of small adenomas and hyperplastic polyps and sessile serrated lesions/polyps with accuracy of approximately 90%, based on differences in surface vascular pattern (Plate 10.2).

All adenomatous polyps by definition are dysplastic. The dysplasia may be classified as high or low grade. They can be subdivided into tubular, tubulovillous, and villous adenomas. The simplest and most common adenomatous polyps have a tubular configuration. Eighty percent of adenomas are less than 10 mm in diameter. Over time, they can grow larger and develop villous components. Larger polyps are usually tubulovillous or villous on histopathologic examination (Fig 10.2). The tendency for malignant degeneration increases as the size and percent of villous elements increases. The presence of high-grade dysplasia is not ominous unless the lesion has been incompletely resected, in which case an underlying malignancy must be considered. If an adenoma containing high-grade dysplasia is completely removed, there is no possibility of spread, as the dysplastic cells are confined to the superficial layers of the polyp. The commonly used term "advanced adenoma" describes polyps that are >10 mm in diameter or that have a villous component.

Serrated polyps include hyperplastic polyps (HPs) and sessile serrated adenomas/polyps (SSAs), and the unusual traditional serrated adenomas (TSAs). SSAs (Plate 10.3) are considered to be more advanced lesions than HPs. Serrated polyps have architectural abnormalities, such as conspicuous infolding of the crypt epithelium and dilation of the base of the crypt, but no cytological dysplasia (Fig 10.3; Video Clips 10.1 and 10.2).

Less frequently, polyps arise from cells in the submucosa. Generally submucosal tumors are recognized by an intact mucosal covering, as well as by atypical characteristics of texture, color, and shape. Lipomas (Plate 10.4; Video Clip 10.3) and carcinoids (Video Clip 10.4) are soft and firm, respectively, and both are yellowish. In many cases, polypectomy is inappropriate for a submucosal tumor, because the tumor has little malignant potential, and/or colonoscopic resection carries a risk of perforation.

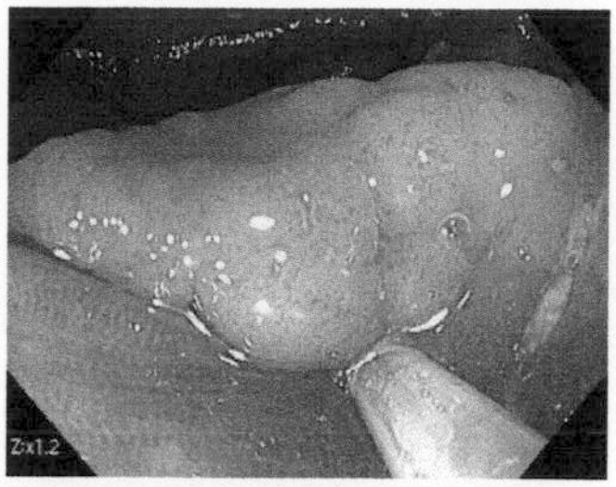

Fig 10.2 A large (3-cm) sessile tubulovillous adenoma (Paris 0–Is). Because this is elevated >2.5 mm above the surrounding mucosa (snare catheter width is 2.5 mm), the lesion is classified as sessile rather than flat. Note the distinct border, lobular surface, absence of central depression or surface ulceration, and cerebriform surface architecture. These characteristics distinguish this adenoma from a carcinoma and from a sessile serrated polyp.

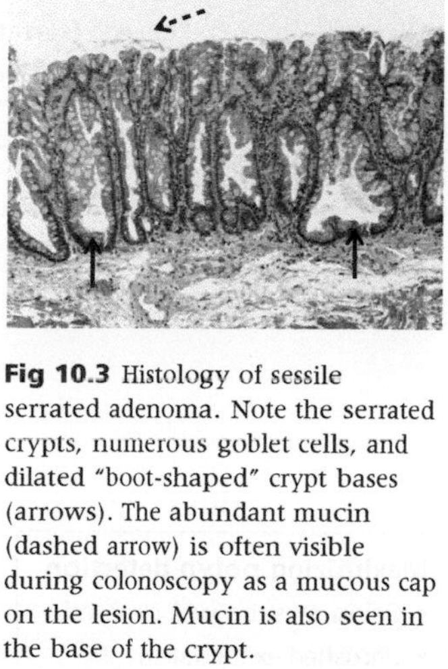

Fig 10.3 Histology of sessile serrated adenoma. Note the serrated crypts, numerous goblet cells, and dilated "boot-shaped" crypt bases (arrows). The abundant mucin (dashed arrow) is often visible during colonoscopy as a mucous cap on the lesion. Mucin is also seen in the base of the crypt.

Detecting polyps

If no adenoma or SSA is found on screening colonoscopy, guidelines suggest that 5–10 years can elapse before the next colonoscopy. However, polyps can be hard to detect, owing to colon spasms, convolutions, telescoping, folds, and debris; many are small, flat (Plate 10.5), or pale. Tandem colonoscopy studies (when a repeat examination immediately follows the first) report polyp "miss rates" of over 20%. Most missed polyps tend to be small and have low malignant potential. However "interval cancers" are reported in patients who have had a negative screening examination within the previous 3–5 years, and death from colorectal cancer may occur within 7 years; some of these cancers presumably arose from precursor lesions that were missed at the previous exam. (Others may be from fast-growing tumors.)

Causes of "interval" cancer

- Missed polyps at prior colonoscopy
  - Polyp overlooked ("missed")
    - Despite excellent colonoscopist technique
    - As a result of suboptimal colonoscopist technique
  - Poor colon cleansing
- Incomplete polypectomy
- Rapid progression to carcinoma
  - Premalignant (adenoma or SSA/P to carcinoma)
  - Normal mucosa to carcinoma

Submucosal polypoid lesions

- Lipoma
- Neuroendocrine (e.g. carcinoid)
- Stromal cell
- Sarcomas (e.g. Kaposi's)
- Granular cell tumor
- Metastatic tumors
- Locally invasive non-GI tumors

During intubation, most colonoscopists focus on passing the scope to the cecum, and during the scope withdrawal phase meticulously inspect the colon mucosa.

Epithelial polyps

	Polyp type	Histological feature		
		Dysplastic epithelial cells ("cytological dysplasia")	Dysplastic crypts ("distorted crypt architecture")	Serration of crypts at base
Adenomatous	Tubular adenoma	✓	✓	
	Tubulovillous adenoma	✓	✓	
	Villous adenoma	✓	✓	
Serrated	Hyperplastic polyp		✓	
	SSA/polyp		✓	✓
	Traditional serrated adenoma	✓	✓	
Mixed	"Mixed" (serrated and adenomatous) polyp	✓	✓	✓

Several principles help maximize polyp detection during withdrawal.

- Systematically examine the full 360° circumference of each colonic haustral segment. This may require scope repositioning and back-and-forth reinspection of a segment.
- Look behind every fold. To do this, deflect the tip maximally and hold it in that position as the scope is withdrawn behind the fold that is being explored. Then advance the scope and torque it and repeat the inspection at 3 and at 9 o'clock.
- Know the blind spots. Missed polyps most commonly occur behind flexures, behind the large folds (valves of Houston) in the rectum, or in between the larger thick sigmoid folds that occur in diverticular disease. Examine these blind spots repeatedly.
- Retroflexion of the scope tip in the rectum and the right colon can help to visualize areas that are difficult to see in the antegrade position (Plate 10.6).
- Suction all fluid pools and wash away debris. Even small amounts of material may conceal polyps. This is tedious and time-consuming but invaluable.
- If a fold "just doesn't look right" go back and examine it. Try washing, looking from a different angle, or removing air. Polyp detection is about pattern recognition and often occurs at a subcortical level.

Maximizing polyp detection

- Colon must be well cleansed
- Unrushed examination
- Complete colon intubation
- Meticulous examination of every haustral fold
- Inspection of far side of each fold
- Several passes through each colon segment
- U-turn maneuvers in rectum, right colon
- Special attention to flexures, rectal valves, large folds, diverticular segments

• Do not rush. The recommended average withdrawal time is at least 6 minutes for a routine, uncomplicated colonoscopy. This does not include time for washing or tissue acquisition. Although some colons are straight and can be surveyed relatively quickly, others are long and convoluted and careful withdrawal may take considerably longer.
• If the preparation is poor and cannot be made satisfactory by washing, the colonoscopy should be rescheduled, even if the cecum was reached. It is not acceptable to wait 5 or 10 years if the inspection was not thorough.

The detection of flat polyps is especially challenging. SSAs are generally pale, so they may not be evident by either protuberance or redness. Often, SSAs are betrayed only by a thin coating of brownish mucus on their surface, produced by their abundant goblet cells. When the mucus is washed away, SSAs appear as minimally elevated, glistening, pale, and slightly nodular, obscuring the underlying mucosal vascular pattern (Plate 10.3; Video Clips 10.1 and 10.2).

Detecting sessile serrated adenomas/polyps

- Increase alertness
  - When scope proximal to the splenic flexure
  - In higher risk populations
    - Females
    - >65
    - Previous or synchronous SSA/Ps
- Look out for
  - Mucous cap
  - Loss of normal vascular pattern
  - Loss of innominate grooves
  - Ring of mucus or debris
  - Red appearance of mucus on NBI

Finding a polyp that cannot be relocated for resection

- Prevent the problem
  - After identifying polyp
    - Keep polyp within endoscopic field of view
    - Keep eyes on monitor
      - Use "no-look" transfer of the snare
    - If polyp seen during insertion, remove it during insertion
    - If polyp hard to see and positioning is tricky, consider "marking" the site by taking a mucosal biopsy adjacent to the polyp
- Review endo-photograph of lesion taken before lesion was "lost" (often provides clues regarding location)
- Request input from endoscopy assistant (often assistant will remember relative location of lesion)
- Use the retroflex view
- Depress adjacent folds with a probe to look behind them (Fig 10.4)
- Do not rely on the centimeter markings on the scope insertion tube

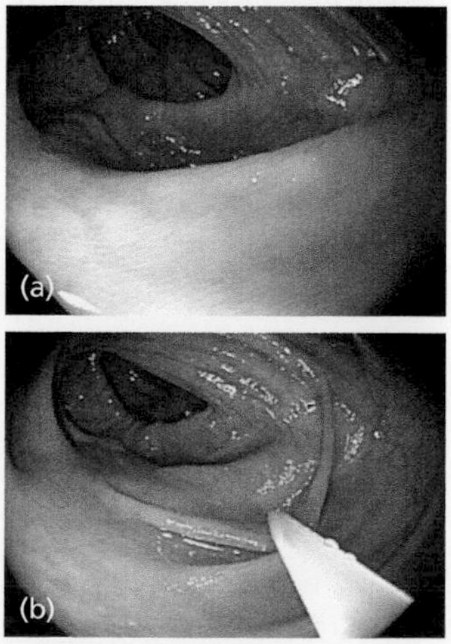

Fig 10.4 Push down a fold to look behind it. (a) Large haustral folds may conceal polyps. The closed snare or a forceps may be used as a probe (b) to expose the concealed area.

When to consider *not* resecting a colon polyp

- Polyp of no consequence (e.g. lipoma)
- Polyp submucosal
- Polyp appears cancerous
- Patient has overriding comorbidity/short life expectancy
- Not confident that complete resection is possible
- High risk and wish to discuss options with patient
- Anticoagulated patient
- Poor colonic cleansing
- Patient clinically unstable
- Proper equipment/staffing not available

Conditions for polypectomy

- Good colon preparation
- Cooperative patient
- Medically stable patient
- No recent anticoagulation
- Adequate time slot in endoscopy unit
- Fully equipped unit
- Polyp positioned at 5 o'clock position

General principles of polypectomy

Because of their malignant potential, most polyps encountered should be removed.

If detected during scope insertion, a small polyp should be removed immediately, because it may be impossible to relocate it during withdrawal. Large polyps are often resected during the withdrawal phase, as they are easy to re-identify.

Depending on the size and architecture of the polyp, severing it from the wall may be achieved simply with mechanical force (avulsion with a forceps or transection with a snare). This technique minimizes tissue damage to the resected specimen and surrounding tissue but may result in bleeding. In general this technique is restricted to polyps less than 5 mm but occasionally up to 10 mm in diameter. For polyps > 8–10 mm in diameter, cautery should usually be used in addition to mechanical force. The principles of electrosurgery are discussed in detail in Chapter 9. Electrocautery provides thermal hemostasis but poses a risk of adjacent mural injury.

Polypectomy: small polyps

If the polyp is diminutive, it can be contained within a single forceps bite and removed by simple avulsion. Following forceps polypectomy, be sure to inspect the site for residual polyp. Polyps in the range of 1–2 mm in diameter can be totally extirpated with one pass of the biopsy forceps, but for polyps larger than 3 mm forceps multiple bites may be required for complete removal. The concern is that adenoma fragments may be left *in situ*; even with small polyps, cancer may be the end result of incomplete polypectomy.

Another option for small polyp ablation is the "hot biopsy forceps." The upper portion of the polyp is grasped in the forceps, "tented" into the lumen, and current applied. A zone of white thermal injury appears, creating a "Mount Fuji effect," whereby blanched mucosa representing the enlarging area of tissue ablation is observed extending gradually from the summit toward the base of the tented polyp. Low power (15–25 watt) settings may be used but most endoscopists do not change the current from those used for standard polypectomy. When this injury zone is 1–3 mm, current is discontinued and the specimen is avulsed. Any residual polyp can be destroyed with the activated closed forceps. The specimen entrapped within the cups of the hot biopsy forceps is not thermally damaged. Because of reported complications, there has been some reluctance to use hot biopsy forceps, but many endoscopists employ them routinely to eradicate polyps in the range of 1–5 mm. An advantage of using forceps rather than a snare is that the resected polyp is preserved within the cup of the forceps and cannot be lost. The activated closed forceps can be used to destroy any visible polyp at the base of the resection site.

Small polyps may also be removed with a wire snare in the absence of electrical current. Cold snare resection is easy and safe (Plate 10.7). The "mini-snare" (30 mm long by 10 mm wide) is typically best suited to this purpose. The snare is placed around the polyp and around a small "collar" of normal tissue at the periphery of the polyp; the collar ensures that the entire polyp is eradicated. The snare is closed slowly, leaving a "button" of denuded submucosa. With cold snare, there is no risk related to thermal injury. Some colonoscopists use cold snare technique for flat polyps up to 8 mm in diameter. With cold snare technique, bleeding is generally insignificant and stops spontaneously. The specimen can be suctioned into a polyp trap. A potential disadvantage of snare polypectomy of diminutive polyps is that the small specimen may be difficult to locate and retrieve.

Safety precautions during electrosurgical polypectomy

- "Tent" the polyp away from the colon wall
- Be sure adjacent tissue is not enclosed in the snare loop
- Consider submucosal fluid injection
  - Increases thickness of submucosa
  - Limits depth of thermal injury
  - Color contrast aids in visualizing polyp contours
    - Methylene blue or indigo carmine
- If endoloop or endoclips are deployed, be alert for concentration of current at the site of the loop or clip
- Avoid "contracoup" thermal injury to opposite wall (rarely a significant problem)

Safety precautions during "hot" polypectomy

• Check the electrosurgical unit (ESU) settings before activating the current

• "Tenting" a polyp into the lumen can decrease the likelihood of full-thickness burn and confirm that the accessory is closed accurately around the polyp and not entrapping adjacent tissue

• Injecting fluid solution into the submucosa elevates the polyp away from the deeper layers of the wall, decreasing the risk of transmural burn. This is especially useful for broad-based right colon polyps

• Staining the submucosal injection fluid with methylene blue or indigo carmine helps to define the margins of flat polyps

• If an endoloop is applied to a pedunculated polyp, the portion of the stalk that has been narrowed by the loop may receive more concentrated current than the site less compressed by the polypectomy snare—thus the major portion of the thermal injury will occur at the loop site, not the snare

• If a metallic clip is applied to a polyp pedicle prior to snare resection or for hemostasis, the activated snare should not touch the clips, lest the current be conducted via the clip into the wall, resulting in transmural burn and perforation.

Polypectomy: recommendations

1. Immediately resect small polyps identified during insertion (do not defer until withdrawal phase)
2. Consider "cold" forceps resection for polyps <5 mm in diameter
3. Consider "cold" snare resection for polyps <8 mm in diameter
4. Check functionality and settings of electrosurgical unit before applications
5. Mark snare handle shaft to show when tip of snare is at tip of catheter
6. Orient polyp at right lower (5 o'clock) position before resection
7. When polypectomy snare is open, carefully position tip of plastic catheter at "near" border of polyp (closing snare will "pull" the polyp toward this point)
8. After closing snare around polyp, deflect scope tip toward lumen to assure no snaring of adjacent wall
9. Check distance between snare handle mark and position after snaring polyp ("gap" should be <1 cm)
10. During cautery application, "tent" snared polyp into lumen
11. Before initiating further closure of the activated snare, wait for coagulation (visible as blanching) to occur
12. Deliver cautery steadily until polyp resected (do not deliver energy in short bursts)
13. Generally, continue cautery until resection completed

Choosing the best snare

- All snares are not appropriate for all polyps
- Have several varieties available
- Thinner wires cut better, and may be preferable for "cold" resection
- Smaller loops are easier to manipulate in narrow segments
- Narrower wires are more flexible
- Smaller loops ("mini-snares") are large enough to encircle the great majority of polyps
- If one snare type is not working, change to another type; often the different design will help entrap the polyp

Snare cautery polypectomy

Safe and effective snare cautery polypectomy requires coordinated use of two forces: shearing, achieved by tightening the wire snare loop around the body of the polyp, which results in tissue cutting; and heating, which results in cauterization (hemostasis). Thermal energy is delivered through the wire loop, heat-sealing the vessels. The mechanical action of closing the snare may be insufficient to transect a polyp, so heat may also be needed to complete the transection. Most polypectomies do not result in significant blood loss. Tightening the snare around the base or pedicle of the polyp interrupts its circulation, requiring little current to seal the coapted walls of the arteriole (Fig 10.5). Coapting the vessel also eliminates "heat sink" (i.e. dissipation of electrocautery heat by flowing blood). This technique is effective for both pedunculated polyps that have a single-vessel blood supply and sessile polyps, which have several nutrient vessels.

(a)

(b)

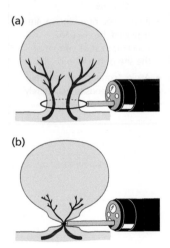

Fig 10.5 Snaring the polyp pedicle. Gently tighten the snare around the stalk before initiating cautery. This coapts the larger vessels, so that blood is no longer flowing into the head of the polyp, improving hemostasis.

Some endoscopists close the snare themselves during current application, whereas others entrust that operation to a trained assistant. Once the endoscopist becomes comfortable with the dial settings, the same setting is used for small or large polyps. Many experienced endoscopists prefer to use only pure coagulation current, and do not change the power output of the ESU during polypectomy or even from one polyp to the next. Others will toggle to cutting current during a difficult polypectomy if adequate coagulation has been delivered and the snare is not progressing through the lesion.

Passing the snare

The snare consists of a long, thin, conductive wire inside a plastic catheter. The action is controlled by a handle. When the slide bar is extended the snare loop opens, and when the slide bar is retracted the loop closes. Before polypectomy, the assistant should mark the point on the handle shaft when the tip of the retracted snare loop

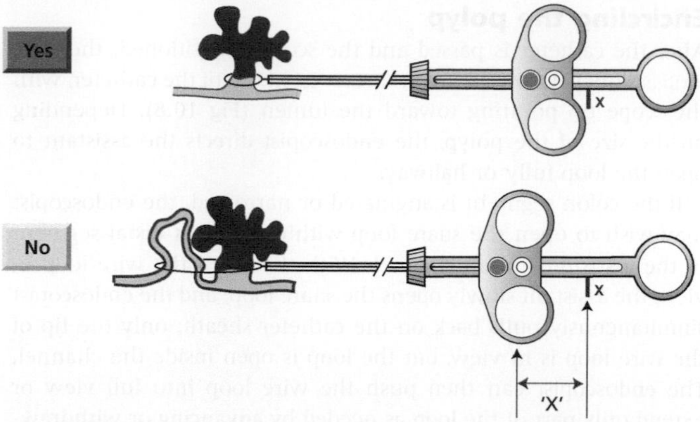

Fig 10.6 Polypectomy: Using the information mark on the snare handle. In some cases, it is difficult to see in the endoscopic image whether the snare has erroneously captured adjacent normal mucosa. The volume of tissue captured in the snare is reflected in the distance ("x") between the slide bar and the mark.

is flush with the end of the plastic catheter (Fig 10.6), check the settings of the ESU and test the functioning of the unit and snare.

To begin snare polypectomy, the catheter with the loop closed is passed through the channel until the catheter tip appears in the endoscopic image. Because the snare exits the scope at the 5 o'clock position in the visual field, this field should be directed toward the colon lumen, preventing trauma to the colon wall.

What to do if you need an "extra hand" during polypectomy

- Have the endoscopy assistant advance and/or withdraw the forceps or snare by manipulating the catheter at the port on the scope handle
- Stabilize the shaft of the scope between the pinky and ring finger of the left hand. This permits the left hand to simultaneously control the dial controls and the insertion tube, when the right hand is manipulating an accessory instrument (see Fig 6.7)

Positioning the scope

Colonoscopic accessories enter the visual field at the 5 o'clock position (the right lower quadrant) of the endoscopic image and progress toward the 11 o'clock position. This engineering results in easy capture of a polyp located in the right lower portion of the field, but more difficulty when the lesion is positioned elsewhere.

An attempt should be made to bring all polyps into the 5 o'clock position prior to snare entrapment (Fig 10.7). This is accomplished by torquing the scope and/or deflecting the instrument tip using the dial controls. These maneuvers, as well as precise tip control, are more difficult when the insertion tube is looped, so before beginning polypectomy the scope should be straightened as much as possible.

At times it may be difficult to straighten the scope and/or position the polyp at 5 o'clock. The sigmoid colon can be particularly tricky in this respect. It may help to rotate the patient, apply abdominal pressure, or to intubate the colon proximal to the polyp and then re-identify the polyp during scope withdrawal. In some cases, the endoscopist may need to perform polypectomy with suboptimal positioning.

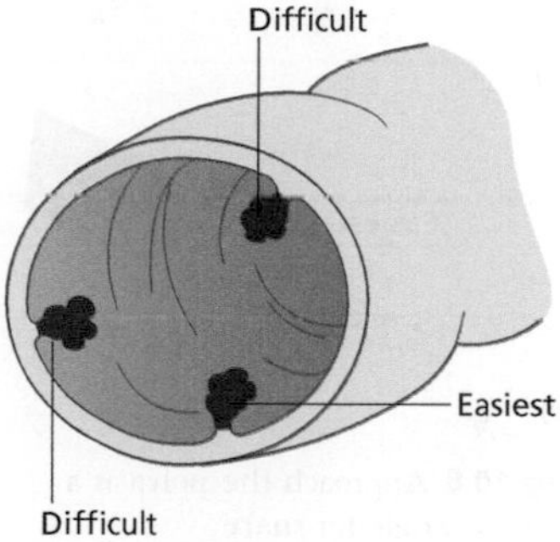

Fig 10.7 Orienting the polyp. Because the snare exits the scope at the 5 o'clock position, polypectomy is easiest if the polyp is at this orientation. The scope can be torqued so that the view of the polyp rotates in order to move it into the 5 o'clock position.

Positioning the polyp at 5 o'clock

- Reduce loops (most useful)
- Apply torque (most useful)
- Roll patient to supine position
- Apply abdominal pressure
- Advance proximal to the polyp and then withdraw the scope

Encircling the polyp

After the catheter is passed and the scope is positioned, the wire loop is slowly delivered under direct vision out of the catheter, with the scope tip pointing toward the lumen (Fig 10.8). Depending on the size of the polyp, the endoscopist directs the assistant to open the loop fully or halfway.

If the colon segment is angulated or narrowed, the endoscopist may wish to open the snare loop within the most distal segment of the instrumentation channel. With the tip of the wire loop in view, the assistant slowly opens the snare loop, and the endoscopist simultaneously pulls back on the catheter sheath; only the tip of the wire loop is in view, but the loop is open inside the channel. The endoscopist can then push the wire loop into full view or extend only part of the loop as needed by advancing or withdrawing the sheath.

The endoscopist maneuvers the open loop around the polyp like a lasso. The goal is to encircle all abnormal tissue, but to avoid entrapping more than a small collar of normal tissue (Fig 10.9). If too much tissue is captured, muscularis propria may be entrapped, which could lead to perforation during transection; and more cautery will be needed, which increases the risk of thermally induced perforation.

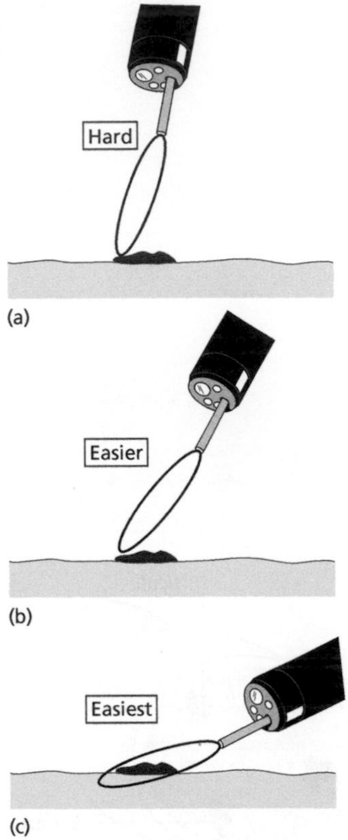

Fig 10.8 Approach the polyp at a shallow angle for snare polypectomy. This will helps stabilize polyp capture.

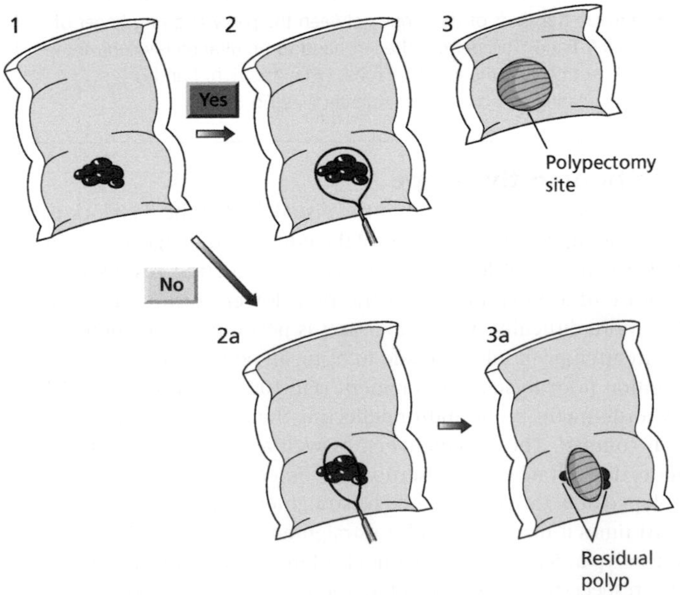

Fig 10.9 Entrap a small "collar" of normal mucosa. This will help prevent incomplete polypectomy.

Note that:

• the opened snare wire is flexible and can safely be pushed against the colon wall, either to anchor the wire tip position or to widen the loop (Fig 10.10)

• the closing snare will "pull the polyp back" to the tip of the plastic sheath; thus, position the sheath tip at the junction of the near side of the polyp and normal mucosa (Fig 10.11)

• after the polyp has been lassoed, it is often possible to pull the open snare back so that the tip of the open wire should be adjacent to the far side of the polyp, to safeguard against entrapping normal mucosa

• to ensure proper seating of the wire loop, loop closure should occur under direct vision, and the endoscopist should confirm at the end of loop closure that the slide handle is at or close to the ink mark on the handle (Fig 10.12)

• to facilitate polyp entrapment during snare closure, the catheter and the plane of the snare wire should be (whenever possible) parallel to the colon surface (Figs 10.13 and 10.14)

• during snare resection of flat or sessile polyps, aspirate some intraluminal air; this causes the colon to decrease in circumference and length. Because the volume of the polyp does not change, the polyp actually protrudes more than when the colon is maximally distended, facilitating capture.

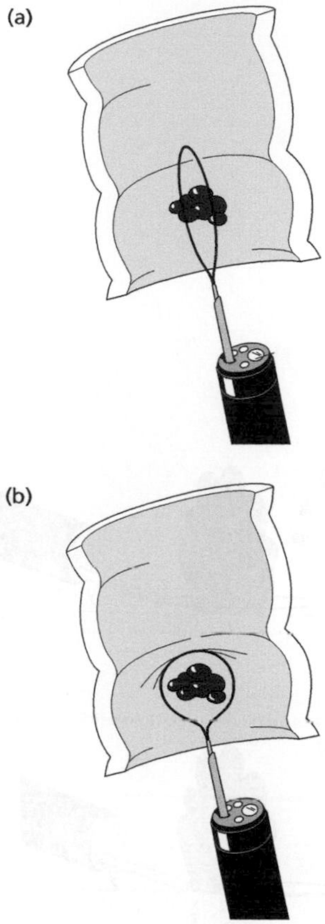

Fig 10.10 Increase the diameter of the snare loop. Most snares are oval, and exit the scope tip with a small diameter, making polyp capture difficult. Pushing with the snare tip against the colon wall increases the snare diameter.

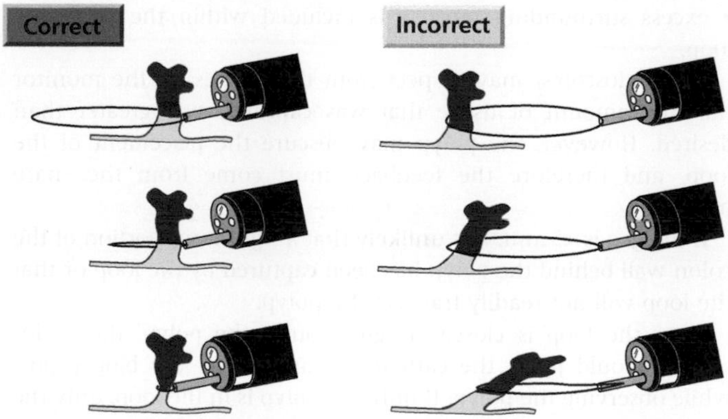

Fig 10.11 Correct position of the tip of the plastic sheath of the snare. The sheath tip is advanced to the polyp edge, at the junction with normal tissue on the colon wall. This promotes stable capture of the entire polyp as the wire loop is closed into the sheath.

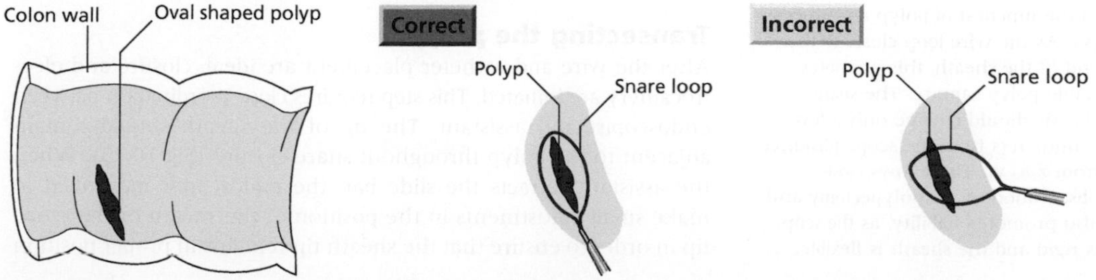

Fig 10.12 Orient the long axis of the snare in the same direction as the long axis of an elliptical sessile or flat polyp. This will make polyp capture more efficient.

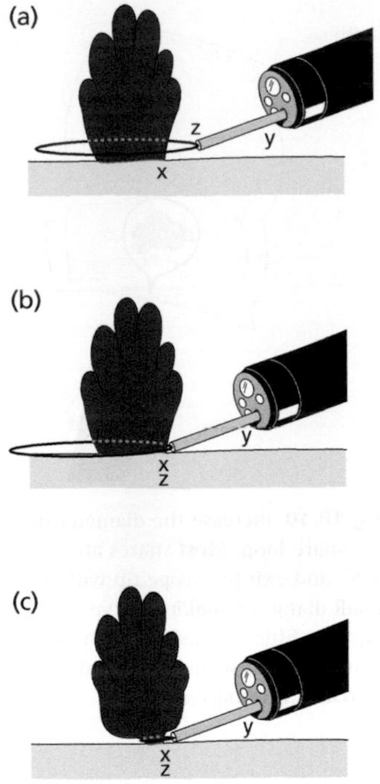

Fig 10.13 Optimizing snare mechanics. Once the snare has encircled the polyp head, the tip of the sheath (z) should be advanced to the junction of polyp and mucosa (x). As the wire loop closes to the end of the sheath, this promotes stable polyp capture. The snare sheath should emerge only a few centimeters from the scope (distance from z to y). This allows close observation of the polypectomy and also promotes stability, as the scope is rigid and the sheath is flexible.

Closing the snare around the polyp

A continuing dialogue between endoscopist and assistant is necessary. Upon the endoscopist's request, snare closure begins, and is slow and continuous. Both participants watch the video monitor. If the snare loop slips to a suboptimal position, the loop is reopened and repositioned.

In order to prevent guillotining polyps, the assistant monitors the snare handle, and stops snare closure when the slide bar reaches the mark. The assistant informs the endoscopist and cautery is activated if desired.

With larger polyps, the assistant often perceives resistance—a "spongy" sensation that impedes easy further retraction of the slide bar—when the wire loop becomes snug. The assistant must communicate this to the endoscopist, and note the distance (the "gap") between the slide bar and the mark on the handle. Management of larger polyps is discussed in Chapter 11.

If the gap is >1 cm and the polyp is large the gap may be deemed appropriate (decision: resect). In other circumstances, the large gap may be deemed inappropriate (decision: open the snare and reposition). This latter situation happens if:

- the snare is seated across a wide head of a pedunculated polyp (instead of at the narrow base);
- the polyp base is too wide for transection with a single cut;
- excess surrounding mucosa is included within the tightened loop.

The endoscopist may suspect from the images on the monitor that the amount of tissue that was captured was greater than desired. However, the polyp may obscure the placement of the loop, and therefore the feedback must come from the snare handle.

If the gap is <5 mm, it is unlikely that a significant portion of the colon wall behind the polyp has been captured by the loop or that the loop will not readily transect the polyp.

After the loop is closed snugly around the polyp, the endoscopist should jiggle the catheter to and fro at the biopsy port while observing the polyp. If only the polyp is in the loop, only the polyp will move; if the polyp and the surrounding wall move simultaneously, a portion of the adjacent mucosa is probably captured within the snare loop, and the loop should be opened and repositioned.

Transecting the polyp

After the wire and catheter placement are ideal, closure and electrocautery are initiated. This step requires close coordination between endoscopist and assistant. The tip of the sheath should remain adjacent to the polyp throughout snare closure (Fig 10.13). When the assistant retracts the slide bar, the endoscopist may need to make small adjustments in the position of the sheath or the scope tip in order to ensure that the sheath tip remains in proper position

(Fig 10.14). As the slide bar is closed, the wire loop closes snugly against the far edge of the polyp, but should not strangulate or guillotine it.

The endoscopist next activates the current with the foot pedal (Fig 10.15). The energy delivery should be continuous, not intermittent. Following start of current application, whitening of tissue adjacent to the electrified snare may be observed, signaling the endoscopist to instruct the assistant to close the snare slowly. Complete transection usually occurs after a few seconds of current

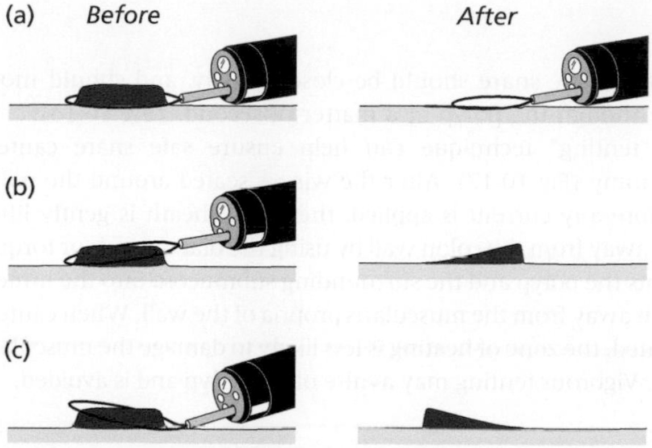

Fig 10.14 Snaring a flat polyp. The snare should be kept parallel to the mucosal surface. If the tip of the sheath is elevated or depressed, the snare may cut across the polyp tangentially, or slide over the polyp altogether.

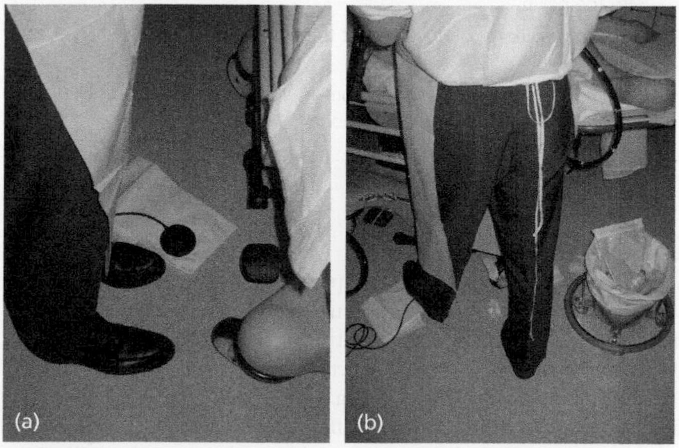

Fig 10.15 Correct positioning of the endoscopist. The examiner stabilizes the shaft of the scope by compressing it with the right leg against the examining table. The left foot activates the pedals that control electrocoagulation or the water jet. The pedals should be placed by the examiner's left foot. A trash receptacle is in position for discarding used materials.

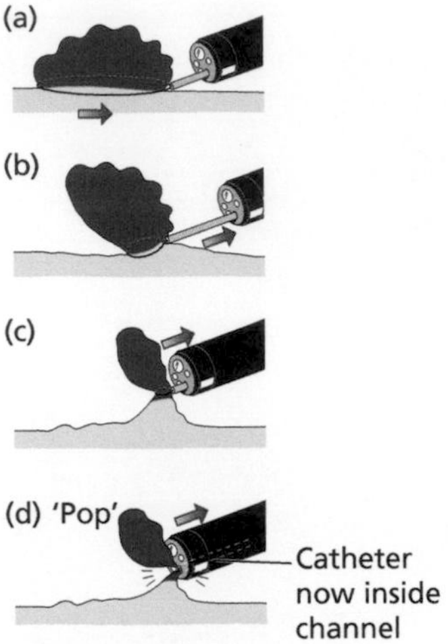

Fig 10.16 Using the scope faceplate during polypectomy. If the tightened snare is not cutting through the polyp after the application of a reasonable amount of cautery, the snare catheter can be firmly pulled back with the right hand. This will shear away the residual tissue, avulsing the polyp from the wall.

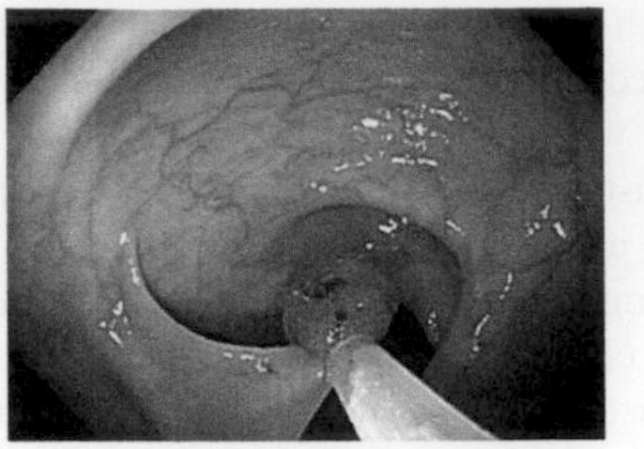

Fig 10.17 Tenting up a polyp. The polyp (1 cm, Paris 0–Is) is "pulled" into the middle of the lumen in order to reduce the risk of transmural burn and to confirm that adjacent mucosa has not been entrapped by mistake.

application. The snare should be closed slowly, and should move steadily though the polyp in a matter of seconds (Fig 10.16).

The "tenting" technique can help ensure safe snare cautery polypectomy (Fig 10.17). After the wire is seated around the polyp and before any current is applied, the snare sheath is gently lifted slightly away from the colon wall by using the dial controls or torque. This tents the polyp and the surrounding submucosa into the lumen, pulling it away from the muscularis propria of the wall. When cautery is activated, the zone of heating is less likely to damage the muscularis propria. Vigorous tenting may avulse of the polyp and is avoided.

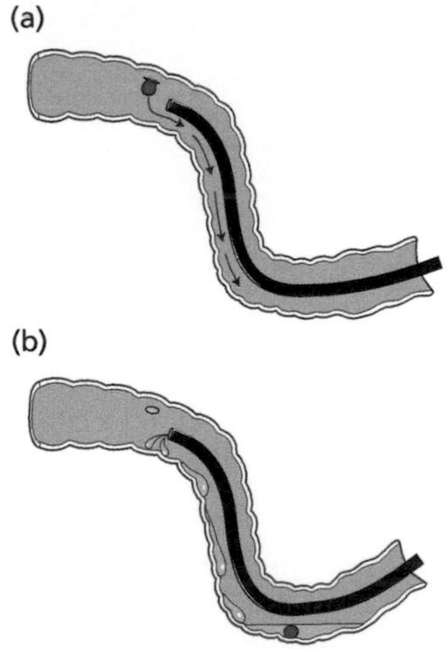

Fig 10.18 Retrieving an elusive polyp after resection. Oftentimes following polypectomy a polyp may disappear from sight. Severed polyps follow the force of gravity. The polyp location can be predicted by looking for nearby fluid pools. If none is apparent, instill a small volume of water through the instrumentation channel and observe the direction of flow.

Ensuring that polypectomy is complete

- Flat and sessile polyps: resect a small collar of normal appearing tissue with the polyp
- Pedunculated polyps: resect a small segment of uninvolved pedicle with the polyp
- After polypectomy, carefully inspect the margin to ensure that no polyp remains
- If there is doubt whether polypectomy is complete, snare-resect the margin, or ablate with a thermal modality

Locating the specimen

With forceps polypectomy the specimen is retained within the jaws. After snare polypectomy, usually the specimen falls onto the mucosa near the site or remains attached to the snare wire. Sometimes gravity and/or colon contractions propel the specimen out of the field of vision, or it falls into a pool of debris, and it is hard to find, particularly if it is small. To find the specimen:

• look systematically between the folds in the area, tip-deflecting into the troughs;

• gently infuse water into the lumen—this will illustrate the direction of gravity (Fig 10.18), and also may "float" the polyp out;

• roll the patient 90 or 180°, so gravity may propel the specimen into an exposed field.

Using these techniques, >95% of specimens can be found.

Retrieving the specimen

If the specimen is small enough to fit through the channel, it is suctioned into a retrieval trap or into a gauze pad that has been placed between the suction nipple of the scope and the suction tubing (see page 12).

To avoid entrapping mucosa when suctioning up the specimen, the scope tip is precisely positioned so that the specimen is visible at the 5 o'clock position at the lower edge of the visual field (where the channel orifice is located; Fig 10.19). Suction is applied and the fragment disappears into the channel. If the fragment does not vanish or if adjacent mucosa is entrapped, then "microadjustments" in the tip position are made and the process is repeated. Many specimens that appear too big to fit through the channel actually do fit because they are deformed by the suction force. Suction force may be maximized using the dials on the suction machine or by removing the suction button and occluding the orifice with a finger.

If the specimen is too big to suction, or there are multiple fragments, it can be removed from the colon in the snare or net or by suctioning it onto the tip of the scope and withdrawing the scope while maintaining continual suction (Fig 10.20). With these techniques, the specimen blocks the view of the mucosa on the way out, so it is necessary to reintubate up to the polypectomy site and repeat a careful withdrawal.

An alternative technique is to transect the resected polyp into smaller pieces, which are then suctioned; this approach may interfere with histological interpretation.

Options for retrieving resected polyps from the lumen

- Suction through colonoscope channel into trap
- Capture in snare or net/basket and pull out scope
- Use snare to cut polyp into smaller pieces for suctioning
- Suction resected polyp onto tip of scope and remove scope
- Capture in forceps or snare and pull through channel

Retrieving polyps after polypectomy

- Attach the polyp retrieval trap *before* polypectomy is performed: this prevents inadvertently suctioning the fragment into the large waste canister
- Wash the segment near a polypectomy site before performing polypectomy: this prevents the polyp from becoming lost in debris
- Ascertain using water where the resected polyp is likely to "fall": this can be done while the assistant is setting up the cautery system
- If the colonic intubation was difficult, cut large resected right colon polyps into smaller pieces that can fit through the suction channel; this is generally preferable to a difficult reintubation
- If the intubation was easy, grasp the polyp in the snare and pull assembly out, and then reintubate
- A basket or net may be useful for retrieving multiple polyp fragments
- After piecemeal polypectomy, retrieve as much tissue as possible (invasive cancer may be present in only a small part of a large polyp)

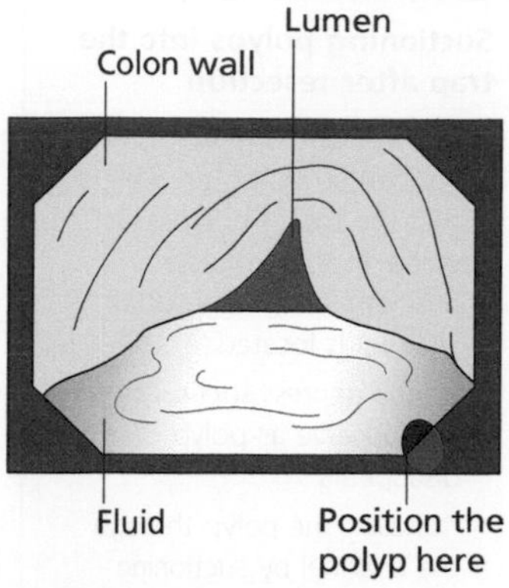

Fig 10.19 Proper orientation of scope for suctioning of polyp. When the tip of the polyp is just visible at the 5 o'clock position, successful aspiration of the polyp without inadvertent suctioning of mucosa is most likely.

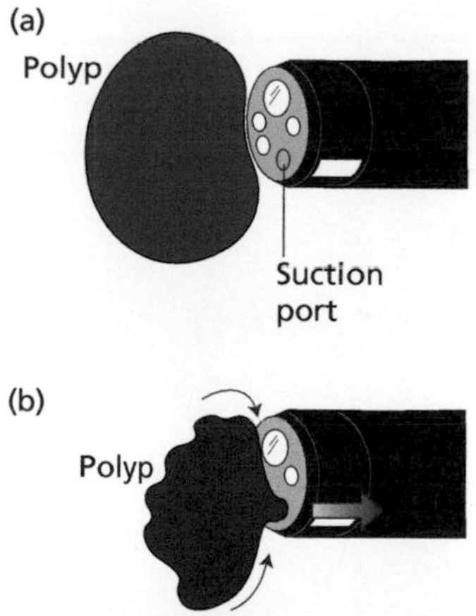

Fig 10.20 Larger polyps may be retrieved by suctioning them onto the tip of the endoscope and withdrawing the scope. A potential problem with this retrieval technique is that the suction channel is relatively small (3.2 mm), so the suction force is relatively small and the polyp can be dislodged from the tip of the scope by a fold as the assembly is withdrawn through the colon. If the polyp is small to medium sized, place a specimen trap on the system, lest the suction unexpectedly pull the polyp through the channel.

Suctioning polyps into the trap after resection

- Make sure the trap is in place!
- Position scope tip precisely, so that the top of polyp is just visible at the 5 o'clock position, where the suction channel is located
- Gently depress suction button and observe as polyp disappears
- "Chase" the polyp through the channel by suctioning some luminal fluid

Retrieving/finding of a polyp that is "lost" after resection

- Instill water onto the resection site and observe where gravity takes the water
- "Blindly" infuse 10 ml water and then suction back into trap (you do not need to see the lost polyp to retrieve it)
- Check the snare catheter
- Check the suction cap
- Push down the adjacent folds with a snare catheter, and look behind into the valleys between them
- Roll the patient, so gravity will move the lost polyp
- Look with tip retroflexed

Polypectomy: Pedunculated polyps

A pedunculated polyp of any size (Plate 10.8) should be removed by a single transection of the stalk. The lasso should be maneuvered over the "head" of the polyp and onto the pedicle. The wire should be seated about midway down the pedicle (Fig 10.11), so that the dysplastic adenomatous head plus a segment of nondysplastic stalk tissue are resected, and leaving behind a short pedicle that can be resnared if bleeding occurs. This residual pedicle, made up of unremarkable mucosa that was elongated by traction on the polyp head from colonic contractions, often quickly retracts when the polyp has been transected. If there is any suspicion that the polyp is malignant, the pedicle should be transected close to the wall.

Large sessile polyps

Techniques for resection of broad-based, larger polyps are discussed in Chapter 11.

Summary

The colonoscopist must know how to perform basic polypectomy and have the equipment available to accomplish it. Polyps usually are removed during the index colonoscopy, and do not require a second colonoscopy for polypectomy. The endoscopist and gastrointestinal assistant must work as a team to maximize safety effectiveness, and efficiency.

Further reading

1. Brenner H, Chang-Claude J, Seiler CM, Rickert A, Hoffmeister M. Protection from colorectal cancer after colonoscopy: a population-based, case-control study. *Ann Intern Med* 2011;154:22–30.
2. Chaput U, Alberto SF, Terris B, *et al*. Risk factors for advanced adenomas amongst small and diminutive colorectal polyps: a prospective monocenter study. *Dig Liver Dis* 2011;43:609–12.

3. Levin B, Lieberman DA, McFarland B, *et al.* Screening and surveillance for the early detection of colorectal cancer and adenomatous polyps, 2008: a joint guideline from the American Cancer Society, the US Multi-Society Task Force on Colorectal Cancer, and the American College of Radiology. *CA Cancer J Clin* 2008;58:130–60.
4. Rabeneck L, Paszat LF, Saskin R, Stukel TA. Association between colonoscopy rates and colorectal cancer mortality. *Am J Gastroenterol* 2010;105: 1627–32. Epub 2010 Mar 2.
5. Repici A, Hassan C, Vitetta E, *et al.* Safety of cold polypectomy for <10 mm polyps at colonoscopy: a prospective multicenter study. *Endoscopy* 2012;44:27–31.
6. Rex DK, Ahnen DJ, Baron JA, *et al.* Serrated lesions of the colorectum: review and recommendations from an expert panel. *Am J Gastroenterol* 2012;107:1315–29.
7. Soetikno RM, Kaltenbach T, Rouse RV, *et al.* Prevalence of nonpolypoid (flat and depressed) colorectal neoplasms in asymptomatic and symptomatic adults. *JAMA* 2008;299:1027–35.
8. Tadepalli US, Feihel D, Miller KM, *et al.* A morphologic analysis of sessile serrated polyps observed during routine colonoscopy (with video). *Gastrointest Endosc* 2011;74:1360–8. Epub 2011 Oct 21.
9. Winawer SJ, Zauber AG, Fletcher RH, *et al.* Guidelines for colonoscopy surveillance after polypectomy: a consensus update by the US Multi-Society Task Force on Colorectal Cancer and the American Cancer Society. *Gastroenterology* 2006;130:1872–85.
10. Winawer SJ, Zauber AG, O'Brien MJ, *et al.* Randomized comparison of surveillance intervals after colonoscopic removal of newly diagnosed adenomatous polyps. The National Polyp Study Workgroup. *N Engl J Med* 1993;328:901–6.
11. Zauber AG, Winawer SJ, O'Brien MJ, *et al.* Colonoscopic polypectomy and long-term prevention of colorectal-cancer deaths. *N Engl J Med* 2012;366:687–96.

Chapter video clips

Video Clip 10.1 Sessile serrated adenoma/polyp
Multiple examples of identification and resection of sessile serrated adenomas/polyps are provided.

Video Clip 10.2 Resection of sessile serrated polyp
Sessile serrated adenoma/polyp identified and resected with saline lift followed by piecemeal snare polypectomy.

Video Clip 10.3 Giant lipoma
Giant, pedunculated lipoma with erythema related to trauma.

Video Clip 10.4 Ileal carcinoid
Intubation of the ileum reveals a 1.5-cm submucosal carcinoid.

CHAPTER 11
Difficult Polypectomy

Reason for difficulty
- Large polyp
- Awkward location of polyp
  - In narrowed segment (e.g. dense diverticulosis)
  - Hard to reach
    - Behind a fold
    - At the end of a long colon
- Flat polyp/hard to entrap

The difficult polyp: Management strategies

A difficult colon polyp can be managed with a number of strategies.

1. Remove now (and possibly mark)
2. Biopsy, mark and schedule polypectomy
3. Biopsy, mark and refer to an expert endoscopist
4. Biopsy, mark and refer to a surgeon
5. Biopsy, mark and follow by colonoscopy

Introduction

Most colonoscopic polypectomies are straightforward; some pose technical challenges; a few are impossible. Some polyps are extremely large; some oriented on the colon wall in a position difficult to access or in a segment with limited maneuverability. Polyps may be flat or wrapped around a fold so the snare slides over the surface. Creativity, strategic thinking, and perseverance usually can overcome these obstacles.

Options when encountering difficult polyps

In general, once a polyp has been identified, "watchful waiting" is not acceptable to most patients or physicians. On the one hand, because colonoscopic resection has lower morbidity than surgery, it is generally preferred; moreover, many "difficult" colon polyps formerly referred for surgical resection can be removed by an expert colonoscopist. On the other hand, the increased availability of laparoscopic segmental colectomy makes a surgical approach a more palatable alternative.

In choosing among the management options the colonoscopist must weigh:
- the characteristics of the polyp;
- the magnitude of the procedure;
- the clinical status of the patient;
- the local surgical and endoscopic expertise and resources;
- the skill set of the colonoscopist

Characteristics of the polyp

Location

Location affects the management decision. For instance, for some large rectal polyps, a transanal, full-thickness resection by a colorectal surgeon may be the simplest and most definitive treatment. Similarly, if the polyp is located in the cecal caput, where the colon wall is thin and the scope may be difficult to maneuver, a surgical

Practical Colonoscopy, First Edition. Jerome D. Waye, James Aisenberg, and Peter H. Rubin.
© 2013 John Wiley & Sons, Ltd. Published 2013 by John Wiley & Sons, Ltd.

approach may be favored, especially because elective ileocolic resection is relatively efficient and straightforward. Conversely, if the polyp is located high in a flexure, and would require extensive surgical mobilization of the colon and a wider resection, a colonoscopic approach may be favorable. For an extremely large, sessile, ascending colon polyp—perhaps encountered after an arduous intubation—the wisest approach may be surgical resection, obviating the necessity of repeated difficult colonoscopic intubations.

Can I completely remove it?

Colonoscopic polypectomy should be initiated with the expectation that the resection will be complete. Otherwise the polyp should be biopsied and marked. An incomplete polypectomy necessitates a repeat procedure to remove residual adenoma and prior incomplete snare cautery polypectomy may cause local fibrosis, making the polyp more difficult to elevate and remove during subsequent colonoscopy. In some instances the site may be difficult to locate again.

Is the polyp a serrated lesion or a conventional adenoma?

Serrated polyps are believed to grow slowly and are more common in the elderly and in the thin-walled right colon. Sessile serrated adenomas may be challenging to resect because they can cover a large surface area of colon and are flat. Some experts argue that under these circumstances a "biopsy and follow" strategy is acceptable. However, an advanced adenoma represents a high risk for cancer and requires more immediate intervention.

Equipment for advanced polypectomy

- Needle injector
- Several different snares
- Endoloop (Video Clip 11.1)
- Clips
- Thermal devices
- Retrieval baskets
- Specimen traps
- Epinephrine for hemostasis
- Vital stains

Characteristics of the procedure

Resection of the difficult polyp mandates excellent technical conditions. This begins with a clean field. If bowel cleansing is inadequate, debris makes the polyp difficult to visualize, resect, and retrieve. The patient must be adequately sedated and cooperative. The equipment for advanced polypectomy must be readily available. If not, the difficult polypectomy may need to be deferred.

Clinical status of the patient

The removal of polyps is not "life or death" and acute clinical problems should be addressed before attempting polypectomy. In patients approaching the end of life, a "biopsy and observe" strategy may be appropriate.

The resources of the endoscopy facility

Successful resection of the difficult polyp may require specialized equipment (e.g. an argon plasma coagulator (APC) for ablation or clips to control bleeding) and an assistant who is experienced with advanced polypectomy. If surgical backup or support is likely to be needed, it is preferable to perform the procedure in a hospital endoscopic unit.

The procedure schedule also impacts decision-making. In some endoscopy units, colonoscopies are scheduled every 20 or 30 minutes, and it is not practical to occupy a room for a prolonged polypectomy and have the entire unit run behind schedule. Removing a difficult polyp takes time and concentration in an unpressured environment. If these conditions are not available, it is appropriate to consider deferring the polypectomy.

Expertise available locally

Approaches to difficult polypectomy may vary in different communities. Referral to a local expert in endoscopic mucosal resection (EMR) or to a skilled laparoscopic surgeon may not be possible in certain localities. Conversely, in a region with a "tertiary referral" endoscopy unit and an expert advanced endoscopist and/or laparoscopist, referral to that facility may be appropriate.

The characteristics of the colonoscopist

Most colonoscopists possess the expertise to resect difficult polyps. In many instances, the colonoscopist who is adept at removal of small and medium-sized polyps will be able to remove large polyps by applying piecemeal resection techniques and approaching each portion of a large polyp as if it were a smaller adenoma. Some colonoscopists are hesitant to attempt complex cases because of the potential impact of a complication, or the amount of time required. Some endoscopists may not possess the ingenuity, perseverance, patience, and technical proficiency that contribute to successful removal of advanced polyps.

Colonoscopic resection of the difficult polyp: Preparation

Discussing management options with the patient

If the patient is referred for management of a previously discovered polyp, discuss the risks, benefits, and alternatives of the colonoscopic approach with the patient and family. The unusual considerations may not adequately be addressed with a standard pre-procedure informed consent. For example, for large sessile polyps, several colonoscopies may be required and there may be a higher rate of local recurrence and complications.

If the large polyp is discovered unexpectedly during routine colonoscopy and the best treatment option is uncertain, it may be necessary to defer the resection to a later date in order to discuss the risks, benefits, and alternatives. Despite the fact that this may entail repeating the colonoscopy, most patients and their families appreciate participating in the decision-making.

Scheduling an elective polypectomy for the difficult polyp

When scheduling an elective polypectomy for a challenging lesion it is reasonable to reserve a longer block of procedure time and to arrange for the most skilled endoscopy assistant to be available. A morning appointment may be best, as complication management (if needed) can be performed during standard work hours.

Should the polyp be removed in the hospital or in an outpatient unit?

Ambulatory polypectomy is safe and expeditious for almost all colorectal polyps. The incidence of perforation during removal of large polyps is approximately 1 in 1000 polypectomies. If the perforation occurs in an ambulatory setting, the patient can be transferred by ambulance to the endoscopy unit's affiliated hospital for management. Most immediate postpolypectomy bleeding can be stopped colonoscopically at the time of polypectomy.

The hospital is suitable for a patient or a lesion that is extraordinarily high risk, when there may be a need for specialized equipment or surgical standby, or if the patient refuses out-of-hospital colonoscopy.

Equipment preparation

A full array of accessory equipment should be available, including an electrosurgical unit, forceps, snares (several sizes and types), injection needles, epinephrine, sterile saline, clips, loops, a retrieval basket or net, and an APC unit or similar cautery option.

Choice of colonoscopes

For difficult polypectomy, a therapeutic adult colonoscope with a 4.2-mm working channel and a separate irrigation channel is often ideal; some experts prefer the more nimble "pediatric colonoscope" with a 3.2-mm suction/biopsy channel for even the most difficult procedures. The presence of a dedicated water jet provides a strong wash capability for cleansing the mucosal surface of fluid, debris, or oozing blood. The large working channel in a standard adult scope allows for enhanced suction during the procedure, even after an ancillary device has already been deployed.

Colonoscopic resection of the difficult polyp: Technique

Snare resection of large sessile polyps

The basic principles used for removal of smaller polyps are followed. The polyp is positioned in the right lower field of view. It

Conditions favoring piecemeal polypectomy

- Polyp is flat or sessile and >2 cm at the base
- Polyp is in the cecum or right colon, where risk of transmural burn is greater
- Unusual polyp shape
  - Polyp cannot safely be encircled with one closure of the snare
  - Polyp is highly lobular
  - Only one polyp segment can be entrapped; often resection of the first piece will make it easier to entrap the next piece

may be helpful to advance the scope to the cecum and address the polyp during withdrawal, as this maneuver straightens the scope and improves the responsiveness of the tip. The field is washed until it is clean and the ancillary equipment is readied.

The thickness of the distended colon wall varies from approximately 1.4 to 2.3 mm. When the polyp site of attachment is broad, the risk of colonic perforation from polypectomy increases. The deeper layers of the wall (including the muscularis propria) may be bunched up and enfolded in the snare as it closes around the base of the polyp. If this happens, deeper layers of the wall may be transected along with the polyp. Broad-based polyps generally also require more cautery application, and the thermal injury may devitalize the muscularis propria. In general, most colonoscopists limit the size of polyp fragments to <2 cm in order to decrease the risk of transmural injury. Larger polyps are removed with serial snare resection of <2-cm fragments—so-called "piecemeal polypectomy" technique (Video Clip 11.2). Although piecemeal technique may hinder histopathologic interpretation, it is standard of care because it decreases the risk of complications.

During piecemeal polypectomy of a large sessile polyp, one edge of the wire loop is positioned at the edge of the adenoma (the junction between adenoma and normal mucosa) and the other edge wire of the loop is sited over a portion of the polyp, encircling a large piece of tissue (Fig 11.1). By checking the snare handle (noting the mark placed prior to the examination), the assistant confirms that the snare is not encircling too large a portion of the polyp. The sheath is advanced to the line of demarcation between adenoma and colon wall. The segment is then resected and the process repeated until the entire polyp is resected (Video Clip 11.3).

If the piecemeal technique is being used to resect the outer portions of a bulky sessile polyp, larger portions can be removed than would be resected by application of the wire loop around a single polyp, because the remainder of the polyp insulates the colon wall from thermal damage or the risk of mechanical perforation.

The decision as to whether large polyps should be removed piecemeal or with one transection is related not only to the size of the polyp, but also to the volume of tissue within the closed snare (as determined by the mark on the snare handle). Some large polyps are soft and spongy, permitting a greater amount of slide bar retraction than is possible with a smaller but firmer polyp.

Occasionally, it is not possible to completely remove a large sessile polyp. In that case the site should be marked with a tattoo for identification on a follow-up examination or for future surgery (see Chapter 12). When marking a polyp site for subsequent polypectomy, the injection of the surgical marker should be made in three or four quadrants near, but not directly into, the residual polyp, as some fibrosis may occur, making the eventual polypectomy more difficult. (Forceps biopsy does not present any technical problems with subsequent polypectomy.) Often the carbon suspension will spill out of the injection site and no tattoo is achieved.

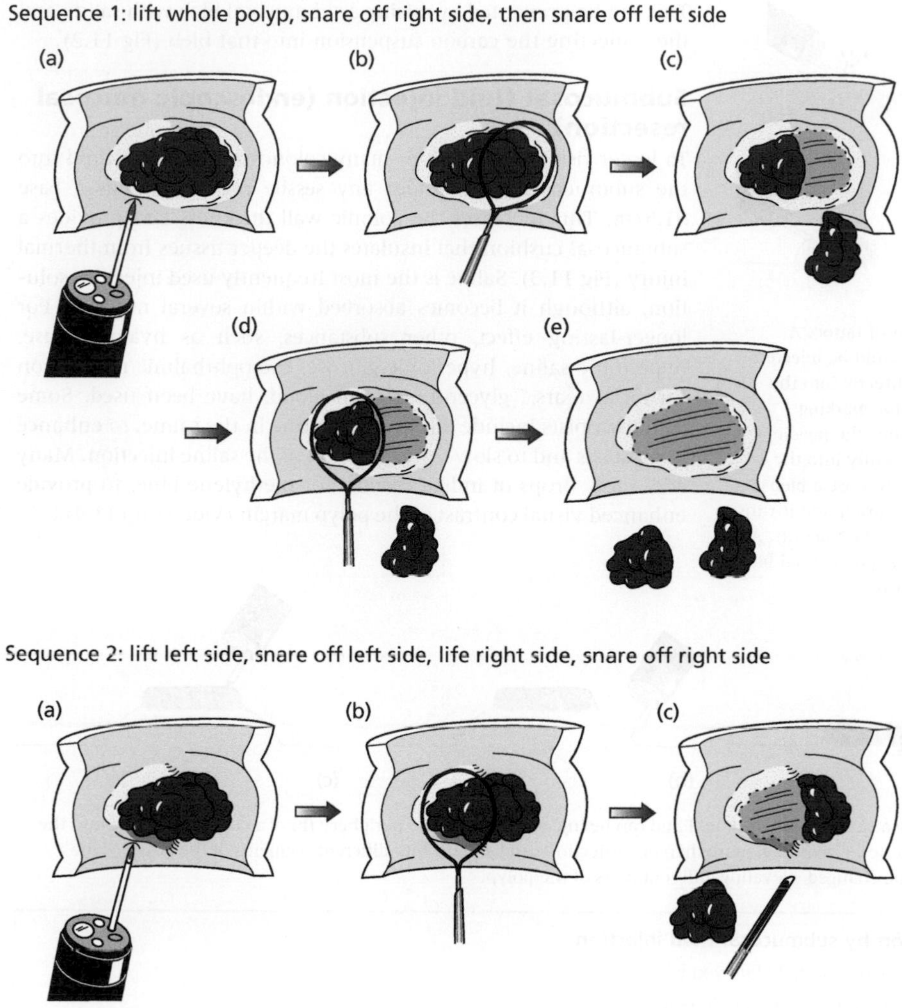

Sequence 1: lift whole polyp, snare off right side, then snare off left side

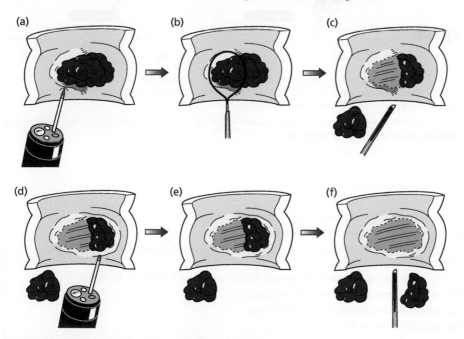

Sequence 2: lift left side, snare off left side, life right side, snare off right side

Fig 11.1 Piecemeal resection of large sessile polyp. Sequence 1 shows removal after saline lift (a) of entire polyp. The snare is placed around a <2-cm section of the polyp (b), which is then resected utilizing cautery (c). The snare is then placed around the second section of the polyp (d), and resection is performed (e). Sequence 2 shows saline lift of the left half of the polyp (a), followed by resection of the left half (b,c), followed by lifting the right half (d), before complete resection (e,f).

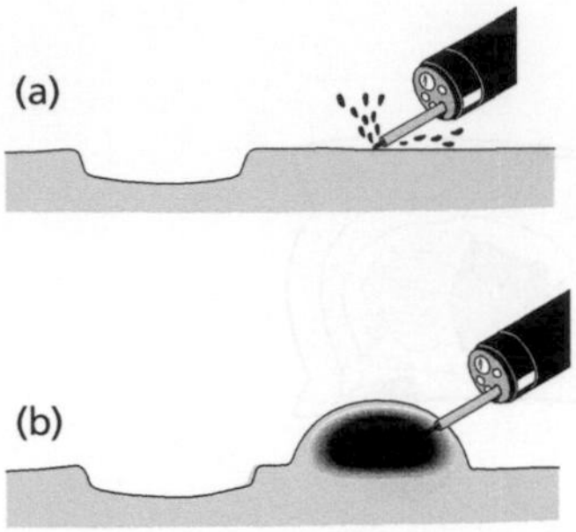

Fig 11.2 Injection of tattoo. A surgical marker should be injected close by but not directly into the polypectomy site for marking purposes. Oftentimes the needle is not inserted sufficiently into the submucosal tissue to raise a bleb with the surgical marker and it runs out through the needle tract (a). An obvious large black submucosal bleb should be visible (b).

This can be prevented by raising a submucosal bleb with saline and then injecting the carbon suspension into that bleb (Fig 11.2).

Submucosal fluid injection (endoscopic mucosal resection)

To lower risk of perforation, many colonoscopists inject fluid into the submucosal space under any sessile polyp that has a base >1.5 cm. This increases the colonic wall thickness and provides a submucosal cushion that insulates the deeper tissues from thermal injury (Fig 11.3). Saline is the most frequently used injection solution, although it becomes absorbed within several minutes. For longer-lasting effect, other substances, such as hyaluronidase, hypertonic saline, hypertonic glucose, the ophthalmic medication "artificial tears," glycerol, or even blood, have been used. Some colonoscopists include dilute epinephrine in the saline, to enhance hemostasis and to slow the absorption of the saline injection. Many add a few drops of indigo carmine or methylene blue, to provide enhanced visual contrast of the polyp margin (Video Clip 11.4).

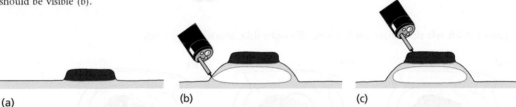

Fig 11.3 Creating a submucosal cushion. Fluid can be injected either at the periphery (b) of a polyp or directly into the center of the polyp (c). If required, more than one injection can be made into different segments of the polyp or the needle angle can be changed, elevating different parts of the polyp.

Polyp elevation by submucosal fluid injection

- Prepare snare and cautery *before* you inject
- Consider elevating any flat or sessile polyp >1.5 cm
- Prime injector needle/catheter before injecting
- Attempt to orient needle tangential to the surface
- Make mucosal puncture adjacent to polyp margin or directly into polyp
- Multiple attempts at needle placement may be required
- With large polyps, use multiple injection sites; make first injection into proximal (far) edge of polyp, raising "back" of polyp toward scope
- Injection may be initiated just before needle penetrates mucosal surface, or immediately thereafter
- When fluid enters submucosa, immediate visible elevation occurs
- Inject enough fluid to see substantial (>5–10 mm) elevation
- If no elevation of polyp or surrounding mucosa
  - Needle is in wrong plane
  - Needle is in peritoneal cavity
  - Needle is too superficial
  - The polyp is fixed to submucosa
- Coloring injection fluid with methylene blue may help visualize polyp margin
- Adding dilute epinephrine to fluid may shrink polyp and promote hemostasis

When performing submucosal injection, the assistant should prime the needle with the saline solution; otherwise air injection into the wall (an iatrogenic pneumatosis) will occur. Whenever possible, the colonoscopist should advance the catheter and the injector needle tangential to the mucosal surface; this decreases the chance of intraperitoneal injection, and favors insertion of the needle into the plane between the mucosa and the muscularis propria. The needle tip should be deliberately implanted under the mucosa. The puncture is made through or immediately adjacent to the polyp. Multiple attempts at needle placement may be required to locate the correct plane. After the tip enters the correct plane, correct positioning is confirmed by injecting a small volume of fluid. If the needle has not adequately penetrated the mucosa, the fluid will stream back out into the colonic lumen. If the needle is too deep, the fluid will go into the peritoneal cavity, and no mucosal elevations will occur. If the position is correct, the injected fluid will visibly expand the submucosal layer and elevate the polyp. Some endoscopists ask the assistant to begin injection just before thrusting the needle into the mucosa and the streaming fluid expands the submucosa as soon as it enters the proper plane.

The portion of a large sessile polyp that is farthest away from the colonoscope tip (the "back" or the anatomically proximal portion of the polyp) is generally the hardest to see and resect. Therefore, the first submucosal injection should be into the back portion of the polyp, elevating this portion and making it easier to visualize and ensnare (Plate 11.1). An injection into the near portion of a polyp will preferentially elevate this part and may render the back portion harder to see and ensnare. The far-side injection is accomplished by passing the scope beyond the polyp and protruding the needle tip so that it is just visible in the endoscopic image. While the scope is withdrawn the needle tip is thrust into the mucosa at the proximal edge of the polyp when it first comes into view (Fig 11.4a,b).

Injections are performed by the assistant upon the request of the endoscopist. If placement is correct, the polyp will elevate after 1 ml of fluid is injected. Inject sufficient fluid to cause a visible and substantial elevation of the entire polyp (Plate 11.2). This may take 3 to 30 ml of fluid, depending on the size and shape of the polyp and the accuracy of needle placement. If the polyp is large, several submucosal injections in different sections in the polyp may be required. Another approach is to perform segmental fluid injections at one edge of the polyp and snare-resect that portion before repeating the inject/resect sequence around the polyp.

If the polyp fails to elevate ("non-lifting sign") (Video Clip 11.5) it means either that needle placement is incorrect or that the polyp is fixed to the submucosal tissues. Fixation may result from scarring due to previous polypectomy attempts, underlying colitis, or malignant infiltration into deeper tissues. Failure to elevate is not an absolute sign of submucosal invasion; occasionally, a benign polyp that is not scarred will not elevate easily. The non-lifting sign occurs when the injection is performed and the polyp does not elevate but the mucosa adjacent to the polyp bulges out with the fluid,

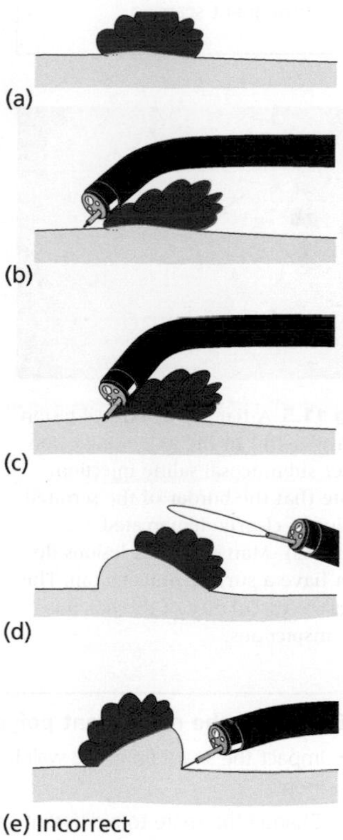

Fig 11.4 Injection on the proximal aspect of a broad-based sessile polyp. The endoscope is passed beyond the polyp (a) and the needle brought into view at the tip of the endoscope (b). With the scope deflected toward the polyp, the scope is slowly withdrawn. As soon as the proximal edge of the polyp comes into view, the needle is extended through the mucosa and injection made on the proximal aspect of the polyp (c,d). The last frame shows a poorly placed injection under the distal part of the polyp, which may actually obscure the polyp behind the mound of saline, making capture considerably more difficult (e).

The "non-lifting" sign: Major causes

1. Incorrect injector needle placement/angulation
2. Active colitis or fibrosis related to healed colitis
3. Malignant infiltration by polyp into submucosa
4. Previous polypectomy with subsequent scarring

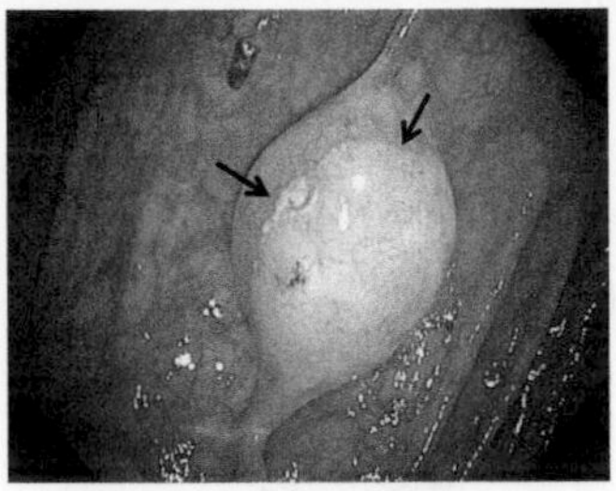

Fig 11.5 A flat 2-cm serrated lesion (Paris 0–IIb) in the ascending colon after submucosal saline injection. Note that the border of the serrated lesion is clearly demarcated (arrows). Many serrated lesions do not have a surface mucous cap. The surface vascularity of the polyp is inconspicuous.

indicating the probability of malignant fixation of the polyp to deeper layers of the submucosa that interdicts colonoscopic resection. If a polyp lifts well during submucosal injection, but is later found to contain cancer, this suggests that there is only a limited degree of invasion into deeper tissues and that the polypectomy may have been curative. If a polyp does not lift as expected, the colonoscopist must decide between proceeding with snare resection or limiting the intervention to biopsy, based in part on whether the lesion otherwise appears potentially malignant.

Saline lifting is generally safe (Fig 11.5). Even if transmural intraperitoneal injection occurs, this does not result in a complication because the fluid is sterile and the tiny puncture seals immediately. On the negative side: submucosal injection may increase the risk of delayed postpolypectomy bleeding, especially after resection of large flat polyps in the ascending colon.

There is a theoretical possibility that injection through a malignant tumor could cause tracking of cancer cells through the bowel wall. Data gained from direct percutaneous needle aspiration of malignant tumors in other sites suggest that this danger is negligible, with the risk of tumor seeding a needle track estimated to be 1 in 10,000 to 1 in 20,000.

Ensnaring the recalcitrant polyp

- Impact the snare tip in the wall beyond the polyp; use this point as a fulcrum to pivot or splay open the snare loop
- Change the snare to a different caliber or different diameter wire
- Reintubate the colonic segment where the polyp is located: this will often reorient the polyp
- Aspirate intraluminal air: this will help ensnare flat polyps
- Use the "reverse lasso" technique, by impacting the snare tip on the near side of the polyp, the catheter end on the far side of the polyp, and then closing the snare
- If maneuverability is limited due to colonic narrowing, switch to a narrower caliber scope
- Use saline lift technique

Techniques to ensure complete polypectomy

The goal of a polypectomy is resection of all adenoma. With large sessile polyps, this can be challenging. Before the polypectomy is begun, the colonoscopist should carefully "map" the extent of the polyp, pushing back adjacent folds, viewing the lesion with narrow band imaging or chromoendoscopy as needed, and noting relevant landmarks. After the tumor is resected, examine the circumference of the site in order to look for residual remnants of polyps. After piecemeal polypectomy, be certain that "islands" of polyp do not remain between the larger segments that were snare resected. Some experts deliberately remove a "collar" of normal mucosa from around the perimeter of the polyp, in the belief that this ensures complete resection. Others routinely "touch up" the perimeter of the polypectomy site using a thermal ablative treatment. The application of thermal energy to fragments of adenoma remaining at the base and edges of a fresh snare polypectomy site can improve the rate of complete resection: studies of "adjuvant" ablation with the APC after snare resection of large polyps have documented reduction of residual adenoma on follow-up colonoscopy. In many cases, a follow-up colonoscopy to inspect the site at 3–6 months is appropriate.

The mucosal defect after endoscopic mucosal resection: What to look for

- Residual polyp (incomplete polypectomy)
  - Located outside margin/circumference of defect
  - Located in "body" of defect, as "island" of residual polyp (especially if resection was piecemeal)
- Bleeding/oozing/large exposed vessels
- Signs of muscularis propria resection
  - In defect ("target sign")
  - In resected specimen ("mirror target sign") (Plate 11.3)

Thermal techniques for ablation and hemostasis

The principles with regard to electrocautery use are similar for small and large polyps. Many colonoscopists select pure coagulation current when resecting large polyps, especially when using piecemeal polypectomy technique, because this approach optimally seals blood vessels. Some experts (and some electrosurgical unit programs) combine bursts of coagulation with cutting current. In theory, this combines the surgical benefits of cutting with the hemostatic benefits of coagulation.

With some large sessile polyps, the progress of closing the snare through the polyp may stop despite the continued use of mechanical force (snare closure) and the application of cautery current. In this situation, some experts toggle to "cutting" current, which may permit the snare to sever the remaining polyp base. Another option is to pull firmly on the catheter at the entry port with the right hand, pulling the ensnared polyp against the rigid faceplate of the scope tip and thereby guillotining the polyp. Electric current can be given during this maneuver.

If bleeding from residual polyp occurs during piecemeal polypectomy, the wisest course is to resect the remaining polyp, as the next application of thermal energy is likely to cauterize the bleeding site. If arterial bleeding occurs, hemostasis may be achieved by injecting dilute epinephrine or by the applying clips.

Some extremely large polyps occupy the entire colon lumen, and during cautery application the polyp's surface may remain in contact with the opposite wall of the colon. In this situation the electrical current can travel from the wire through polyp to the opposite wall of the colon and then to the return plate, instead of following the desired circuit through the base of the polyp. This

Transecting large sessile polyps: Six recommendations

1. Optimize scope position before grasping the polyp—loops and torque forces should be minimal
2. Optimize snare position before initiating cautery
3. Begin the burn with the wire snug around the polyp but not embedded in the polyp (i.e. do not overtighten the snare); this optimizes the physics of the burn
4. Close the snare slowly after the white of the coagulation zone is visible (with large villiform polyps, no blanching may be evident)
5. If the snare ceases to progress through the polyp despite a sustained burn and loop closure, pull the catheter back with the right hand, pulling the polyp against the faceplate of the scope tip; this will shear off the polyp in most cases
6. If the polyp is >2 cm and flat, strongly consider saline lift and/or piecemeal polypectomy

aberrant pathway may cause a minor *"contra coup"* burn of the opposite wall, but this is generally of minor consequence.

Special situations and techniques

The giant polyp

When a polyp is so large that it fills the lumen of the bowel (Video Clip 11.6), it may be difficult to pass the scope beyond it. Occasionally, the polyp must be "debulked" in piecemeal fashion using snare cautery technique. Fluid injection is generally not necessary (or possible), as the polyp base is rarely identified until substantial portions have been resected. Pure coagulation current should be used, and a jiggling motion of the scope will indicate whether the nearby wall has been caught in the snare. After debulking, it may become evident that the polyp is pedunculated with the stalk folded under the bulky head. If a large stalk is noted, it should be encircled midstalk and a sustained burn delivered before the snare is closed; this will heat seal the large artery in the stalk.

Another strategy that may help with very large polyps is to inject the polyp with epinephrine. This causes vasoconstriction, which minimizes bleeding, and may actually shrink the polyp.

Using the mini-snare

In some tightly angulated segments of colon, the snare loop can be extended only a few centimeters beyond the scope and may not spread sufficiently to enable polyp capture with the standard polypectomy snare, which must be extended to its full length (5 or 6 cm) in order for the loop to completely expand. In this circumstance a mini-snare is used, which will open fully when extended only 3 cm beyond the sheath (Fig 11.6). The vast majority of colon polyps are less than 1.5 cm in diameter, and can be captured with this mini-snare.

Using auxiliary scopes

Gastroscopes can be used to intubate difficult and narrowed segments, and reach a previously inaccessible polyp. The nimbler

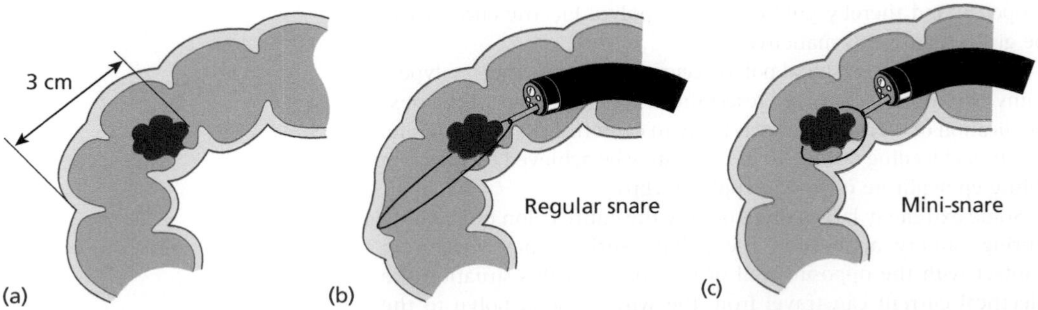

Fig 11.6 A "mini-snare" may be useful for polypectomy. Note that the smaller snare requires less space to achieve a wide radius.

gastroscope may also allow easier snare positioning in a narrowed or angulated colonic segment (e.g. a narrowed, diverticular sigmoid colon, where the anatomy can interfere with positioning polyps for resection). The gastroscope can be of use in the rectum, where its tip deflection capability and short "nose" may facilitate removal of a polyp on the proximal surface of a rectal valve. When using a snare through a gastroscope, the accessory channel is located at the 7 o'clock position in the field of view. Rarely, a two-channel colonoscope may be useful. In this technique, a snare is passed through the first channel and placed loosely around the polyp like a lasso. A forceps is passed through the second channel and is used to grasp the center of the polyp and tent it up. Once the forceps lifts up the polyp, the snare is tightened to capture the polyp.

Polypectomy in retroflection

Many right colon polyps are located on the back (proximal) side of folds. These may be best resected from the proximal aspect after carefully retroflexing the scope tip (Video Clip 11.7). Right colon retroflexion can be performed safely with either a standard adult colonoscope or a pediatric colonoscope in most patients. Ancillary tools can be passed as usual through the working channel even with a retroflexed scope; the resistance to passage through the tip may be somewhat increased, but this does not incur undue risk of channel damage. Electrocautery and other techniques are performed in the standard manner. The polyp specimen can be retrieved after the scope is returned to the forward viewing position.

Flat polyps

Flat or minimally elevated (<3 mm above the surface) polyps represent a special challenge (Video Clip 11.8). They can be difficult to entrap in the snare—often the closing wire will slip over the "curb" where polyp adjoins normal mucosa. Several tactics may prove useful in this situation (Fig 11.7). With the snare opened around the polyp, aspirate intraluminal air. This collapses the colon, causing the flat polyp to become more elevated and easier

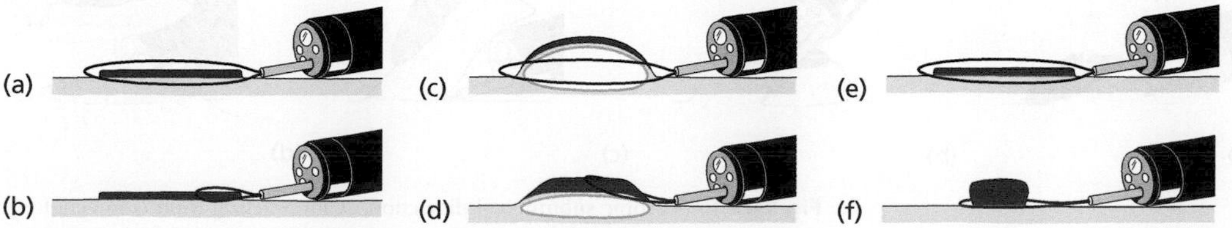

Fig 11.7 Snaring a large flat polyp. These may be extremely challenging to entrap. The snare may slide over the flat polyp (a,b). The use of submucosal saline may in fact make capturing the polyp more difficult (c,d). Aspirating air before closing the snare may be helpful (e,f).

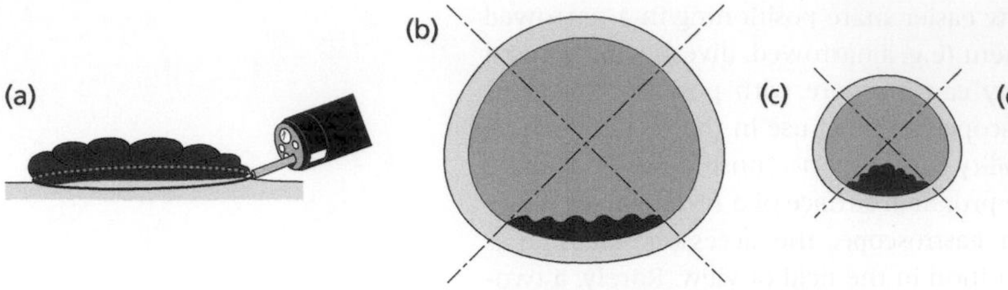

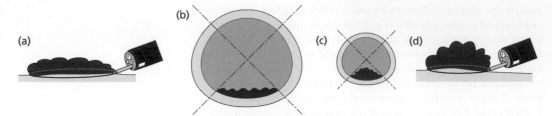

Fig 11.8 Intraluminal air aspiration to help capture flat polyps. The open snare is placed around the flat polyp (a). As the colon circumference decreases, the "footprint" of the polyp also decreases, but the polyp volume does not change, so the polyp "rises up" into the open snare (b,c). This makes capture considerably easier (d).

to entrap (Fig 11.8a). The ensnared tissue should be tented away from the colon wall before current is applied, to ensure that the muscularis propria has not been caught. Sometimes simply switching from a standard to a mini-snare or vice versa will be useful. Another strategy is to use submucosal injection. Once a cushion is created, the open snare is placed around the polyp and then the snare loop and catheter are pushed down, creating a circumferential doughnut-shaped indentation in the fluid cushion. The loop is then closed. (Occasionally, fluid injection may cause a very flat polyp to become even *more difficult* to ensnare because the effect of air aspiration is negated.) It may be necessary to switch to a "barbed" or "spiral" snare, which in theory should help "bite" into the mucosa as the snare is tightened. Sometimes very flat polyps may require primary ablation with the APC or other thermal device, preferably after biopsy. More often thermal ablation is used to "touch up" the site after snare resection.

Resecting flat polyps

- Before opening snare, optimize orientation of scope and sheath with respect to polyp
- With snare loosely around polyp, aspirate air
- Beware of snaring adjacent mucosa
- After snaring lift ("tent") polyp into lumen
- Consider submucosal injection
- Use appropriate snare
- If first snare not working, consider switching snares
- Consider suctioning flat polyp into suction channel before resection; this may "tent" the mucosa into the lumen and facilitate polyp entrapment

Endoscopic submucosal dissection

Developed in Japan, endoscopic submucosal dissection (ESD) is a novel technique first used to remove polyps in the stomach. ESD is performed using modified needle knives instead of snares. The procedure begins with injection of a long-lasting fluid cushion under the lesion. The knives are then used to incise the mucosa and dissect through the submucosa, tunneling under the polyp (Fig 11.9).

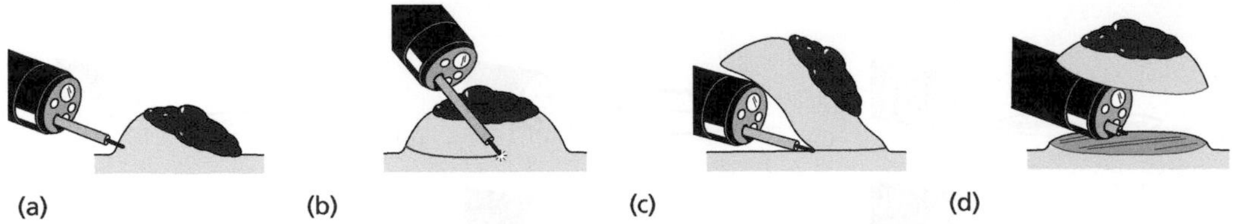

Fig 11.9 Endoscopic submucosal dissection. A long-acting fluid is injected into the submucosa from punctures around the edge of a polyp. The mucosa around the polyp is incised, and specialized electrosurgical cutting tools are used to dissect through the fluid-filled submucosal plane underneath the polyp, undermining it completely. The specimen is obtained in one large piece and the tumor is not touched.

With ESD, polyps are resected in one large, well-oriented piece, providing the pathologist with the optimal specimen. Compared with EMR, ESD takes longer and is more challenging technically, often taking an hour or more. In the colon, the perforation rate is about 5%; most of these defects can be closed with endoscopic clips. Because of its high morbidity, technical difficulty and steep learning curve, ESD is mainly being performed in Japan.

Residual fragments of adenoma after polypectomy

Incomplete polypectomy may occur despite meticulous technique, particularly after piecemeal resection. For this reason, it is generally recommended that the patient return to have the resection site reexamined colonoscopically approximately 3–6 months following a piecemeal polypectomy. If appropriate, the site should have been marked endoscopically for future surveillance. For large polyps, the scar is usually, but not invariably, visible.

The defect at the site of polyp resection heals and retracts concentrically, from the edges toward the center. For this reason, residual adenomatous tissue usually results in only one polypoid excrescence, even if several small islands of adenoma remained at the periphery of the initial resection base (Fig 11.10a,b). Generally this residual polypoid tissue can be removed easily. Scarring may prevent mucosal elevation with saline. On occasion, there may be granulation tissue at the scar site that is endoscopically difficult to distinguish from residual adenoma.

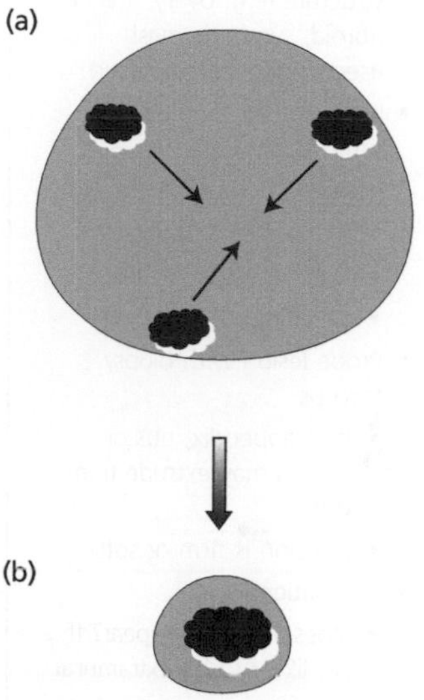

Fig 11.10 Healing at the polypectomy site. (a) The defect heals concentrically, not from the bottom up. If fragments of polyp remain at the polypectomy site, complete healing usually results in a single residual polyp, as the pieces tend to coalesce as the polypectomy site gradually contracts as it heals (b).

The impossible polyp

These include polyps with a giant base (e.g. >4 cm), polyps that can be only partially visualized or reached, and polyps that extend into the appendix or a diverticulum or the ileum. In these instances, surgical resection is appropriate after colonoscopic marking.

What to do when a polyp involves the appendix (Plate 11.4)

- Serrated or adenomatous polyps may extend into appendiceal orifice
- Confirm that "lesion" is not inverted appendiceal stump
- When considering resection, inspect lesion to ensure that margin is visible
- If margin is evident, resect using conventional strategies
- If margin is not visible, grasp lesion with forceps and gently pull it into cecal caput; this maneuver will often invert the appendix and reveal the margin of the lesion, allowing complete resection
- If lesion extends into the appendix and margin cannot be exposed, biopsy and consider surgical resection (colonoscopic polypectomy will probably be incomplete)

Cap-assisted resection

A special EMR kit consisting of a thin snare that can be seated at the tip of a short clear plastic cylinder affixed to the end of a colonoscope is available. It is used to suction mucosa and submucosa into the cap, as is done during esophageal varix banding. As the polyp tissue is suctioned into the cap the snare is closed, encircling then transecting by electrocautery current the base of the aspirated tissue. It is advised that this device be used only below the peritoneal reflection, as the full thickness of the thin colon wall could be gathered into the cap and perforation could ensue.

Nonmucosal elevated lesions in the cecum

- May reflect submucosal polyp, or indentation by extraluminal structure (e.g. ovary, uterine fibroid, synthetic mesh used during hernia repair)
- If located at appendiceal orifice, consider
  - Inverted appendiceal stump
  - Mucocele of appendix
  - Chronic appendicitis
  - Carcinoid of appendix
- Probe lesion with biopsy forceps
  - If at appendix, pus or mucus may extrude from orifice
  - Is lesion is firm or soft?
- Roll patient
  - Does lesion disappear? If so, likely to be extramural
- Consider CT scan (often diagnostic)

The polyp that involves the Ileocecal valve

- Inspection or resection in retroflex position may be useful
- Ensure that lesion is polyp and not part of the valve
- May be difficult to determine exact margin between villous small bowel mucosa and villous polyp endoscopically
- Inspect lesion carefully to determine "proximal" margin of polyp (i.e. the margin involving the valve)
- Valve can often be evaginated with forceps, facilitating resection
- Saline injection into small bowel mucosa may be helpful
- If proximal margin cannot be identified (very rare), consider surgical resection
- Resection proceeds using convention methods
- No unusual perforation/stricture risks if usual polypectomy precautions are followed

Summary

The resection of difficult polyps requires creativity, careful planning, and effective endoscopist/assistant collaboration. Very few colon polyps are unresectable in expert hands, and referral centers that offer specialized tools and expertise in "advanced polypectomy" are emerging. With appropriate training most colonoscopists can resect most difficult polyps. The risks, benefits, and alternatives to colonoscopic resection must be continuously weighed.

Further reading

1. Ahlawat SK, Gupta N, Benjamin SB, Al-Kawas FH. Large colorectal polyps: endoscopic management and rate of malignancy: does size matter? *J Clin Gastroenterol* 2011;45:347–54.
2. Ferrara F, Luigiano C, Ghersi S, *et al*. Efficacy, safety and outcomes of 'inject and cut' endoscopic mucosal resection for large sessile and flat colorectal polyps. *Digestion* 2010;82:213–20.
3. Gallegos-Orozco JF, Gurudu SR. Complex colon polypectomy. *Gastroenterol Hepatol* (*NY*) 2010;6:375–82.
4. Iishi H, Tatsuta M, Iseki K, *et al*. Endoscopic piecemeal resection with submucosal saline injection of large sessile colorectal polyps. *Gastrointest Endosc* 2000;51:697–700.
5. Morson BC. Histological criteria for local excision. *Br J Surg* 1985;72(Suppl.):S53–4.
6. Moss A, Bourke MJ, Williams SJ, *et al*. Endoscopic mucosal resection outcomes and prediction of submucosal cancer from advanced colonic mucosal neoplasia. *Gastroenterology* 2011;140:1909–18. Epub 2011 Mar 8.

7. Ponsky JL, King JF. Endoscopic marking of colon lesions. *Gastrointest Endosc* 1975;22:42–3.
8. Rex DK, Khashab M. Colonoscopic polypectomy in retroflexion. *Gastrointest Endosc* 2006;63:144–8.
9. Sanaka MR, Thota PN. Efficacy of colonoscopic polypectomy in removing large polyps. *Gastrointest Endosc* 2010;72:906.
10. Uno Y, Munakata A. The nonlifting sign of invasive colon cancer. *Gastrointest Endosc* 1994;40:485–9.

Chapter video clips

Video Clip 11.1 Detachable loop and pedunculated polypectomy
The detachable loop is used to promote hemostasis before resection of this large, pedunculated polyp.

Video Clip 11.2 Piecemeal polypectomy, argon plasma coagulation, and net retrieval of fragments
The sequence of saline injection, piecemeal polypectomy, and argon plasma coagulation and net retrieval of polyp fragments is used to eradicate this 3-cm adenoma.

Video Clip 11.3 Piecemeal resection of sessile adenoma
Large sessile adenoma removed piecemeal following saline lift.

Video Clip 11.4 Saline-assisted polypectomy
Multiple injection sites are used to elevate the polyp with methylene blue and saline.

Video Clip 11.5 The non-lifting sign
This polyp does not lift with saline injection, suggesting the presence of malignancy.

Video Clip 11.6 Giant villous adenoma
This enormous sigmoid adenoma occupied the entire lumen and is debulked. Water immersion is used to examine the defect for signs of residual polyp, which are ablated with the argon plasma coagulator.

Video Clip 11.7 Cecal retroflexion with polypectomy
A large, right-colon polyp is hidden behind a fold and identified and removed in retroflexion.

Video Clip 11.8 Flat right colon polyp
A flat right-colon polyp is seen and resected in retroflexion.

CHAPTER 12
Management of Malignant Polyps

Introduction

A "malignant polyp" contains malignant cells that invade through the muscularis mucosa into the submucosal tissue, gaining the potential to enter lymphatics and/or blood vessels and spread to lymph nodes or other organs. If these cells invade deeply into the submucosa or the muscularis propria, eradication by polypectomy may not be safe due to the risk of transmural perforation. The term "malignant polyp" is distinct from "carcinoma *in situ*," an obsolete histological descriptor for high-grade dysplasia in the absence of invasion, and "intramucosal carcinoma," which describes invasion across the epithelial basement membrane into the lamina propria without invasion across the muscularis mucosa (Fig 12.1). In these latter situations, the risk of spread is minimal.

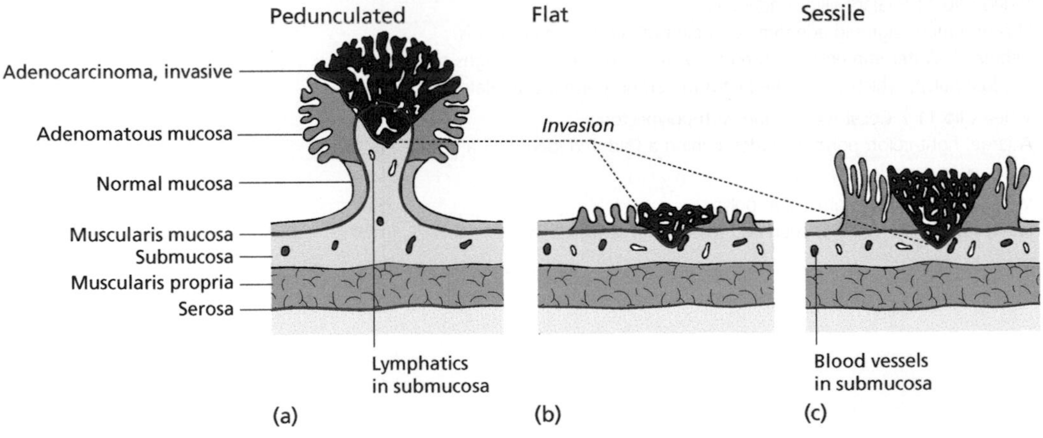

Fig 12.1 The malignant polyp. A malignant polyp that contains dysplastic crypts that invade the muscularis mucosa. There are no lymphatic channels above the muscularis mucosa. A malignant pedunculated polyp (left) is less prone to metastasis, as the head of the polyp is at a distance from the submucosal layer of the colon wall. Malignant polyps may be pedunculated (a), flat (b) or sessile (c).

Practical Colonoscopy, First Edition. Jerome D. Waye, James Aisenberg, and Peter H. Rubin.
© 2013 John Wiley & Sons, Ltd. Published 2013 by John Wiley & Sons, Ltd.

Advanced polyps: Understanding the pathology report					
Language in report	**Microscopic finding**				**Risk of spread**
	High-grade epithelial cell dysplasia ("cytological dysplasia")	High-grade dysplasia of crypt morphology ("architectural dysplasia")	Invasion of malignant cells into lamina propria	Invasion of malignant cells through muscularis mucosa into submucosa	
"High-grade dysplasia" "Carcinoma *in situ*"	✓	✓			Extremely low
"Intramucosal carcinoma" "High-grade dysplasia with invasion of lamina propria"	✓	✓	✓		Extremely low
"Invasive adenocarcinoma"	✓	✓	✓	✓	Extremely low to very high (depending on adequacy of polypectomy and histological criteria)

Malignant polyps may be pedunculated, sessile, or flat, and may arise anywhere in the colon. They are relatively rare, with an incidence of less than 1% in the screening population. The incidence is not related to gender, and increases with age. Some studies suggest a left-sided predominance. Most arise in tubular, tubulovillous, or villous adenomas; it is rare for malignant polyps to arise via the "serrated pathway."

The goal of the management is cure. The discussion that follows pertains to the management of the malignant polyp in the average-risk patient. The management of malignant polyps in high-risk settings such as colitis or hereditary polyposis (e.g. familial adenomatous polyposis (Video Clip 12.1), present other considerations.

Can I recognize a malignant polyp by its gross appearance?

In some cases macroscopic clues differentiate malignant polyps from their benign counterparts. Larger, irregularly shaped polyps are more likely to harbor carcinoma. A dense, hard texture may be appreciated during biopsy, and/or during polypectomy, when the electrocautery snare wire cuts haltingly through the base of a malignant polyp. Invasion into deeper layers of the submucosa may

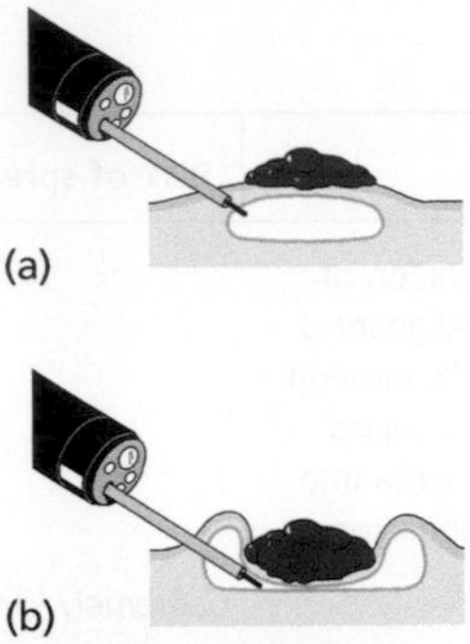

(a)

(b)

Fig 12.2 The non-lifting sign. Ordinarily, when fluid is injected into the submucosal space beneath a polyp, the polyp will elevate (a). If a previous attempt at polypectomy has created scarring, or if the polyp is malignant and is tethered to deeper layers of the wall, the polyp may not be elevated. Fluid may flow under the polyp and elevate mucosa adjacent to the polyp.

result in the "non-lifting sign," which describes the failure of a polyp to elevate when fluid is injected into the submucosa (Fig 12.2a) (Video Clip 12.2). Subtler signs include: ulceration of the mucosal surface; concave rather than convex polyp contour; central depression; deformity ("tethering") by the polyp of the adjacent mucosa; and spontaneous surface bleeding. In the case of flat polyps in particular, a depressed center (Paris Classification 0-IIc or 0-III) may be a clue to submucosal invasion (Plate 12.1).

If I think it may be malignant, should I still undertake polypectomy?

Polyps that appear highly likely to be malignant should be biopsied to confirm the diagnosis and resection deferred. To minimize sampling error, numerous biopsies should be obtained. Colonoscopy should be performed to the cecum and any synchronous polyps should be removed. To optimize future management the polypectomy site should be marked (see below).

Non-lifting sign: Causes

- Cancer invades into deep submucosa
- Scarring from prior polypectomy
- Needle in wrong tissue plane
- Chronic colitis

Resection of a polyp that might be malignant

If the polyp appears likely to be benign, and logistically favorable for resection, then colonoscopic polypectomy may be the strategy of choice. Operator-level factors, such as experience, aggressiveness, and risk-tolerance impact the decision. If the colonoscopist decides to proceed with polypectomy, it should be performed at the index colonoscopy, rather than postponed until a second procedure. Exceptions to this may include the patient receiving an antiplatelet or anticoagulant agent, or a polyp that appears to pose an especially high risk for removal; here, a discussion of the risks, benefits, and alternatives is advisable.

The principles of colonoscopic resection of the possibly malignant polyp and a benign polyp are the same. Partial polypectomy should be avoided whenever possible, as the submucosal fibrosis from the previous partial attempt at polypectomy can make complete colonoscopic polypectomy impossible. For pedunculated polyps, resection closer to the base of the stalk will increase the likelihood of a clear margin between the invasive cancer and the resection margin. For sessile malignant polyps, incomplete resection is of special concern (Video Clip 12.3). Deliberate inclusion in the resection of a small "rim" of normal appearing mucosa helps to ensure complete resection and aids pathological interpretation. Submucosal saline injection promotes a "clean" resection. After polypectomy, carefully inspect the mucosa at the immediate perimeter of the mucosal defect, with the colonoscope lens close to the mucosal surface. At times, it may be difficult to distinguish residual polyp from normal mucosa that is erythematous and edematous from thermal injury. In this situation, thermal ablation or snare resection of an additional few millimeters of mucosa may be prudent. Rarely, the snare wire may become embedded in the hard stroma of a malignant polyp; toggling from blended to cutting current may facilitate transection. For sessile polyps, the endoscopist can aid the pathologist by identifying the base of the polyp, and by gently flattening or pinning the polyp onto a substrate such as gelatin sponge or cellulose before placing the polyp in formalin. If a polyp is possibly malignant, it is imperative that all resected fragments be retrieved for histological analysis. The endoscopist should report that the polypectomy appeared complete and photograph the defect.

Marking the site

Unless the polyp is located near the cecum or the rectum, estimation of polyp site location is notoriously inaccurate. "Localization" using the centimeter markings of the colonoscope or other "landmarks" such as the colonic flexures may be erroneous. At worst, incorrect localization of a malignant polyp can lead to surgical resection of the wrong segment of colon. Scars from polypectomy arc difficult to locate colonoscopically and are not visible at laparoscopy or laparotomy (Fig 12.3). Therefore, if the colonoscopist suspects that a polyp may be malignant, the site of polypectomy should be permanently marked—typically with submucosal injection of a bioinert substance such as a carbon particle tattoo (Plate 12.2). Injections should be made circumferentially to ensure that they are visible to the surgeon during the examination of the serosa. The site of the tattooing (i.e. whether it is distal or proximal to the tumor) should be recorded in the procedure report and in endoscopic photographs.

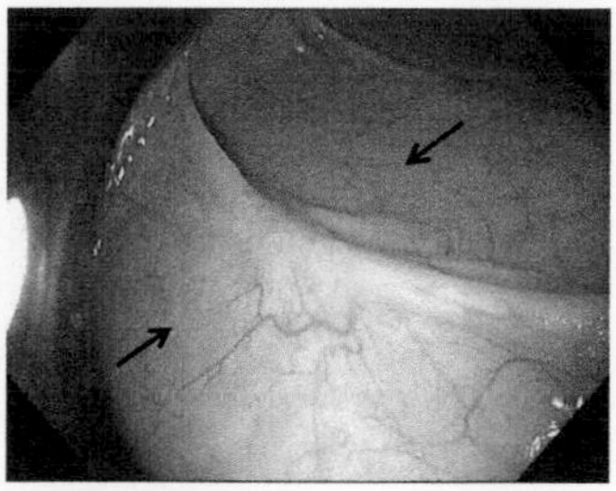

Fig 12.3 Scar after polypectomy. Note the stellate appearance, decreased vascular pattern (pallor), and deformity of fold due to scar contraction.

The unsuspected malignant polyp

Occasionally, histological examination of a seemingly benign polyp reveals that it is malignant. The colonoscopist should carefully review the procedure report, the photographs taken at the time of the endoscopy, and confirm the presumed location of the malignant polyp. This is particularly important if several polyps were removed during that exam. At this point, discussion with the patient of the findings and management options (see below) should occur. Assuming the site was not tattooed, it is usually advisable to re-colonoscope the patient within a week or two of the index examination and mark the site, because during the first few weeks after polypectomy a conspicuous eschar usually makes identification of the site secure.

Decision-making after resection of a malignant polyp

Two options are available: colonoscopic surveillance or surgical resection of the involved colonic segment. The optimal choice is often not clear. Even when the resected specimen meets favorable criteria, a small chance exists that the tumor has spread to adjacent or distant tissues. The risk of recurrence must be weighed against the immediate morbidity and mortality of colectomy. The age, overall health and functional status of the patient are important considerations. Death from colonic surgery may occur within 30 days of surgery, and rates range from 0.1 to 1%. The risk of spread of a malignant polyp is in the same range of magnitude, but death from such an endoscopically removed lesion occurs at a much later time.

Factors favoring colonoscopic approach

- Patient prefers this approach
- Patient is elderly
- Patient has significant comorbidity
- Endoscopist considers that polypectomy was complete
- Resection specimen allows clear histological interpretation
- Margin is clear
- The tumor is well differentiated, and does not invade lymphatics or blood vessels
- The focus of malignant tissue within the polyp is small
- The polyp is pedunculated
- The polyp removed in one piece
- Shallow invasion (<2 mm) of the submucosa

Factors favoring consideration for surgical resection

- Patient requests surgical resection
- Patient is young
- Patient is otherwise healthy (no significant comorbidities)
- Endoscopist uncertain that polypectomy was complete
- Specimen is fragmented and difficult to interpret histologically
- Adequate tissue margin not evident histologically
- Lymphatic or vascular invasion is present
- Cells are poorly differentiated
- Polyp is sessile
- Polyp was removed piecemeal
- Deep submucosal invasion is present

Decision-making must involve close collaboration among patient, patient's family, gastroenterologist, and pathologist. Malignant polyps in the distal rectum pose unique considerations, because they may be amenable to trans-anal techniques, radiotherapy, and may require colostomy.

Many experts believe that the risk of spread is lower for pedunculated than sessile polyps because "clean" colonoscopic resection is easier to achieve and because the stalk of the pedunculated polyp distances the submucosa of the polyp head from the colonic wall, thus in theory providing an additional obstacle to tumor spread (Fig 12.4(a–c), 12.5 (a–d)). Some experts favor surgical resection for all sessile malignant polyps, particularly for those that are removed piecemeal.

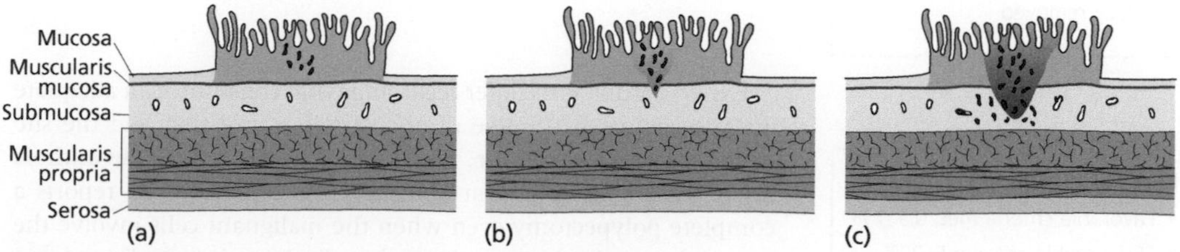

Fig 12.4 **(a)** Sessile polyp (adenoma). Dysplastic cells do not cross muscularis mucosa (no invasion). Detection of abnormal crypts in the lamina propria alone, without invasion of the submucosa, does not constitute malignancy. **(b)** Sessile polyp (adenocarcinoma). Dysplastic cells cross muscularis mucosa, but do not invade lymphatics or vessels, or reach the resection margin. Likelihood of lymph node metastasis is very low. Colonoscopic polypectomy alone is usually adequate treatment. **(c)** Sessile polyp (adenocarcinoma). Dysplastic cells cross muscularis mucosa, and cross the resection margin. Surgery indicated if patient is reasonable candidate.

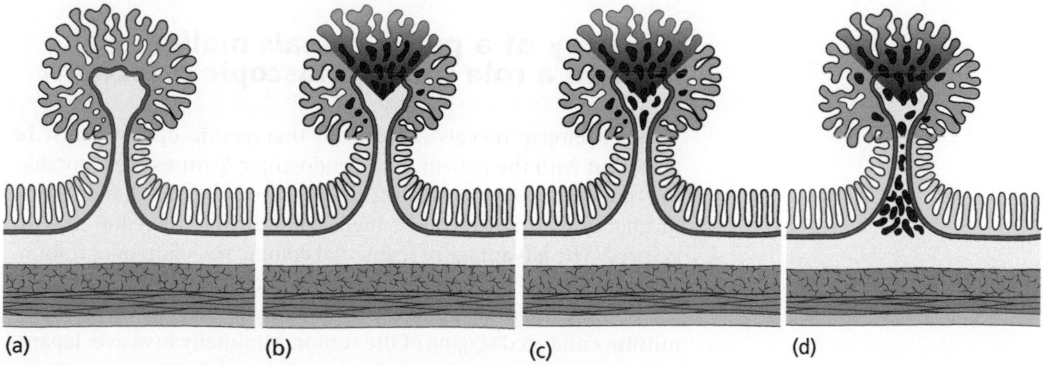

Fig 12.5 **(a)** Pedunculated polyp (adenoma). Dysplastic cells do not cross muscularis mucosa (no invasion). Detection of abnormal crypts in the lamina propria alone, without invasion of the submucosa, does not constitute malignancy. **(b)** Pedunculated polyp (adenocarcinoma). Dysplastic cells cross muscularis mucosa, but do not invade lymphatics or vessels, or reach the resection margin. Likelihood of lymph node metastasis is very low. Colonoscopic polypectomy alone is usually adequate treatment. **(c)** Pedunculated polyp (adenocarcinoma). Dysplastic cells cross muscularis mucosa, and invade lymphatics or vessels, but do not reach the resection margin. Likelihood of lymph node metastasis is not low. Surgery indicated if patient is reasonable candidate. **(d)** Pedunculated polyp (adenocarcinoma). Dysplastic cells cross muscularis mucosa, and cross the resection margin. Surgery indicated if patient is reasonable candidate.

Favorable criteria in the malignant polyp

- Well or moderately well differentiated cancer
- No lymphatic or vascular invasion
- Margin clear
- Endoscopist declares it is totally removed

Adverse outcome (residual cancer in colon or nodes) in malignant adenomas with favorable pathology*	
Pedunculated adenomas	0.3%
Sessile adenomas	1.5%

*Well differentiated, no vascular or lymphatic invasion, clear margins.

Risk for cancer recurrence

- Favorable criteria met: 0.5–1%
- Unfavorable criteria: 5–20%

Expert pathologists differ regarding what constitutes an adequate distance between the line of endoscopic transection and the site of malignant invasion (i.e. an adequate "margin"). Some authors report favorable long-term outcomes if the endoscopist reports a complete polypectomy even when the malignant cells involve the resection margin, hypothesizing that the burn has eradicated any possible residual tumor. Others argue that a 2-mm margin of healthy tissue is necessary to ensure cure. Newer pathological characteristics, including tumor genetics, may help guide decisions.

If the patient chooses the nonsurgical approach, baseline computed tomography scanning and measurement of carcinoembryonic antigen (CEA), a blood marker associated with colon cancer, are reasonable, although of unproven benefit. Endoscopic ultrasound is usually of little benefit because of artifact related to the polypectomy. Likewise, repeat colonoscopy in 3 months' time with inspection and biopsy of the polypectomy site is reasonable.

If biopsy of a polyp reveals malignancy, is there a role for colonoscopic resection?

When a biopsy reveals cancer, the therapeutic options must be discussed with the patient. If the endoscopic features are favorable, the patient prefers a minimally invasive approach, and/or the morbidity of surgery will be high, colonoscopic resection may be favored. The advantage of segmental colonic resection over colonoscopic resection of malignant polyps is that the specimen contains the entire colonic wall and the underlying lymph nodes, thus permitting enhanced staging of the tumor. Minimally invasive, laparoscopic, colon surgery may reduce surgical morbidity.

Summary

The management of malignant polyps represents a unique challenge for the colonoscopist. Careful intra-and post-procedural decision-making promotes the likelihood of cure with minimal morbidity. In certain instances, colonoscopic polypectomy will represent the treatment of choice, whereas in others surgical resection is favored. Careful collaboration among colonoscopist, surgeon, pathologist, and patient is mandatory.

Further reading

1. Butte JM, Tang P, Gonen M, *et al.* Rate of residual disease after complete endoscopic resection of malignant colonic polyp. *Dis Colon Rectum* 2012;55:122–7.
2. Cooper HS. Pathology of the endoscopically removed malignant colorectal polyp. *Curr Diagn Pathol* 2007;13:423–37.
3. Cooper GS, Xu F, Barnholtz Sloan JS, Koroukian SM, Schluchter MD. Management of malignant colonic polyps: a population-based analysis of colonoscopic polypectomy versus surgery. *Cancer* 2011;118:651–9. Epub 2011 Jul 12.
4. Morson BC, Whiteway JE, Jones EA, Macrae FA, Williams CB. Histopathology and prognosis of malignant colorectal polyps treated by endoscopic polypectomy. *Gut* 1984;25:437–44.
5. Muller S, Chesner IM, Egan MJ, *et al.* Significance of venous and lymphatic invasion in malignant polyps of the colon and rectum. *Gut* 1989;30:1385–91.
6. Pizarro-Moreno A, Cordero-Fernández C, Garzón-Benavides M, *et al.* Malignant colonic adenomas. Therapeutic criteria. Long-term results of therapy in a series of 42 patients in our healthcare area. *Rev Esp Enferm Dig* 2009;101:830–6.
7. Rembacken BJ, Fujii T, Cairns A, *et al.* Flat and depressed colonic neoplasms: a prospective study of 1000 colonoscopies in the UK. *Lancet* 2000;355:1211–4.
8. Ueno H, Mochizuki H, Hashiguchi Y, *et al.* Risk factors for an adverse outcome in early invasive colorectal carcinoma. *Gastroenterology* 2004; 127:385–94.
9. Wasif N, Etzioni D, Maggard MA, Tomlinson JS, Ko CY. Trends, patterns, and outcomes in the management of malignant colonic polyps in the general population of the United States. *Cancer* 2011;117:931–7.
10. Winawer SJ, O'Brien MJ. Management of malignant polyps. In: Waye JD, Rex DK, Williams CB, editors. *Colonoscopy. Principles and Practice*. 2nd ed. Chichester: Wiley-Blackwell; 2009.

Chapter video clips

Video Clip 12.1 Familial adenomatous polyposis
Innumerable adenomas seen in a patient with familial adenomatous polyposis.

Video Clip 12.2 The Non-Lifting Sign
3 cm malignant polyp in ascending colon which exhibits the non-lifting sign upon sub-mucosal saline injection.

Video Clip 12.3 Malignant sessile polyp
A 2-cm sessile malignant polyp removed with saline injection and snare polypectomy.

CHAPTER 13
Therapeutic Colonoscopy

Life-threatening colonic dilation: Etiologies
- Mechanical obstruction
  - Colonic adenocarcinoma
  - Extrinsic compression by non-colonic carcinoma
  - Benign stricture (diverticular, anastomotic, inflammatory bowel disease)
  - Severe fecal impaction
- Non-mechanical
  - Volvulus
  - Pseudo-obstruction

Introduction

Colonoscopy has multiple therapeutic applications in addition to management of polyps and thermal treatment of bleeding.

Relief of colonic obstruction

Acute colonic obstruction is life-threatening and requires prompt diagnosis and treatment. Endoscopic intervention can decompress both benign and malignant colonic obstruction; it can be definitive, or serve as a bridge to surgery. Compared with surgical diversion, endoscopic treatment is minimally invasive and cost-effective. Additionally, colonoscopic decompression is recommended for patients who are too ill for surgery, unwilling to undergo surgical diversion, or with widespread metastatic disease. The colonoscopic approach confers risk, requires expertise, is contraindicated in certain clinical situations, and may fail. Of particular concern, the obstruction may function as a one-way valve and air insufflation may result in a proximal "blow out" of the distended colon. Air insufflation needs to be minimized during intubation.

For each patient with colonic obstruction the endoscopic approach should be tailored to the clinical situation and local expertise, involving the collaboration of gastroenterologist, surgeon, and radiologist. The immediate goal is decompression of the high-pressure segment to resolve the clinical emergency. With this achieved, the attention shifts to longer-term treatment. Even if surgery eventually will be required an initial colonoscopic intervention can provide three specific advantages:

1. the previously obstructed colon can be lavaged with a cathartic, making it more feasible to perform one-step surgery without the need for diverting colostomy;
2. the patient can be stabilized medically, converting emergency surgery into elective surgery;
3. in the case of malignant obstruction, proximal synchronous lesions can be excluded by total colonoscopy or retrograde contrast study.

Malignant colonic obstruction

Approximately two-thirds of malignant colonic obstructions result from colonic adenocarcinoma; the remainder are caused by extrin-

Practical Colonoscopy, First Edition. Jerome D. Waye, James Aisenberg, and Peter H. Rubin.
© 2013 John Wiley & Sons, Ltd. Published 2013 by John Wiley & Sons, Ltd.

sic compression or colonic invasion by noncolonic (usually gynecological) malignancies. The most common colonic site of malignant obstruction is the sigmoid colon, and obstruction is the presenting feature in 10–20% of cases of colon cancer. Endoscopic treatment of malignant obstruction can involve tumor debulking, transanal placement of decompression tubes, and/or placement of self-expanding metal stents.

Debulking is achieved endoscopically by using thermal ablation with laser or argon plasma coagulation. Relief of obstruction may be achieved in approximately two-thirds of patients, but repeat sessions may be required to maintain luminal patency. Transanal placement of a decompression tube is used in some centers as a bridge to surgery. In this approach, a guidewire is passed through the obstructing lesion under both direct vision and fluoroscopic control. A colon decompression tube is then passed over the guidewire through the lesion, resulting in decompression. The tube may be used for irrigation of the colon proximal to the stricture, although this procedure is labor-intensive, and plagued by obstruction of the tube and the risk of tube dislodgement.

Self-expanding metallic stents (SEMS) have emerged as a valuable approach to malignant colonic obstruction. Using a narrow-diameter delivery system, these stents are placed across the malignant obstruction under direct and/or fluoroscopic visual guidance; an outer sheath is then withdrawn, and the stent expands, due to its "shape memory." A fluoroscopic "waist" in the radiopaque stent confirms accurate placement. Some wire mesh stents are engineered with a plastic membrane intended to discourage tumor ingrowth, prevent the wire mesh from embedding into tissue, and allow the stent to be removed at a later date. A variety of stent technologies are available: covered versus uncovered; through-the-scope (TTS) versus non-TTS; fluoroscopically guided; nitinol versus stainless steel. For each stent design, different lengths (ranging from 40 to 120 mm) and widths (20–25 mm) are available (Fig 13.1). There are few comparative data to guide the choice among the different technologies, and the choice will often be

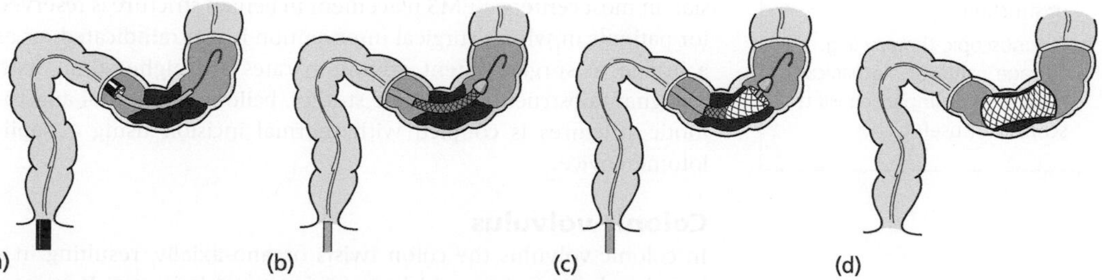

Fig 13.1 Stent placement for malignant obstruction of the colon. Under fluoroscopic control, a guidewire and then a sheath containing the stent system are passed across the obstructing lesion (a,b). The sheath is gradually withdrawn (c), allowing the stent to deploy. After the assembly is removed (d) the stent deploys fully, restoring luminal patency. Characteristically a "waist" is observed in the middle of the stent.

Indications for SEMS

- Malignant obstruction
  - Colon adenocarcinoma
  - Noncolonic extrinsic tumor (e.g. gynecological)
- Benign obstruction
  - Postoperative stricture
  - Inflammatory stricture
  - Diverticular stricture
- Fistula

driven by the colonoscopist's experience and the institution's inventory. If the lesion is at a flexure, an angulation, or is proximal, stent placement may be technically challenging.

Most data from SEMS placement involve left-sided tumors. In skilled hands stents can relieve left-sided malignant obstruction and obviate the need for emergency surgery in approximately 90% of cases. SEMS are particularly useful for palliation of obstruction in individuals with advanced incurable colorectal cancer, who would not otherwise require colonic resection. The reported incidence of serious complications with SEMS placement is <5%; however, colonic perforation (with intraperitoneal seeding of malignant cells) and death may occur. Other complications include stent migration (10%) and stent occlusion (10%). It is not known whether uncomplicated SEMS placement can disseminate cancer. Dilation or thermal ablation of malignant strictures before stent placement, or immediately after stent deployment (by using a TTS balloon) may increase the perforation rate. Covered stents migrate more frequently than uncovered stents. The reported experience of SEMS placement in the right colon or for extracolonic tumors is smaller, the procedure technically more difficult, and the success rate less certain.

Benign colonic obstruction

Management of fecal impaction

- Primary treatment
  - Enemas
  - Oral cathartics
  - Digital disimpaction
  - Close clinical observation
  - Supportive care
- Colonoscopy on rare occasion useful diagnostically to rule out other causes of obstruction
- Colonoscopic therapy (e.g. "lavage" and/ or mechanical disruption of impaction via the scope) not useful

Benign colonic obstruction in Crohn's disease may be primary or postsurgical. If the stricture is short in length (i.e. <5 cm), and fibrotic rather than inflammatory, endoscopic hydrostatic balloon dilation may relieve symptoms. Balloon dilation is typically performed under direct visualization, utilizing a TTS balloon. The balloons range in length (5–8 cm) and maximal diameter (10–25 mm). Such endoscopic balloon dilation in Crohn's (with or without steroid injection) is reported to be effective in approximately three-quarters of patients, but recurrence is common.

Anastomotic stricturing complicates ileo-colonic or colo-colonic anastomosis in up to 30% of cases. These strictures are usually quite short and respond well to TTS balloon dilation (Video Clip 13.1). Perforation rates are reportedly <1%. The use of SEMS in the management of benign colonic obstruction remains controversial. In most centers, SEMS placement in benign stricture is reserved for patients in whom surgical intervention is contraindicated, or as a bridge to surgery. Stent migration rates are higher than with malignant obstruction. In some studies, balloon dilation of anastomotic strictures is coupled with thermal incision using a papillotome device.

Colonic volvulus

In colonic volvulus the colon twists organo-axially, resulting in a functional obstruction and in some instances ischemia. It is most common in males, the elderly, in patients with flaccid or dilated colon, chronic laxative dependency, and in those receiving narcotic analgesics. Rarely, it may occur in pregnancy. It typically involves either a redundant loop of sigmoid colon or an unusually mobile cecum. Cecal volvulus occurs in a younger age group of patients.

Volvulus presents with pain and abdominal distension, and classic radiological findings on plain film (the "bent inner tube" or "coffee bean" sign) and/or CT scanning (the "bird's beak" sign). If not treated promptly, the mortality of sigmoid volvulus may be as high as 20%.

For sigmoid volvulus, colonoscopy is the gold standard for diagnosis and treatment. The flexible endoscope is cautiously advanced through the distal colon; a minimum amount of air is insufflated. Typically, the distal colon has no stool, because of the obstruction. When the obstruction is reached, typically at 20–30 cm from the dentate line, a twisted, pinpoint narrowing (the "whirl" sign) is identified. The mucosa should be assessed for evidence of ischemia (e.g. dusky blue discoloration). If the mucosa appears viable, the endoscope tip is introduced gently into the "eye" of the narrowing. Usually the twist can be undone with minimal resistance. This characteristically results in a rush of air and fluid, with immediate relief to the patient. The scope tip is then passed above the twist for aspiration of more air and fluid. A decompression tube is often inserted, although the value of this is unproven. A similar technique can be performed using a rigid sigmoidoscope. The recurrence rate after endoscopic decompression may be 40–70%. Although decompression generally results in correction of the torsion, depending on the clinical setting (severity, recurrence, comorbidities) a more definitive surgical approach may be indicated. If the colon appears necrotic, the patient is rushed to surgery. For cecal volvulus, colonoscopic diagnosis is valuable, but decompression is technically more difficult, and at most temporizing.

Common predisposing factors to pseudo-obstruction ("Ogilvie syndrome")

- Advanced age
- Critical comorbid illness
- The postoperative period
- Intra-abdominal or retroperitoneal tumor
- Chronic use of tricyclic antidepressants, antiparkinsonian agents, and narcotic analgesics

Treatment of pseudo-obstruction

Under certain circumstances, the colon may become atonic and progressively dilated in the absence of a mechanical obstruction.

"Pseudo-obstruction" is believed to result from an imbalance in autonomic nervous system tone. It can be acute, arising over several days, or chronic. Of gravest concern is cecal perforation due to progressive dilation and consequent transmural ischemia, with mortality rates as high as 40%. The risk for perforation rises as the cecal diameter increases, and generally a radiologic cecal diameter >12 cm is believed to be a reasonable threshold for intervention.

Colonoscopic decompression of pseudo-obstruction is technically challenging. If there is evidence of peritonitis, colonoscopy is contraindicated. Sedation with narcotics should be avoided, as narcotics inhibit colonic motility. As the colon is dilated and flaccid, large loops often form. Because of the colonic inertia, the patient cannot be prepared with oral purgatives or enemas, so the lumen is typically filled with liquid stool. The patient is often severely ill, perhaps in the intensive care unit. Air insufflation must be kept to a minimum during the scope insertion. For an effective procedure, the scope must be advanced at least to the ascending colon.

Retrospective series suggest that placement of a long decompression tube in the proximal colon helps to prevent recurrence. A

Pseudo-obstruction: Management

- Supportive care
  - Intravenous fluids and electrolytes
  - Stop narcotics/anticholinergics
  - Rotate/mobilize patient
- Close observation
  - Abdominal exam
  - Plain abdominal x-rays
- Directed intervention
  - Pharmacotherapy (intravenous neostigmine)
  - Colonoscopic decompression
  - Percutaneous cecostomy

14-French plastic catheter with multiple vent holes is available. With the tip of the scope in the proximal colon, a flexible guidewire is passed through the working channel of the scope. The scope is then withdrawn with the wire left in place (as can be confirmed by fluoroscopy). The plastic tube is then passed over the wire until its tip is located in the proximal colon. Tube placement is technically successful in 60–90% of cases, although it is not uncommon for the tube to fall out of position. The tube is left in place, draining to gravity. Unfortunately, in either circumstance, the recurrence rate is reported to be approximately 40%, and may necessitate subtotal colectomy.

In some medical centers intravenous neostigmine, administered under careful cardiopulmonary monitoring, is a safe and effective alternative to endoscopic intervention in as many as two-thirds of patients with colonic pseudo-obstruction. In those who relapse after neostigmine administration, colonoscopic decompression is the usual alternative approach.

Intralesional drug injection

A sclerotherapy-type injection catheter may be utilized to deliver a high concentration of a therapeutic agent colonoscopically to a diseased area of bowel. The most widely applied usage of this approach relates to steroid injection of strictures in fibrostenotic Crohn's disease. The literature is mixed as to the lasting efficacy of this approach, either as primary treatment or to prevent restricturing.

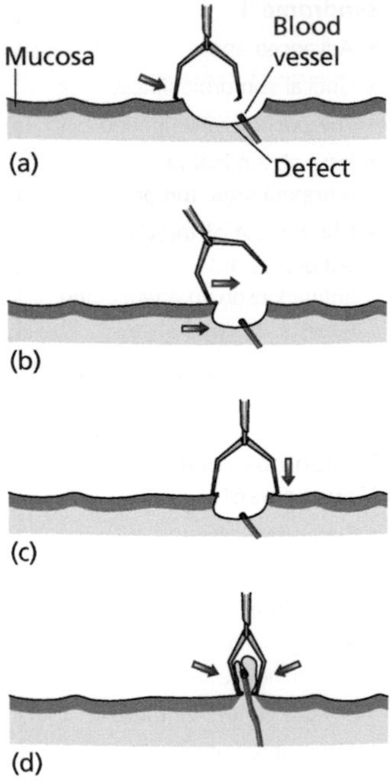

Fig 13.2 Clipping a large defect after polypectomy. The objective is to "patch" the defect with normal mucosa. The first edge of the polyp is grabbed with one jaw of the clip (a) is "pulled" toward the other side (b). The opposite edge of normal mucosa is then "grabbed" (c). When correct positioning is confirmed, the clip is fired (d).

Closure of perforation or fistula

Endoscopic clips, deployed through the colonoscope, may seal communications between the colonic lumen and either the peritoneal cavity or other organs (see Chapter 1). Clipping is quick and low risk (Fig 13.2).

If a localized perforation occurs during a therapeutic intervention, clips may be placed immediately across the defect. If the defect is small (i.e. <1 cm) and promptly identified, clipping may obviate the need for surgery in over two-thirds of patients. Air insufflation should be minimized; a first clip is used to juxtapose the walls of the defect, and then further clips are placed to reinforce the closure. The popularity of this strategy is growing. The strategy has been used in all segments of the colorectum. The presence of radiographic free air is not a contraindication.

Clipping has also been utilized to treat sigmoid lacerations related to diagnostic colonoscopy, although these defects are larger and therefore less amenable to clipping. Reports exist of successful closing of iatrogenic perforation up to 3.5 cm in length. In noniatrogenic colonic perforation (e.g. related to diverticular disease), clipping is not a viable option because of the inevitability of peritoneal contamination. In the postoperative setting, clipping has been used to manage staple line dehiscence.

Symptomatic fistulas between the colon and the skin, vagina, small bowel, stomach, and bladder, may occur postoperatively, or as a result of Crohn's disease or infection. The orifice of the fistula is not always apparent at colonoscopy. In Crohn's disease the fistula often originates from diseased small intestine; in this case the colonic opening may be heralded only by a small mound of granulation tissue in a background of normal mucosa. Because of fibrosis, epithelialization of the tract, and bacterial contamination, the success rate for closure of fistulas is lower than for acute perforations; nonetheless, clipping (in some instances coupled with fibrin glue or other adjunctive strategies) has been used successfully in the management of colo-cutaneous, colo-enteric, colo-vesical and recto-vaginal fistulas. In some centers, covered SEMS have also been used.

Potential indications for clips

- Prophylaxis against bleeding
  - Pedicle of large pedunculated polyp
  - Large mucosal defect (or exposed vessel) after resection of sessile polyp
- Tamponade of bleeding vessel
  - Postpolypectomy
    - Immediate
    - Delayed
  - Noniatrogenic (e.g. in neck of a diverticulum or Dieulafoy lesion)
- Closure of iatrogenic perforation
- Closure of fistula

Non-thermal treatment of bleeding sites

Clips or loops can be placed on the stalk of a pedunculated polyp during polypectomy. Clips can be placed over a mucosal polypectomy defect to promote a tamponade effect. Endoscopic intervention may safely and effectively control diverticular hemorrhage. After whole-gut lavage, early colonoscopy is used to identify the bleeding diverticulum. Meticulous withdrawal technique is required, with irrigation of individual diverticular orifices, and careful attention for stigmata of bleeding such as pigmented spots and erosions. Inversion of the diverticulum using a translucent mucosal cap on the tip of the endoscope may be useful; this allows visualization and clipping of lesions at the dome of the diverticulum. Once identified, tamponade of the culprit vessel is achieved with clip or rubber-band placement. A radiopaque clip also marks the site for radiologist or surgeon in the event of recurrent bleeding.

Removal of foreign body

Rarely, a patient presents with a foreign body in the colorectum or distal ileum. In the case of gallstone ileus, a stone may impact at the ileocecal valve. This can be removed with a basket, or fragmented using endoscopic lithotripsy. Fish bones or toothpicks may become embedded in the colon wall, and may be removed with a biopsy forceps or a snare (Video Clip 13.2). Rectal and rectosigmoid foreign bodies, including contraband materials and devices used in sexual practices, can be removed during flexible endoscopy or with a rigid instrument during examination under anesthesia.

Summary

Colonoscopy provides a means for resecting neoplasms, preventing and treating bleeding, treating benign or malignant obstruction, relieving volvulus and pseudo-obstruction, intralesional drug injection, closure of perforation or fistula, and removal of foreign body. A variety of technologies, including thermal devices, clips, stents, and decompression tubes enable these interventions.

Further reading

1. ASGE Standards of Practice Committee, Harrison ME, Anderson MA, *et al.* The role of endoscopy in the management of patients with known and suspected colonic obstruction and pseudo-obstruction. *Gastrointest Endosc* 2010;71:669–79.
2. Baron TH, Wong Kee Song LM, Repici A. Role of self-expandable stents for patients with colon cancer (with videos). *Gastrointest Endosc* 2012;75:653–62.
3. Bonin EA, Baron TH. Update on the indications and use of colonic stents. *Curr Gastroenterol Rep* 2010;12:374–82.
4. Di Nardo G, Oliva S, Passariello M, *et al.* Intralesional steroid injection after endoscopic balloon dilation in pediatric Crohn's disease with stricture: a prospective, randomized, double-blind, controlled trial. *Gastrointest Endosc* 2010;72:1201–8. Epub 2010 Oct 16.
5. Feo L, Schaffzin DM. Colonic stents: the modern treatment of colonic obstruction. *Adv Ther* 2011;28:73–86. Epub 2011 Jan 6.
6. Kaltenbach T, Watson R, Shah J, *et al.* Colonoscopy with clipping is useful in the diagnosis and treatment of diverticular bleeding. *Clin Gastroenterol Hepatol* 2012;10:131–7. Epub 2011 Nov 2.
7. Lal SK, Morgenstern R, Vinjirayer EP, Matin A. Sigmoid volvulus an update. *Gastrointest Endosc Clin N Am* 2006;16:175–87.
8. Magdeburg R, Collet P, Post S, Kaehler G. Endoclipping of iatrogenic colonic perforation to avoid surgery. *Surg Endosc* 2008;22:1500–4. Epub 2007 Dec 11.
9. Parra-Blanco A, Kaminaga N, Kojima T, *et al.* Hemoclipping for postpolypectomy and postbiopsy colonic bleeding. *Gastrointest Endosc* 2000;51:37–41.
10. Paspatis GA, Paraskeva K, Theodoropoulou A, *et al.* A prospective, randomized comparison of adrenaline injection in combination with detachable snare versus adrenaline injection alone in the prevention of postpolypectomy bleeding in large colonic polyps. *Am J Gastroenterol* 2006;101:2805; quiz 2913.

Chapter video clips

Video Clip 13.1 Dilation of strictured anastomosis
Strictured ileocolic anastomosis dilated with a through-the-scope balloon.

Video Clip 13.2 Foreign body in sigmoid
A chicken bone is identified embedded in the colon wall, and is removed with the snare.

CHAPTER 14

Complications of Colonoscopy

Introduction

If the indication is appropriate and the standard of care is met, the benefits of colonoscopy dominate the risks. Most complications are minor and self-limited, a few are serious, and very rarely a colonoscopy can result in death (approximately one in every 20,000 procedures). The rate of serious complications can be minimized by fastidious adherence to best practices. The important risks must be enumerated to the patient during the pre-procedure informed consent discussion. The rate of serious adverse events is higher in therapeutic procedures, in the elderly, and in patients with multiple comorbidities.

Principal colonoscopic complications

- Cardiac
  - Hypotension (volume depletion, drug-related, or vagally mediated)
  - Arrhythmia
  - Ischemia
- Pulmonary
  - Central hypoventilation
  - Aspiration
  - Laryngospasm
- Colonic perforation
  - Early
  - Delayed
- Postpolypectomy coagulation syndrome
- Hemorrhage
  - Early
  - Late
- Other
  - IV site infiltration or infection
  - Renal injury
  - Splenic rupture or hemorrhage
  - Electrolyte imbalance

Factors associated with complications

- Therapeutic colonoscopy
- Elderly patient
- Multiple comorbidities
- Active colitis
- Previous abdominal or pelvic surgery
- Extensive diverticulosis/diverticulitis
- Internal hernia

Practical Colonoscopy, First Edition. Jerome D. Waye, James Aisenberg, and Peter H. Rubin.
© 2013 John Wiley & Sons, Ltd. Published 2013 by John Wiley & Sons, Ltd.

Cardiopulmonary care during colonoscopy

- Evaluate the cardiopulmonary risk status before starting the case
- Use the minimal effective drug dosages
- Monitor the patient carefully during the case
- Inspect monitoring devices regularly
- Institute appropriate "rescue" systems for emergency management
- For high-risk patient, consider anesthesiologist
- Train and re-certify staff and endoscopists regarding best sedation and monitoring practice
- Require advanced cardiovascular life support (ACLS) training where appropriate
- Stock and quality-control a readily available "crash cart"

Cardiopulmonary complications

Colonoscopy poses a "triple threat" to the cardiovascular and pulmonary systems: the bowel preparation causes fluid and electrolyte shifts, the sedative drugs impact cardiovascular tone and respiratory function, and the instrumentation and distention of the colon can induce vagally mediated hypotension. The risk of death is greater with serious cardiovascular or respiratory adverse events than with hemorrhage, or even perforation. Serious cardiopulmonary complications during colonoscopy are rare, occurring in approximately 1/500 to 1/1,000 cases. In high-risk patients, most experts recommend that an anesthesiologist participate. In most studies, the risks are comparable for propofol versus benzodiazepine/opioid-based sedation regimens. The risks are independent of procedure venue (hospital versus outpatient setting).

Primary hypoventilation is a result of sedative drugs, and can usually be prevented by careful drug titration. Management depends on prompt recognition, use of reversal agents where possible, and ventilatory support. Upper airway obstruction, which is more common in patients with obstructive sleep apnea, and laryngospasm, is usually triggered by microaspiration of secretions, and can be recognized by the presence of stridor and/or ineffective cough. These are generally treated with upper airway maneuvers or positive pressure ventilation. Significant aspiration will occur only if the stomach has residual fluid. Sedation-related cardiopulmonary complications account for 40–50% of the serious adverse events that occur during all types of endoscopic procedures. The risk is lower during colonoscopy than gastroscopy, as the instrument does not perturb the upper airway.

Ischemic cardiac complications during colonoscopy are extraordinarily rare. Hypotension is common, owing to the vagal stimulation, vasodilatation, negative inotropy related to the sedative drugs, and dehydration related to the laxative and fasting. Typically, hypotension is readily remedied with fluid administration and the use of vasopressive drugs if necessary. Serious ventricular arrhythmias are extremely rare, but atrial arrhythmias such as atrial fibrillation, probably brought out by fluid and electrolyte shifts in susceptible patients, are encountered periodically.

Mild hypoxemia, hypotension, hypertension, hypopnea, sinus tachycardia and bradycardia, and premature ventricular contractions are common during colonoscopy. Cough, related to microaspiration, and hiccupping, related to central nervous systemic actions of the sedative drugs or to diaphragmatic perturbation by the scope are frequent and are usually transient and insignificant. However, these minor events should trigger a pause and assessment of the situation: Might this problem become more serious? Is the patient oversedated? Would intravenous fluid be useful? Does the patient need suctioning?

Procedure-related complications such as syncope may occur after discharge. To minimize these risks, patients should be monitored in the suite until they are approaching their baseline cognitive function, reevaluated by a member of the care-giving team, and discharged in the presence of an adult companion.

Perforation

Perforation is a potentially life-threatening complication. Fortunately it is rare, and often avoidable. A high index of suspicion and early diagnosis will minimize morbidity. The reported incidence of colonoscopic perforation ranges from 1/1000 to 1/10,000 procedures. Perforation is approximately seven times more likely during a therapeutic than a diagnostic procedure. Risk factors include acute colitis, previous pelvic surgery, colonic dilation, diverticulitis, obstruction, connective tissue disorders such as Ehlers–Danlos syndrome, and chronic steroid use. Many times, perforation is not recognized until the case is over, or even hours or days later. It must be considered in any post-colonoscopy patient who has persistent severe pain or marked abdominal distention, or develops significant abdominal complaints within days of the procedure.

Causes of colonoscopic perforations

- Tip of scope (rare)
- Shaft of scope
- Cecal blow-out
- Postpolypectomy or coagulation

Colon perforations

When recognized	Cause	Symptoms	Signs
During the procedure	Mechanical (scope/ snare)	Pain None, if patient sedated	Non-luminal view Failure of colon to distend Visible tear Inordinate abdominal distension Cardiopulmonary instability
In recovery room	Mechanical	Persistent abdominal pain Distension (unrelieved by usual maneuvers) Nausea	Inordinate tenderness/peritoneal signs Distension Failure to expel gas Failure to take p.o./nausea/vomiting Cardiopulmonary instability
<24 hours later	Mechanical or cautery	Persistent pain Anorexia Nausea Fever	Tenderness and peritoneal signs (may be localized) Inordinate distension
>24 hours later	Cautery	New and increasing abdominal pain, nausea, distension, etc.	New tenderness (may be localized) Peritoneal signs Inordinate distension

Types of perforation

Because the colon wall is compliant and the tip of the scope blunt, it is unusual for the tip of the endoscope to cause a perforation. Intra-abdominal adhesions that "fix" the colon raise this risk. More commonly, perforation occurs when the radial pressure created by a large "loop" of the scope exceeds the tensile strength of the

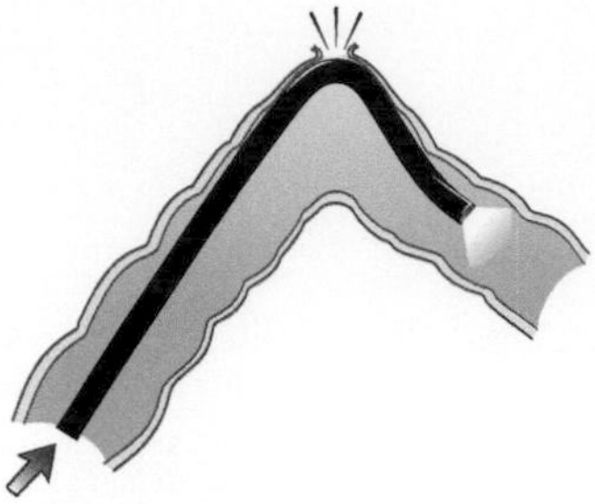

Fig 14.1 Perforation may occur from an expanding loop. As the loop stretches the colon wall, a tear due to radial force may occur at the bend of the scope. Because the injury is not at the scope tip, it will not be immediately visualized in the endoscopic image. If the scope does not advance despite reasonable axial force, the examiner should always withdraw and utilize another maneuver.

muscularis propria (Fig 14.1). This causes a longitudinal split along the antimesenteric surface, most commonly in the sigmoid colon. To minimize this risk, it is essential never to push against a fixed resistance. These perforations may go undetected during insertion because they occur in a portion of the colon that the scope has already passed (i.e. distal to the viewing lens). In some cases, during scope withdrawal the examiner will actually see structures in the peritoneal cavity when the scope tip protrudes through the rent in the wall.

Rarely, air insufflation can cause a barotrauma-related "blow out" in the cecum. The cecum is the thinnest-walled and largest diameter segment of colon; thus the muscular resistance is least and the radial pressures generated by air insufflation are greatest. Cecal barotrauma may occur during attempted passage through a narrowed sigmoid colon when air is given continuously but the tip fails to negotiate that segment (see Fig 6.12). The narrowing functions as a one-way valve. The air passes through, causing a marked rise in proximal intraluminal pressure, resulting in a right colon perforation although the scope may not have been inserted past the sigmoid colon.

Polypectomy can result in immediate perforation from transecting the muscularis propria or entire colon wall during snare closure (Fig 14.2).

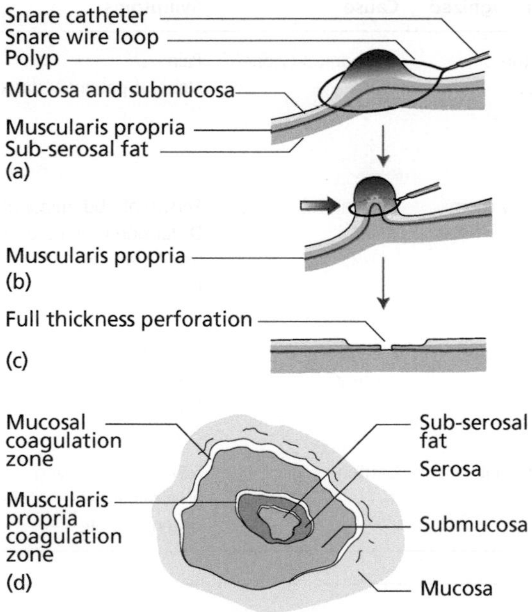

Fig 14.2 Perforation during snare transection of large sessile polyps. If the closing snare entraps muscularis propria (a,b) a transmural injury (c) may occur. This injury may occur despite the use of saline lift technique. Examination of the postpolypectomy defect (d) may disclose a characteristic pattern (the "target" sign). Note the presence of three white rings representing three distinct coagulation zones (mucosa, muscularis propria, and serosa) When promptly identified, the perforation may be repaired endoscopically with clips.

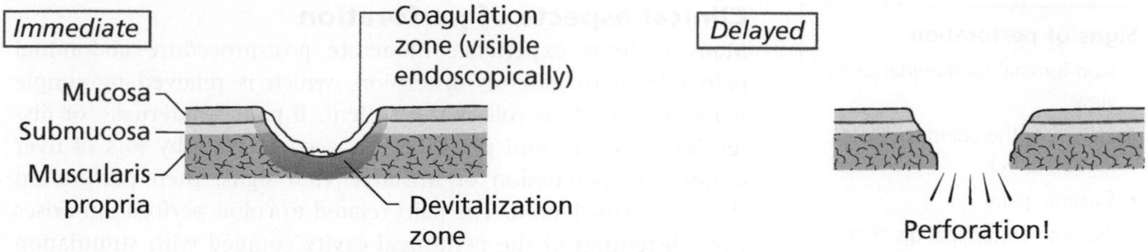

Fig 14.3 Delayed perforation. If the devitalization zone involves the entire colonic wall, delayed necrosis of this zone may result in perforation.

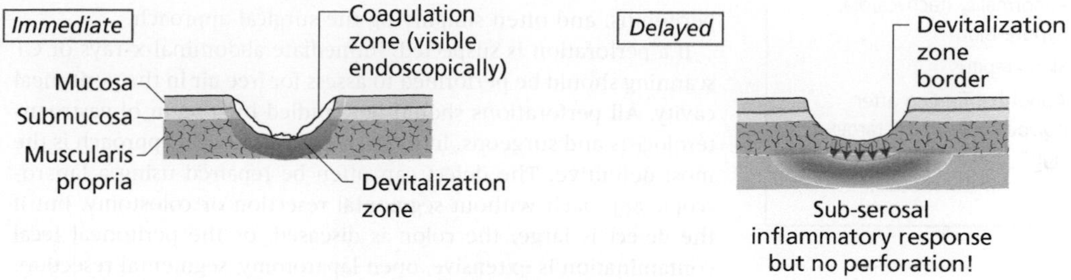

Fig 14.4 Post-polypectomy syndrome. This clinical presentation may result if the devitalization zone involves the entire wall but the structural integrity of the wall is not lost, or if the subserosal tissues contain the defect.

Delayed postpolypectomy perforation, which can occur hours or days later, typically results from full thickness thermal injury and subsequent devitalization of the colon wall (Figs 14.3 and 14.4). Polypectomy performed by endoscopic submucosal dissection is associated with an approximately 5% incidence of perforation; the majority of these perforations are small and immediately recognizable as a black hole in the defect that replaces the expected glistening white matrix of the muscularis propria fibers. Often, this complication can be managed by immediately clipping the defect. Forceps biopsy rarely captures sufficient tissue to create a full thickness excavation of the colon wall. There are case reports of biopsy-induced perforation, and this complication intuitively should be more likely in a colitic or dilated colon, in a thin-walled portion of the colon such as the cecum, or with larger forceps.

Reducing perforation risk

- Do not push against a fixed resistance
- Do not exert undue axial force; if scope tip is not advancing readily, change strategies (e.g. reposition the patient)
- Reduce loops
- In severe colitis, minimize extent of colonic intubation (or postpone procedure)
- Use saline lift for large flat polyps
- In narrowed diverticular sigmoid, avoid overinsufflation, and/or switch to narrow-caliber scope
- In patient with colonic obstruction/dilated proximal colon, minimize air insufflation
- If colonoscopy cannot be completed despite appropriate efforts, refer for "completion" CTC
- Check electrocautery settings before applying
- Avoid overly prolonged application of electrocautery

Signs of perforation

- Non-luminal (abdominal cavity) view
- Failure of the colon to "hold" insufflated air
- Extreme pain
- Extreme abdominal distension/tympany (e.g. loss of liver dullness)
- Sustained hemodynamic abnormality (tachycardia, hypotension)
- Skin crepitus
- Abnormal finding after polypectomy (e.g. "target sign" or black hole in the center of the mucosal defect)

Managing an acute perforation: Steps

1. Identify perforation promptly (from clinical and/or endoscopic signs)
2. Call for help
3. Stabilize patient
   a. Hemodynamic support
   b. Ventilatory support
   c. Analgesia/sedation
4. If defect small and situation amenable, clip shut colonoscopically
5. If occurs outside hospital, arrange emergency transfer and mobilize appropriate teams (Surgery, Emergency Department, etc.)
6. Inform patient's family/companion
7. Determine with consultants appropriate definitive management strategy

Clinical aspects of perforation

Many patients experience moderate post-procedure abdominal pain related to gaseous distension, which is relieved by simple maneuvers such as rolling the patient. If pain, tenderness, or distension is severe and persistent, or accompanied by loss of liver dullness to percussion or unstable vital signs, then perforation should be considered. The pain related to colon perforation arises from distention of the peritoneal cavity coupled with stimulation of peritoneal membrane pain chemoreceptors by spilled intraluminal contents. Colon cleansing in preparation for the colonoscopy decreases fecal contamination, decreasing the risk of florid bacterial peritonitis, and often simplifying the surgical approach.

If a perforation is suspected, immediate abdominal x-rays or CT scanning should be performed to assess for free air in the peritoneal cavity. All perforations should be handled by a team of gastroenterologists and surgeons. In most cases, the surgical approach is the most definitive. The defect can often be repaired using a laparoscopic approach without segmental resection or colostomy, but if the defect is large, the colon is diseased, or the peritoneal fecal contamination is extensive, open laparotomy, segmental resection, and diversion may be life-saving. If the perforation is extremely small and localized, a conservative approach (i.e. antibiotics, bowel rest, and close observation) may be effective, but the team must be prepared to convert to a surgical approach if the clinical situation dictates. On occasion, acute perforations may be addressed during colonoscopy by placing clips across the defect. This approach is useful when the defect is small and readily identified, such as during endoscopic submucosal dissection. Perforations that present hours or days after the procedure are more likely to require surgical intervention.

If the perforation occurs on the mesenteric side of the colon or in a retroperitoneal location, air can track through the retroperitoneal tissues. The patient may develop evidence of soft tissue air, such as neck and facial and scrotal swelling or crepitus, as well as pneumothorax and pneumomediastinum. A pneumothorax often prompts endotracheal intubation, and chest tube placement may be life-saving. Emergency evacuation of intraperitoneal gas using blind insertion of a wide-bore needle into the tensely distended abdomen may be required. However, if the air is in the soft tissues and not in the abdominal cavity, then a conservative approach, using antibiotics, bowel rest, and observation, may be successful.

Postpolypectomy coagulation syndrome

On occasion, a patient will present hours to days after polypectomy with localized abdominal pain, fever, and leukocytosis but imaging studies show no free intra-abdominal air. CT may reveal marked edema of the polypectomy site with localized peri-colonic inflammation. This is the result of full-thickness burn injury to the colon wall. Patients with mild pain and little fever can be managed outside of the hospitalization with oral antibiotics, restricted diet, and close communication with the physician. Those with more severe pain and fever should be observed in the hospital with bowel rest, intravenous antibiotics, and frequent physical examinations and radiographs to assess for a perforation. In general, this syndrome resolves in 2 to 5 days.

Hemorrhage

Bleeding related to colonoscopy is most often associated with a therapeutic intervention, most commonly polypectomy. The incidence of bleeding after polypectomy may be as high as 1 in 200, and is higher with larger polyps and polyps in the right colon. Bleeding can occur during the procedure, immediately afterward, or it may be delayed. Early bleeding is a result of inadequate cauterization of nutrient vessels and can usually be readily remedied endoscopically. Late hemorrhage occurs when the clot or coagulum on a vessel has dislodged or the zone of thermal necrosis has excavated into a blood vessel. Late bleeding most often presents with blood per rectum and/or the signs and symptoms of acute blood loss, and can occur any time from a few hours to 21 days after polypectomy. Late bleeding is always a therapeutic challenge and accounts for about one-third of all bleeding episodes.

Because the biopsy forceps avulses superficial tissue, which contains very small-caliber blood vessels that normally clot within seconds of disruption, significant bleeding after forceps biopsy is extremely rare, even in the setting of antiplatelet drugs or anticoagulants. Not infrequently, a biopsy causes a blue intramucosal hematoma, but this invariably self-tamponades.

Approach to delayed postpolypectomy bleeding

- Obtain targeted history (e.g. How many bloody bowel movements? Estimated amount of blood passed, lightheadedness? Comorbidities, use of antiplatelets or anticoagulants?)
- Hold nonsteroidal anti-inflammatories, aspirin, anticoagulants?
- Observation vs. intervention
- Observation
  - Close communication between patient and endoscopy team
  - Companion with patient
- Colonoscopy (consider rapid prep)

Polypectomy-related bleeding: Colonoscopic interventions

- Prevention of bleeding related to polypectomy
  - Use of cautery
  - Inject polyp with dilute epinephrine
  - Place loop around stalk or clip over site
- Treatment of bleeding during polypectomy
  - If residual polyp is bleeding: complete polypectomy
  - Cauterize
  - Inject epinephrine
  - Place clip
- Treatment of post-polypectomy bleeding from site
  - Electrocautery
  - Inject epinephrine (1 : 10,000)
  - Endoscopic clip
  - Arteriography + embolization
  - Surgical segmental resection

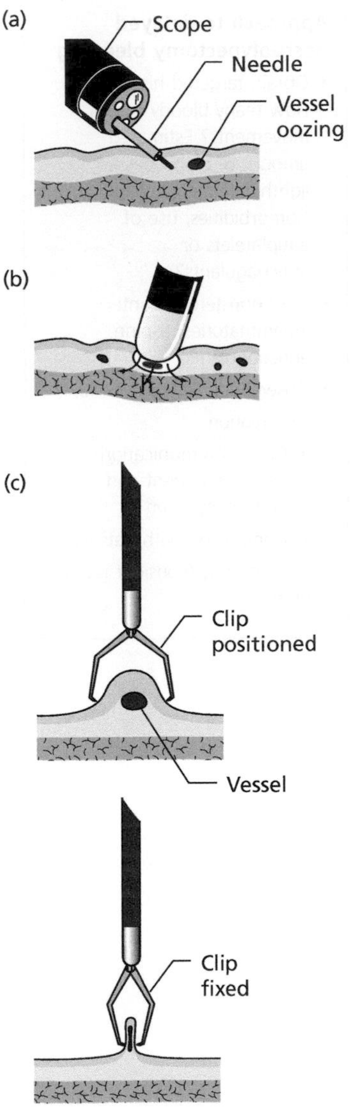

Fig 14.5 Endoscopic treatment of postpolypectomy bleeding. The bleeding site may be injected with dilute epinephrine (a), which can induce transient hemostasis. Definitive hemostasis requires coaptive coagulation treated with a thermal modality (b), and/or clipping (c) of the culprit vessel.

Prevention of bleeding

The guidelines for antiplatelet and anticoagulant drug management around the time of colonoscopy should be followed. The use of cautery during polypectomy is the principal modality used to prevent bleeding. If submucosal fluid is injected, some endoscopists add epinephrine to the solution. Large pedunculated polyps have a large vessel in the stalk, so some endoscopists inject the stalk with epinephrine prior to removal; this may also shrink the size of a polyp.) Another approach is to encircle the pedicle with a detachable nylon loop, which, when tightened, functions as a tourniquet. As a practical matter, however, the plastic loops are rather floppy and may become enmeshed in the interstices of the polyp, which makes positioning the loop around the pedicle a challenge. Following resection, in the presence of a conspicuous visible vessel, many colonoscopists will prophylactically clip the site, even if the site is dry.

Management of immediate postpolypectomy bleeding

Although a small amount of blood may be seen after polypectomy, most of the time the site is fairly dry. A small amount of bleeding may also be seen after "cold snare" resection of small polyps, but this is almost always self-limited and can simply be observed until the bleeding has ceased. During piecemeal polypectomy, minor bleeding can be adequately controlled by snare removal of the remainder of the lesion. Rarely, polypectomy can be transiently interrupted in order to stop bleeding. Bleeding can be addressed by injecting dilute epinephrine solution (1 : 10,000), which vasoconstricts and tamponades vessels; applying a clip, which pinches the bleeding vessel shut; or cauterizing the bleeding site, which heat-seals the vessel (Fig 14.5 and Video Clips 14.1, 14.2, and 14.3). Often these techniques are used in combination. Epinephrine injection offers a less enduring and thus less definitive benefit than the other techniques, but may slow bleeding so that the endoscopist can better visualize the field and precisely use cautery or a clip.

Management of delayed postpolypectomy bleeding

After colonoscopy, minor rectal bleeding is common as a result of anal irritation from the bowel preparation or the scope, hemorrhoidal inflammation, or minor oozing from a polypectomy or biopsy site. The significance of the bleeding can be assessed by targeted questions: Do you feel weak or dizzy? Did the blood fill the toilet bowl? Did this happen once or several times?

If the clinical significance of the bleeding is not clear, the colonoscopist must decide whether the patient should return immediately to the endoscopy unit or hospital for management. Blood is a potent cathartic, so significant intraluminal bleeding results in multiple, rapid, bloody bowel movements. If a patient reports only one or two bloody bowel movements, and has no further bowel activity, there may be no need for further intervention other than ongoing patient–physician communication. Bleeding is generally more troubling if the polypectomy site was on the right side of the colon (as it takes more or faster bleeding from the right colon to cause bright red blood per rectum) or if the patient is elderly, has multiple comorbidities, uses antiplatelet or anticoagulant agents, or lives alone.

Most postpolypectomy bleeding will stop with supportive care. Therefore, if the clinical situation will allow it, a period of close observation is reasonable. Commonsensical factors favoring observation include stable vital signs, a limited number and volume of bloody bowel movements, and relatively stable hemoglobin. If these criteria are not met, repeat colonoscopy should be performed.

If a physician who did not do the index polypectomy performs the emergency colonoscopy, information regarding the original polypectomy is useful. In some circumstances, it may be reasonable to attempt a look into an unprepped colon, particularly if the bleeding site is known and if the bleeding is not torrential (Video Clip 14.4). Although frequent bowel activity usually cleanses the distal colon of any potentially explosive gas concentrations, it is safest to avoid a spark-generating electrosurgical modality for treatment. More acceptable options in this setting are: epinephrine injection, clips, heater probe, or bipolar thermal device. In many cases, however, it is preferable to administer a rapid whole-gut lavage (via nasogastric tube, if necessary) to optimize visualization of the site.

In general, if the colon is reasonably clean, it is almost always possible to identify the bleeding site. If brown stool is encountered in the proximal colon, it is a clue that the bleeding site is distal. If the patient underwent numerous snare polypectomies, the bleeding may (surprisingly) not be from the biggest site or from the site of the polyp that was most difficult to resect. In some cases, active bleeding is noted, whereas in others, an eschar, red spot, vessel, or clot at the site will identify the culprit lesion. If the bleeding area is identified but blood flowing from the site obscures its precise origin, irrigation should be used to clear the field and permit visualization. It is important to pinpoint the bleeding site because precisely targeted treatments are more effective and lower risk. In general, if the bleeding has been significant, the benefits of treatment of the bleeding site outweigh the risks, even if active bleeding is not occurring.

When colonoscopic management of bleeding fails

Rarely, the postpolypectomy bleeding is so torrential that the site cannot be localized, or cannot be stopped with endoscopic therapy. In this circumstance, arteriography with embolization may be a good treatment option, especially if the approximate location of the resection site is known. When all other approaches fail, segmental resection of the affected colon is indicated.

Rare complications of colonoscopy

Severe abdominal pain accompanied by peritoneal signs after colonoscopy does not always portend colonic perforation. Splenic rupture or hemorrhage may be caused by traction on the splenocolic ligament, by direct pressure on the spleen by a distended loop of the colonoscope, or by inherent disease of the spleen. Symptoms and signs are often delayed for several hours and imaging modalities (ultrasound or CT scan) are required to make this diagnosis. More than one-half of patients will require splenectomy.

Systemic infectious complications such as infective endocarditis are extremely rare. Antibiotic prophylaxis for colonoscopy is no longer widely recommended. Acute bacterial peritonitis after colonoscopy in patients with ascites is extraordinarily rare.

Intra-abdominal bleeding from rupture of mesenteric vessels is extremely rare. Acute appendicitis, acute cholecystitis, and renal colic can all be seen after colonoscopy. These sequelae may result from fluid shifts, fasting, perturbation of the colonic flora, or other factors. Chemical colitis can occur from incomplete rinsing of disinfectant solution during equipment processing.

Complications related to the bowel preparation

Most complications related to the bowel preparation are minor—e.g. nausea, bloating, malaise, vomiting, or mild dehydration. Rarely a patient will experience syncope related to the bowel preparation, which can result in a fall and potentially a significant injury. In general, maintaining hydration minimizes this.

Phosphate-based bowel preparations can cause renal injury—including chronic renal failure and dialysis dependency—owing to the precipitation of phosphate crystals in the renal tubules. This complication is more common in individuals with comorbid conditions or concurrent medications that impact kidney function, but may occur idiosyncratically. As a result, phosphate-based preparations, despite their convenience, have fallen out of favor.

The OTC PEG 3350-based bowel preparation (MiraLax) is not osmotically balanced and has been associated with electrolyte abnormalities and generalized seizure.

How to prevent patient falls

- Put side rail up immediately after case is over
- Make sure patient is fully recovered before allowing patient to walk and leave endoscopy center; make sure patient leaves with escort
- Utilize safety belt during every case
- Train assistant to observe patient throughout sedation and recovery period and regarding risk of sedation-related falls

Immediate post-procedural abdominal pain due to intraluminal gas

Post-colonoscopy pain due to intraluminal gas is common. This problem can be minimized by evacuating air during scope withdrawal. Insufflating CO_2 (which is rapidly absorbed into the bloodstream across the mucosa) rather than room air into the colon decreases post-procedure pain, but this approach has not been widely adopted. To aid in expelling air, the patient should roll from the left decubitus to the right decubitus position to have the sigmoid area uppermost and allow air to rise and be evacuated. The prone position is preferred by some endoscopists and the knee-to-chest prone position may also be effective. Sometimes, the only solution is time.

Summary

Properly performed, colonoscopy is an extremely safe procedure. Rarely, serious and even life-threatening complications occur, including bowel perforation, hemorrhage, and cardiopulmonary adverse events. Some of these are avoidable with scrupulous technique and management, but some are unavoidable. Every colonoscopist must be familiar with the important risks, identify complications promptly, and be prepared to manage them.

Further reading

1. ASGE Standards of Practice Committee, Fisher DA, Maple JT, *et al.* Complications of colonoscopy. *Gastrointest Endosc* 2011;74:745–52.
2. Day LW, Kwon A, Inadomi JM, Walter LC, Somsouk M. Adverse events in older patients undergoing colonoscopy: a systematic review and meta-analysis. *Gastrointest Endosc* 2011;74:885–96.
3. Lüning TH, Keemers-Gels ME, Barendregt WB, Tan AC, Rosman C. Colonoscopic perforations: a review of 30 366 patients. *Surg Endosc* 2007;21:994–7.
4. Metz AJ, Bourke MJ, Moss A, Williams SJ, Swan MP, Byth K. Factors that predict bleeding following endoscopic mucosal resection of large colonic lesions. *Endoscopy* 2011;43:506–11.
5. Panteris V, Haringsma J, Kuipers EJ. Colonoscopy perforation rate, mechanisms and outcome: from diagnostic to therapeutic colonoscopy. *Endoscopy* 2009;41:941–51.
6. Rabeneck L, Paszat LF, Hilsden RJ, *et al.* Bleeding and perforation after outpatient colonoscopy and their risk factors in usual clinical practice. *Gastroenterology* 2008;135:1899–1906.
7. Rotholtz NA, Laporte M, Lencinas S, Bun M, Canelas A, Mezzadri N. Laparoscopic approach to colonic perforation due to colonoscopy. *World J Surg* 2010;34:1949–53.
8. Rutter CM, Johnson E, Miglioretti DL, Mandelson MT, Inadomi J, Buist DS. Adverse events after screening and follow-up colonoscopy. *Cancer Causes Control* 2012;23:289–96.
9. Singh H, Penfold RB, De Coster C, Au W, Bernstein CN, Moffatt M. Predictors of serious complications associated with lower gastrointestinal endoscopy in a major city-wide health region. *Can J Gastroenterol* 2010;24:425–430.
10. Swan MP, Bourke MJ, Moss A, Williams SJ, Hopper A, Metz A. The target sign: an endoscopic marker for the resection of the muscularis propria and potential perforation during colonic endoscopic mucosal resection. *Gastrointest Endosc* 2011;73:79–85.

Chapter video clips

Video Clip 14.1 Giant rectal polyp with bleeding
Snare resection of giant rectal polyp complicated by post-polypectomy hemorrhage, managed colonoscopically.

Video Clip 14.2 Immediate postpolypectomy bleeding: sessile polyp
Arterial bleeding seen following snare polypectomy. Clip placement used to achieve hemostasis.

Video Clip 14.3 Immediate postpolypectomy bleeding: pedunculated polyp
Bleeding from pedicle of polyp is controlled with compression and with clip placement.

Video Clip 14.4 Delayed postpolypectomy bleeding
Unprepped colonoscopy used for identification and treatment of bleeding site several days following ascending colon polypectomy.

SECTION 4
Current and Future Considerations

CHAPTER 15

Quality in Colonoscopy

Introduction

A high-quality colonoscopy, when appropriately indicated, results in accurate diagnosis and proper therapeutic intervention, and confers minimal risk. Colonoscopy quality, as measured by adenoma detection, complications, and adherence to guidelines, varies widely among colonoscopists. This impacts effectiveness, safety, and cost.

Colonoscopy continuous quality improvement (CQI) initiatives are designed to identify and correct underperformance. In these initiatives, a quality end point (e.g. adenoma detection rate) is measured, and the performance of the individual is compared to published external benchmarks (e.g. national published standards) and/or to internal practice data (e.g. comparison to peers). If an underperforming colonoscopist is identified, an intervention (e.g. enforcing a scope withdrawal time of >6 minutes) is made. The end point is then remeasured.

CQI programs are imperfect. For example, the commonly utilized numerical cutoffs for appropriate performance (e.g. adenoma detection rate >25%) are not validated and may vary depending on the practice's patient demographics. CQI programs are also at times unpopular. On balance, however: they improve quality; the endoscopy professional societies promote them; third-party payers have instituted financial rewards if quality benchmarks are met (so called "pay-for-performance"); and increasingly, patients request quality data of their colonoscopist, and such data can also serve as a marketing tool.

Today's colonoscopist has many tools to help measure quality: entire colonoscopies can be easily and inexpensively video-recorded for peer review; endoscopic photography techniques allow photodocumentation of cecal landmarks and all relevant pathology; cardiopulmonary monitoring devices electronically capture data regarding the patient's clinical status throughout the procedure; electronic medical record databases permit easy analysis of a large number of variables for a large number of procedure.

In colonoscopy (as in other fields) the simple act of measuring quality improves it. For example, videotaping a colonoscopy for the purposes of quality review increases scope withdrawal time. Unfortunately, the benefit of quality reviews or even linking physician reimbursement to quality metrics is variable. It is not easy to turn a low polyp detector into a high polyp detector. In some studies, improvement is only temporary. CQI programs must monitor quality end points episodically throughout the lifetime of the practice.

Specific quality metrics in colonoscopy

For colorectal cancer screening and surveillance, the most important clinical quality end points are *major complication rate* and *"interval" cancer incidence rate*. An "interval cancer" can be defined as a cancer that occurs between surveillance colonoscopies or within a specified interval (e.g. 3 years) after a "clearing" colonoscopy. Interval cancers can occur because of missed polyps or cancers, incompletely resected polyps, or *de novo* polyps with unusually rapid progression. Unfortunately, neither major complication rate nor interval cancer rate is routinely reported, in part because they are not simple to track. For example, if a patient develops a late post-polypectomy bleed, the management may fall to a different provider, and the first provider never learns about the complication. Likewise, a patient who develops a colorectal cancer 2.5 years after a colonoscopy may not report the development to the original colonoscopist. Nevertheless, all endoscopy units should attempt to track and analyze major complications and interval cancers.

Practical Colonoscopy, First Edition. Jerome D. Waye, James Aisenberg, and Peter H. Rubin.
© 2013 John Wiley & Sons, Ltd. Published 2013 by John Wiley & Sons, Ltd.

Practitioners are encouraged to track two *validated* "surrogate" end points that correlate with the effectiveness of colorectal cancer prevention: cecal intubation rate and adenoma detection rate. During each colonoscopy, cecal intubation should be documented in the written report and by endo-photographs of the cecal and/or ileal landmarks and in the narrative report. Cecal intubation rate should exceed 90–95%. *Adenoma detection rate* is more cumbersome to measure, as the colonoscopy report must be correlated with the pathology report. The appropriate target adenoma detection rate is a matter of some debate. The most widely quoted guidelines suggest that a rate of >25% in men and >15% in women over 50 years of age may be a reasonable starting point, although many experts suggest that this bar is set too low.

There are many other quality end points that can routinely and usefully be measured within any colonoscopy practice. These include:

1. *Time intervals for surveillance examinations.* Guidelines exist for the appropriate age for initiation of colonoscopic polyp detection (screening), as well as the timing for a follow-up colonoscopy (surveillance). Such guidelines exist also for screening and surveillance in patients with chronic ulcerative and Crohn's colitis.

2. *Procedure indications and informed consent.* Guidelines exist regarding appropriate indications for colonoscopy. Likewise, each colonoscopy requires documentation of informed consent, and this too can be measured.

3. *Scope withdrawal time* (cecum to anus). Withdrawal time correlates with adenoma detection rate. In general, withdrawal time should average >6 minutes, excluding the time taken to biopsy, clean the colon, or remove polyps. Withdrawal time is clocked by many endoscopy systems and electronic medical records. Of course the ideal withdrawal time varies from colon to colon (depending on colon length, tortuousness, etc.).

4. *Withdrawal technique.* This can be evaluated by real-time peer observation or review of videotapes. Criteria such as whether the colonoscopist systematically looked behind each fold, cleaned away debris, and took appropriate time to examine and reexamine each colonic segment, can be evaluated.

5. *Adherence to biopsy protocols.* In a 70-year-old woman with watery diarrhea and a normal appearing mucosa, forceps biopsies should have been obtained from the left and right side of the colon. In the patient with chronic ulcerative colitis undergoing surveillance, four-quadrant biopsies should have been taken every 10 cm. Rates of adherence to these and other standards can be analyzed.

6. *Serrated lesion detection rate.* Like adenomas, serrated lesions may be precursors to colorectal cancer. Several studies suggest that a "serrated lesion detection rate" of >5% is a reasonable quality benchmark.

7. *Quality of sedation and analgesia.* Patient satisfaction regarding the adequacy of sedation and analgesia can be readily measured by a simple exit interview survey. The quality of the sedation and analgesia can also be measured by assessing such variables as patient intraprocedural hemodynamics, gas exchange, depth of sedation, and minor adverse events (e.g. need for bag–mask ventilation).

8. *Patient satisfaction.* This can be measured using simple written satisfaction surveys, administered either at the time of departure from the office or a day or two later. Sample surveys are available through the endoscopic societies from online resources. Surveys address such issues as: Was the patient taken on time? Was the facility pleasant and clean? Was the staff courteous and friendly? Was the analgesia adequate? Before discharge, was there a reevaluation and discussion about diet, medication, warning signs, how pathology reports will be communicated, and follow-up?

9. *Quality of the colonoscopy report.* The colonoscopy report records and communicates the procedure. It may be difficult from the endoscopy report to determine whether an expert endoscopist or a person with little experience or training did the procedure. Unfortunately, some reporting is inadequate—illegible, unaccompanied by photographs, incomplete, superficial, and/or inaccurate. A sample of reports should be reviewed and compared to a "quality report checklist."

10. *Quality of nurse/anesthetist charting.* The nurse and/or anesthetist records the vital signs, medications, level of sedation, and other clinical parameters on the procedural flow sheet. The written record is often augmented by electronic data recorded by cardiopulmonary monitoring systems. The quality of the flow sheet can be readily evaluated.

11. *Timeliness of communication.* After colonoscopy, the patient and the referring physician expect to receive a timely communication regarding the results. The interval between procedure and communication with patient and with referring physician can be measured.

12. *Pathology turnaround time.* This is often the rate-limiting step in reporting. It is an important quality metric for pathology laboratories, and the colonoscopist should require timely service. In most centers, a turnaround time of 3 workdays or fewer is a reasonable starting point, unless special stains or additional sections are needed for definitive reporting.

13. *Bowel preparation quality.* The quality of the bowel preparation predicts procedure effectiveness. It can be easily measured using validated bowel preparation scales. Published benchmarks vary considerably, and results will vary according to the demographics of the patient population. Nonetheless, bowel preparation should be good or excellent in at least 70% of subjects.

Risk management

- Always obtain informed consent
- Informed consent is best obtained by the gastroenterologist
- Explain that polyps can be missed despite excellent technique
- Explain that interval carcinomas may occur; document this—e.g. "colonoscopy does not prevent all colorectal cancer"
- If the preparation is suboptimal, explain the implications to patient and where appropriate repeat colonoscopy
- Explain unavoidable rare major risks of bleeding and perforation
- Avoid phosphate-based cathartics
- Obtain signed documentation from the patient that they are ready for discharge
- Document withdrawal time
- Photo-document the cecum and ileum
- Collect personal adenoma detection rate
- Adhere to surveillance interval guidelines
- Use a computerized recall system
- Call the patient the day following the procedure

Endoscope reprocessing and infection control

Published guidelines establish the proper methods for cleaning and disinfection of endoscopes and the accessory instruments. Every major medical and nursing association concerned with gastrointestinal endoscopy has endorsed these guidelines. Unwavering adherence to these guidelines is essential, and careful, periodic review of instrument reprocessing policies and procedures is vital. All accredited facilities are subject to close scrutiny of the policies and procedures related to infection control during the accreditation inspections.

"High-level" disinfection is defined as destruction of all vegetative microorganisms, mycobacteria, small or non-lipid viruses, medium or lipid viruses, fungal spores, and some but not all bacterial spores. "Sterilization" is defined as destruction of all microbial life. For "semi-critical" devices, (such as flexible endoscopes) that come into contact with mucous membranes but do not have direct contact with sterile tissue (i.e. do not penetrate the epithelial barrier), "high-level" disinfection must be achieved. For, a critical device (such as a biopsy forceps or snare) that crosses the epithelial barrier and comes into contact with the bloodstream and the normally sterile subepithelial tissues, sterilization is required. Most accessory devices used during colonoscopy can be obtained as single-use instruments to be discarded after use in one patient, although some centers sterilize and reutilize forceps and snares.

Computer-controlled scope reprocessing machines ("scope-washers"), have become increasingly popular. However, much of the process remains in human hands. Cleaning requires careful training of personnel, fastidious adherence to protocols, and regular quality monitoring. High-level disinfection requires strict attention to mechanical cleansing. The outside of the scope and each interior channel is washed thoroughly, wiped with detergents, and brushed with cleaning instruments. The endoscope is then soaked for a predetermined amount of time and the channels are flushed repeatedly with a chemical that destroys the bacteria and viruses (including HIV and hepatitis viruses) known to infect humans. Following high-level disinfection, the instrument is rinsed and suspended to drain and dry.

When accepted guidelines are followed, the risk of transmission of infection is practically eliminated: infection is estimated to occur in 1 in 10 million endoscopic procedures. Every reported case of transmission of an infectious disease during an endoscopic procedure has been found to be the result of non-adherence to guidelines.

Quality metrics: Examples

- Indication for colonoscopy
- Quality/rate of documented informed consent
- Adherence to recommended surveillance intervals
- Rate of good to excellent bowel preparations
- Quality of procedure report
- Cecal intubation rate
- Photo-documentation of landmarks
- Adenoma detection rate
- Withdrawal time
- Biopsy specimens obtained in patients with chronic diarrhea
- Number and distribution of biopsy samples in ulcerative colitis and Crohn's colitis surveillance
- Rate of resection of large polyps at index colonoscopy (or documentation of the reason for non-resectability)
- Incidence of perforation
- Incidence of postpolypectomy bleeding
- Postpolypectomy bleeding managed nonoperatively
- Interval cancer rate
- Pathology turnaround time

Interventions designed to improve quality end points: Examples

Observation	Intervention
Poor-quality bowel preps	Implement split dosing Improve patient instructions Implement patient videos Contact patients the night before the procedure Use patient "navigator"
Low adenoma detection rate	Increase withdrawal time (use stopwatch; document) Peer review of colonoscopy videotapes Peer observation by high performer Improve bowel preps
Low cecal intubation rate	Peer observation by high performer Improve bowel preps Allow more time per colonoscopy Require that cecal landmarks be photographed Mid-career training regarding technique
High complication rate (colonoscopist related)	Peer observation by high performer Improve bowel preps Allow more time per colonoscopy Mid-career training regarding patient selection Mid-career training regarding technique
High complication rate (anesthesiologist related)	Change anesthesiologist Target shallower sedation Change monitoring methods Change medications utilized
Poor or delayed reporting and communications of results	Change pathology provider Enforce guidelines for proper procedure report Require immediate data entry at the time of the case Implement peer review

The endoscopy report and flow sheet

The medical record includes the procedure report and the pathology report, which are communicated to the patient and the referring physician, and the clinical flow sheets. A well-composed procedure report effectively communicates the findings of the case to all involved parties; it also serves as an important legal protection, an effective practice-marketing tool, and a searchable element in a database for clinical research or quality analysis. The report should include photo-documentation of the relevant normal and abnormal findings. The referring physician should be contacted and provided with a synopsis of the procedure, a diagnosis, how to handle anticoagulants and other medications, and when the patient should return for follow-up examination.

Relevant data that should be recorded in the procedure report and/or the flow sheet include the following.

- Pre-procedure
  - Patient identification
  - Names of endoscopist and other participants
  - Pertinent medical and surgical history and physical exam
  - The indication
  - The informed consent
  - Standing medications, including the timing of the last dose
  - The pre-procedure clinical parameters (e.g. vital signs)
- Intraprocedure
  - The instrument used
  - Extent of the exam (was the cecum/ileum reached?)
  - Quality of the bowel preparation
  - All abnormal findings (in the order that they are encountered)
  - Whether tissue was obtained
  - Medications administered
  - All specific characteristics of the case (time of procedure, hemodynamics, etc.)
  - For polyps, the size, location, shape, method of resection, and completeness of resection
  - All other interventions (dilation, carbon particle tattooing, etc.) and the results of these interventions
  - The diagnostic impression
  - The interpretation of abnormalities
  - Complications (if any)
  - Patient tolerance of the procedure
  - Withdrawal time
- Post-procedure
  - Post-procedure vital signs and recovery data
  - Documentation of readiness for discharge (signed by the patient)
  - Disposition
  - Pathological findings
  - Recommendations for further care

Optimizing the colonoscopy report

- Create it immediately following completion of colonoscopy (when fresh in the mind)
- Use a standardized format
- Report all recommended parameters (preparation quality, completeness, limitations, recommendations)
- Report common "incidental" findings (e.g. diverticulosis, hemorrhoids, etc.)
- Describe "problem" lesions (e.g. polyps in colitis) in meticulous detail (i.e. location, size, site, quality of resection, site of inking, etc)
- Photograph landmarks and important findings

The electronic colonoscopy record

- Advantages
  - Creates searchable database
    - For quality assessment
      - By individual provider
      - By group
      - By procedure type
    - For research
    - For practice management
  - Allows immediate paperless transmission of report to referring physician
  - Allows paperless storage of report and photographs
  - Enforces standardized reporting
  - Enhances compliance with coding
  - Legible
  - Easily accessible
- Disadvantages
  - May be challenging to master
  - Descriptive nuances may be lost due to use of template descriptors
  - Back-up of hard drive required
  - Cost

Summary

Quality in colonoscopy varies widely. Numerous metrics and tools are available to measure quality. Quality assessment in colonoscopy is increasingly emphasized by external parties and within the profession. All colonoscopy units should implement quality assessment measures.

Further reading

1. Adler A, Wegscheider K, Lieberman D, *et al.* Factors determining the quality of screening colonoscopy: a prospective study on adenoma detection rates, from 12 134 examinations (Berlin colonoscopy project 3, BECOP-3). *Gut* 2012. Epub ahead of print.
2. ASGE Standards of Practice Committee, Banerjee S, Shen B, *et al.* Infection control during GI endoscopy. *Gastrointest Endosc* 2008;67:781–90. Epub 2008 Mar 19.
3. ASGE Quality Assurance In Endoscopy Committee, Petersen BT, Chennat J, *et al.* Multisociety guideline on reprocessing flexible gastrointestinal endoscopes: 2011. *Gastrointest Endosc* 2011;73:1075–84.
4. Barclay RL, Vicari JJ, Doughty AS, Johanson JF, Greenlaw RL. Colonoscopic withdrawal times and adenoma detection during screening colonoscopy. *N Engl J Med* 2006;355:2533–41.
5. de Jonge V, Sint Nicolaas J, Cahen DL, *et al.* Quality evaluation of colonoscopy reporting and colonoscopy performance in daily clinical practice. *Gastrointest Endosc* 2012;75:98–106. Epub 2011 Sep 10.
6. Kaminski MF, Regula J, Kraszewska E, *et al.* Quality indicators for colonoscopy and the risk of interval cancer. *N Engl J Med* 2010;362:1795–803.
7. Moritz V, Bretthauer M, Ruud HK, *et al.* Withdrawal time as a quality indicator for colonoscopy - a nationwide analysis. *Endoscopy* 2012;44:476–81. Epub 2012 Apr 24.
8. Palmer LB, Abbott DH, Hamilton N, Provenzale D, Fisher DA. Quality of colonoscopy reporting in community practice. *Gastrointest Endosc* 2010;72:321–7, 327.e1. Epub 2010 Jun 29.
9. Rex DK, Petrini JL, Baron TH, *et al.* Quality indicators for colonoscopy. *Am J Gastroenterol* 2006;101: 873–85.
10. Winawer SJ, Zauber AG, Fletcher RH, *et al.* Guidelines for colonoscopy surveillance after polypectomy: a consensus update by the US Multi-Society Task Force on Colorectal Cancer and the American Cancer Society. *CA Cancer J Clin* 2006;56:143–59; quiz 184–5.

CHAPTER 16

Teaching and Training in Colonoscopy

Introduction and background

The current challenge in colonoscopy training is to produce a cohort of endoscopists who are capable of meeting both the increased demands for colonoscopy and the rising standards for procedure quality. Upon completion of training they must be comfortable handling large sessile polyps, obstructing colorectal tumors, dysplasia in inflammatory bowel disease, and other procedural and cognitive challenges that arise commonly in the endoscopy suite. Teaching colonoscopy is intrinsically difficult and costly, requiring significant time and endoscopy unit overhead, skilled mentors who can verbalize complex motor and cognitive skills and provide ongoing support to the trainee, and repetitive hands-on practice involving live human subjects whose interests must at all times be protected.

Unfortunately, as a result of rising health-care costs, the resources allotted to training are shrinking in many centers. Compounding the challenge is the lack of standardization of training methods or goals, and the great variability in aptitude among both trainers and trainees. Beyond the burden of training new endoscopists is the need to update the knowledge of already trained colonoscopists, so that they are made proficient in the newer advances in imaging technologies and accessories. To meet these challenges both students and educators recognize the importance of skilled, live training and take advantage of enhanced learning technology such as Internet-based sites and simulators.

Broadly speaking, colonoscopy training occurs in phases. The first phase occurs during post-graduate residency and fellowship training programs. Here the goal is to achieve a "core competency," defined as that level of skill, knowledge, and proficiency at which the provider is able to perform colonoscopy safely and efficiently and achieve the community standard of care. The second phase involves acquisition of expertise. This process occurs through continuous practice, and has been estimated (like other complex learning, such as that required to master a musical instrument) to take at least 10 years. During the first phase, the learning curve is steep; during the second phase, the learning curve continues to rise, but

Practical Colonoscopy, First Edition. Jerome D. Waye, James Aisenberg, and Peter H. Rubin.
© 2013 John Wiley & Sons, Ltd. Published 2013 by John Wiley & Sons, Ltd.

more gradually. Most experts recognize that this second phase is life-long, especially in view of the evolving knowledge and technology within the field.

In the USA, colonoscopy is performed by gastroenterologists, surgeons, family practitioners, and (less frequently) nurse practitioners or physician assistants. The intensity of colonoscopy training within the training programs for these different groups varies considerably. Endoscopy training programs are offered in academic teaching centers for fellows in gastroenterology programs, as well as for surgeons undergoing general or colorectal surgery training. Under close supervision, the trainee typically performs hundreds of colonoscopies, admixed with sigmoidoscopy and many complex endoscopic procedures. There is considerable evidence that the intensity of training and the subspecialty of the trainee correlates with the mid-career proficiency of the colonoscopist.

The process of learning to do colonoscopy is in many respects similar to learning to drive a car or fly a plane: the student begins with didactic lessons, may advance to simulators, but eventually, under the close supervision of an experienced teacher, must take over the controls in a real-life situation. There is no teaching aid that can reproduce the navigational challenge of: the contracting, twisting, convoluted colon; the stress created by the breathing, stirring, vocalizing human subject; or the varying resistance of the scope as the practitioner pushes through a tight, tortuous sigmoid colon. Colonoscopy requires hand–eye coordination and interdependent actions of the limbs and torso, while multiple judgments are made in real time. The bulk of learning must occur by performing the procedure on a real patient.

Costs of training: safety and economic issues

An "efficient" endoscopy unit, in which cases are performed as quickly as possible, is incompatible with the needs of a training program. Because the training involves human subjects, patient safety must be protected. Adverse events occur more frequently during training colonoscopy than when performed by mid-career endoscopists. In training centers, endoscopy unit protocols must monitor adverse outcomes carefully and institute specific protections. These include: strict supervision requirements; training protocols (e.g. standards dictating when the trainer should "take the scope" during a difficult case); ethical informed consent policies (i.e. the patient is aware that a trainee is participating in the case); carefully selected and well-trained instructors; adequate time allocation for procedures; up-to-date, well-maintained instruments; and early and frequent trainee feedback and competency assessment programs.

Colonoscopy training is inherently financially costly. These costs relate to: the increased length of training procedures (estimated to last at least 30% longer than non-training cases); the increased physician and non-physician labor hours (i.e. the need for a high-level supervising instructor, perhaps an anesthesiologist, and a nurse or endoscopy assistant for the entirety of the longer case); the inevitable delays in endoscopy unit scheduling related to the unpredictable time requirements of novices; the increased use of ancillary equipment (e.g. imaging equipment to visualize the scope location); the cost of any adverse events related to the procedure; and perhaps the need for a larger room to accommodate extra personnel. Unfortunately, these economic costs are generally underestimated and certainly under-reimbursed. Thus, teaching unit budgets are becoming increasingly strained.

Principles for successful hands-on colonoscopy training

The following are helpful tips that promote successful hands-on colonoscopy training.

- *Schedule adequate time per case.* Inevitably, training cases take longer than non-training cases, and a rushed novice will become flustered and unable to learn. It is reasonable to allocate 1 hour per colonoscopy teaching case, especially at the beginning of the academic year.
- *Create a culture in the endoscopy unit that values training.* The training of novices adds stress and risk to a procedure that is stressful to begin with. If the unit values throughput over teaching, the tension will only rise.
- *Engage ancillary personnel as well as physicians in the teaching mission.* Colonoscopy should be collaborative: nurses and assistants should be encouraged to support the teaching mission, to share their experience and knowledge with trainees, and to take pride in their accomplishments.
- *Carefully select patients for training.* In the initial novice training, an "easy colon" should be the target, although in many units the trainee must perform the procedure for whichever patient is "next on the list." Where possible, select younger, healthy patients, or patients undergoing surveillance who are known to have normal colonic anatomy or have had no prior abdominal or pelvic surgery.
- *Choose the trainers carefully.* Some experienced endoscopists as well as some just having completed fellowship are natural trainers who receive high ratings from the trainees, and derive satisfaction from training. Others view training as onerous or do not have the patience or ability to be an effective teacher of the fledgling colonoscopist.
- *Train the trainers.* Teaching colonoscopy involves translating the "unconscious competence" of the trainers into "conscious competence." This requires educators to analyze and articulate the behaviors that have made them successful. The less-effective or less-experienced instructors can learn a great deal by being paired with an expert teacher during routine teaching sessions.
- *The instructors must always consider that their primary responsibility is to the patient and that the teaching aspect is secondary.*

- *Like most challenging skills, colonoscopy is best taught by regular, sustained, practice, rather than as a "crash course."* For example, three 2-hour teaching sessions per week over 2 years is preferable to full-day teaching on consecutive days packed into 3–6 months. The training curriculum should be designed accordingly.

The actual performance of colonoscopy consists of a myriad of subskills, which can be taught individually by separating the procedure into component parts. During a training procedure, each of these skills should be identified as the opportunity presents itself. For example, trainees inevitably suction mucosa into the suction channel because the tip of the scope is not positioned correctly. When this occurs, stop and take a moment to explain to the trainee how to properly avoid this error. Another example is that often trainees translate the stress during colonoscopy into tense muscles, body contortions, and poor posture. This is not perceived by the student but is readily observed and easily corrected by demonstrating a relaxed, ergonomically sound body position. If the trainee is struggling and repeating an unsuccessful maneuver the instructor should call a pause and encourage consideration of alternative tactics.

During the early phases of instruction, a teacher's constant monologue will serve to form a mental matrix of possibilities to the student. Eventually, the student will internalize this monologue, and independently conduct it either privately or out loud. This can be modified as the learning curve progresses and the student performs the necessary actions spontaneously and thus moves from the state of conscious incompetence into conscious competence. The trainee's learning is compromised if the trainer dons gloves and takes over each time a frustrating colonoscopic problem arises. However, if the trainee is allowed to struggle for too long, trainee confidence, unit morale, and patient safety may suffer. The astute instructor can usually verbally steer the student into the correct movements to "self-adjust" the problem. As experience progresses, the verbal interventions can diminish while encouraging the student to explain what processes are being considered while maneuvering the instrument. When a difficult situation arises, the teacher may physically stand alongside the novice trainee demonstrating engagement and solidarity. This will facilitate communication and allow the trainer to use touch as well as words to teach positioning, posture, and scope handling.

During the progress of the case, the teacher should be enthusiastic and supportive, as most trainees are self-critical. This includes providing encouragement, good humor, and letting the student know that mistakes and frustrations are inevitable. The trainee must be told to be attentive to the remarks of others in the endoscopy suite, such as colleagues, nurses or endoscopy assistants (who are usually more experienced than the trainee) as their suggestions (e.g. Should we roll the patient onto the back? Would abdominal pressure help? What is that bump?) are often helpful. Casual chat among faculty or staff, background music, and other distractions should be discouraged. A laser pointer helps the instructor point out important findings on the endoscopic monitor. The instructor should stand to the right of the trainee in order to observe hand movements, while able to view the same endoscopic image as the student (Fig 16.1). When interesting findings are encountered, they should be video-recorded so they can later be shared at a divisional conference.

At every juncture, it is important to teach versatility. If one approach to a problem is not working, it should not be repeated. Instead, another technique should be attempted. There are usually several alternatives to solve a problem, and the student should be encouraged to think about these and enumerate them to the endoscopic instructor. Likewise, when confronted with a difficult problem many trainees will perform low-yield, non-purposeful, or (worse yet) needlessly forceful scope motions, rather than using creativity and finesse to solve the problem. The instructor should step in verbally at this point, and return the trainee to the logic-based algorithm. It is also important to impart strict, compulsive habits. For surveillance/screening colonoscopy to be maximally effective, every haustral fold and recess of the colon must be examined. This scrutiny, usually occurring during scope withdrawal, although at times tedious, must be meticulous and repetitive. The instructor must also teach finesse. Colonoscopy should be gentle. The trainee must be taught never to push through a fixed resistance, as this can cause perforation.

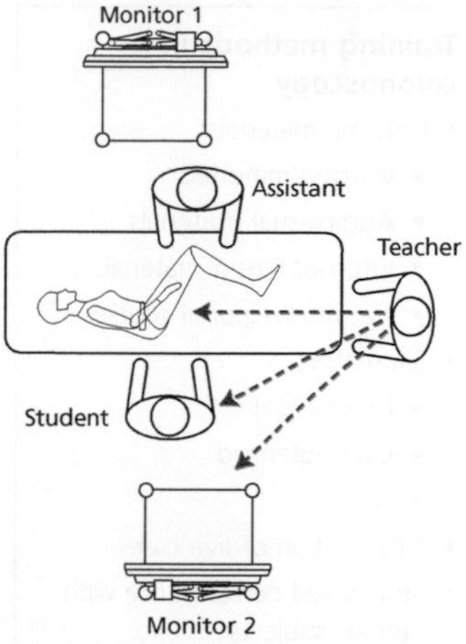

Fig 16.1 The teacher stands at the foot of the examining table. The instructor can watch the hands of the student and also the monitor situated behind the trainee.

After the procedure, the teacher should provide encouraging, constructive feedback to the trainee. A directed critique immediately after the procedure will be more effective than an end-of-month assessment. Each case will provide special learning opportunities, and these should be exploited. If there is a difficult diverticular sigmoid, it is best to take time to discuss the nuances of solving this problem and spend relatively less time on other aspects of the case. An expansion of the learning potential will occur if other students are present during the performance of each case and at the post-colonoscopy critique. During these teaching sessions, when the case is fresh in everyone's mind, the decisions and alternatives should be publicly discussed. If the prep was poor or there was a tight stricture, would it have been better to switch to a smaller caliber scope or to abort the procedure? Perhaps a large villous lesion could be more definitively resected by the colorectal surgeon. Perhaps the cecum should be imaged by computed tomographic colonography (CTC) because the risk of "soldiering on" is too great. Part of learning colonoscopy is identifying the point at which the challenge or the risk of continuing outweighs the benefit.

Continuing education

In an evolving discipline such as colonoscopy, it is obvious that ongoing education is essential. Unfortunately, mid-career training of colonoscopists is often neglected. Recent evidence suggests that quality (as measured by metrics such as adenoma detection rates or complication rates) varies widely among mid-career providers, further reinforcing the importance of ongoing education of this cohort. In most cases, the training of mid-career colonoscopists

Training methods in colonoscopy
- Didactic materials
  - Written materials
  - Audiovisual materials
  - Internet based materials
  - National/regional courses
- Simulators
  - Mechanical
  - Computerized
  - Animal
- Observation of live cases
- Supervised performance with human subjects

occurs privately, through seminars and direct observation by a colleague/expert. Unfortunately, this type of continuing education occurs rarely, although in general learning experts regard this strategy favorably. Expert review of video-recorded colonoscopy may be another untapped strategy for mid-career training. Currently, directed continuing education in colonoscopy occurs mainly through live courses, national meetings, Internet-based courses, and other digital and Internet-based vehicles.

Other learning tools

In addition to hands-on training, a wide and increasing variety of helpful teaching aids is available. These can provide a valuable supplement to hands-on training, particularly regarding the development of the trainee's knowledge and skill base. These include traditional written materials, atlases of colonic pathology, and a wide variety of electronic learning tools (e-tools). Many e-tools are interactive, involve movies rather than still images, and allow unprecedented, instantaneous dissemination of knowledge. They can be accessed in a variety of formats, such as CD-ROM and DVD, and some are available through the Internet. The DAVE project (DAVEProject.org), for example, is a multinational, collaborative, Internet-based, endoscopy learning tool that is free of charge.

Live demonstration courses featuring expert colonoscopists undertaking basic or especially challenging cases also provide another forum for learning. Such courses can be simulcast to off-site venues, leveraging their teaching power. The gastrointestinal (GI) societies have published guidelines regarding proper conduct and ethical distribution of material from these types of courses.

Simulation-based learning represents another option. Simulators help beginning trainees to familiarize themselves with endoscope manipulation, and with the basic challenges and findings of colonoscopy. Animal models have been a traditional teaching tool in surgical techniques, and within colonoscopy the isolated porcine colon has been used for this purpose. In the past decade, computer-based simulation has generated considerable excitement within gastroenterology. It is hoped that such simulation will offer the potential for decreased training costs: fewer trainers may be needed; training can be undertaken during off-hours; lessons learned from simulators might complement the training provided during live colonoscopy. It is also hoped that simulators could decrease errors made during live cases, and thus lead to increased patient safety. However, studies of computer-based simulation thus far have yielded conflicting results, and the long-term role of simulation in colonoscopy training remains uncertain.

Measuring competence

"Core competency" in colonoscopy can be divided into cognitive and technical components. Cognitive proficiency requires the trainee to acquire the requisite knowledge on such topics as: indications and contraindications; patient preparation; principles of informed consent, common visual landmarks and pathology; risks and benefits; screening and surveillance guidelines; principles of sedation, monitoring, and recovery; recognition of complications; principles of use of all ancillary equipment, including electrocautery; reporting and communication of findings; and analysis of findings making recommendations for follow-up examination, other diagnostic studies, and therapy.

Technical proficiency requires achieving deftness with: the mechanical function of the scope (switches, knobs, dials); scope maintenance and cleaning; colonic intubation; scope withdrawal and mucosal inspection; common interventions such as biopsy, polypectomy, injection, treatment of bleeding; administering and monitoring sedation.

Assessment tools that measure competence are a necessary adjunct to training. They can monitor both the effectiveness of the training program and the performance of individual trainees. The measures by which competency in colonoscopy is assessed vary widely, and have not been well validated. One traditional measure involves a simple requirement for numbers of cases performed. This number varies according to the organization that created it: surgery and family practice residencies require >50 cases, whereas GI fellowships require >140. Clearly, these numbers represent a bare minimum. Furthermore, defining competency by numbers of cases does not necessarily take into account the considerable variability in trainees' innate dexterity, hand–eye coordination, and speed of knowledge and skill acquisition. Nor does it embrace the tremendous added effect of one-on-one instruction by an expert teacher. More recent data utilizing more sophisticated measures of competency have suggested that in fact core competency is achieved only after 300–500 colonoscopies. Other measures of competency, such as cecal intubation rate, intubation time, polyp detection rate, and complication rate have been proposed.

More comprehensive, semiquantitative instruments measuring colonoscopy competence also exist. One such is the Mayo Colonoscopy Skills Assessment Tool. This tool requires an expert review of a trainee's live performance, and includes a variety of specific technical measures (e.g. adequacy of luminal view) and cognitive measures (e.g. interpretation of findings). A numerical score is generated and can be tracked and compared to benchmarks.

Summary

Training in colonoscopy is as formidable a challenge as the procedure itself. Time and economic pressures are forcing educators to achieve more with less. Standardized curricula, improved teaching techniques, and increased utilization of teaching surrogates such as simulators and the Internet may be useful in overcoming these obstacles.

Further reading

1. ASGE Training Committee, Adler DG, Bakis G, *et al.* Principles of training in GI endoscopy. *Gastrointest Endosc* 2012;75:231–5. Epub 2011 Dec 7.
2. Cohen J, Cohen SA, Vora KC, *et al.* Multicenter, randomized, controlled trial of virtual-reality simulator training in acquisition of competency in colonoscopy. *Gastrointest Endosc* 2006;64:361–8.
3. Desilets DJ, Banerjee S, Barth BA, *et al.* Endoscopic simulators. *Gastrointest Endosc* 2011;73:861–7.
4. Gupta S, Bassett P, Man R, Suzuki N, Vance ME, Thomas-Gibson S. Validation of a novel method for assessing competency in polypectomy. *Gastrointest Endosc* 2012;75:568–575.
5. Leyden JE, Doherty GA, Hanley A, *et al.* Quality of colonoscopy performance among gastroenterology and surgical trainees: a need for common training standards for all trainees? *Endoscopy* 2011;43:935–40. Epub 2011 Oct 13.
6. Loren DE, Azar R, Charles RJ, *et al.* Updated guidelines for live endoscopy demonstrations. *Gastrointest Endosc* 2010;71:1105–7.
7. Sedlack RE. Training to competency in colonoscopy: assessing and defining competency standards. *Gastrointest Endosc* 2011;74:355–366. e1–2. Epub 2011 Apr 23.
8. Sedlack RE. The Mayo Colonoscopy Skills Assessment Tool: validation of a unique instrument to assess colonoscopy skills in trainees. *Gastrointest Endosc* 2010;72:1125–33.
9. Sedlack RE. Colonoscopy. In: Cohen J, editor. *Successful Training in Gastrointestinal Endoscopy.* Chichester: Wiley-Blackwell; 2011.
10. Thomas-Gibson S, Bassett P, Suzuki N, Brown GJ, Williams CB, Saunders BP. Intensive training over 5 days improves colonoscopy skills long-term. *Endoscopy* 2007;39:818–24.

CHAPTER 17

Computed Tomographic Colonography ("Virtual" Colonoscopy)

Introduction

Although colorectal carcinoma is largely preventable through screening, many adults are not being screened at all. "Virtual colonoscopy" is a radiologic technique whereby thin slices of the abdomen are viewed radiographically with computed tomography (hence "computed tomographic colonography," or CTC), and the air-filled colon is reconstructed using imaging software. When reconstituted and run in sequential fashion, it appears as if the viewer is inside the colon, whizzing around folds and bends and seeing polyps in a movie consisting of multiple still images stacked together. CTC gained recognition when US President Barack Obama underwent it in order to avoid the need for sedation and the transfer of presidential power. CTC is an effective screening tool when properly performed. It should not be viewed as a replacement for optical colonoscopy, but as an additional effective option that has the potential to increase screening rates.

The CTC procedure

The patient must be prepared for CTC with a restricted diet and a cathartic. The colon is distended with air or CO_2 via a rectal catheter. A multidetector CT scanner takes images over an interval of 10–15 minutes and the large intestine is displayed in two-dimensional (2D) and three-dimensional (3D) projections. The 3D endoluminal projection provides a virtual reality navigational view that simulates conventional (optical) colonoscopy.

The 3D endoluminal view is very sensitive, readily permitting detection of polypoid lesions. CTC, however, cannot be interpreted from the 3D display alone, as low specificity would render almost every examination positive. Therefore, 2D correlation is required to distinguish true soft-tissue polyps from retained stool, pills, and other debris. Diagnostic redundancy is the key to accurate polyp detection with CTC. The more chances one has to detect a lesion, the less likely it will be missed. Conversely, examining a potential lesion in multiple ways will lead to fewer false positives. As a result, most interpretive approaches emphasize 3D detection but retain complementary 2D imaging. The more sensitive display (3D) is best for initial lesion detection, whereas the more specific display (2D) confirms suspected polyps and achieves secondary polyp detection. Reader fatigue is less with the 3D mode. As CTC systems improve, 2D polyp detection is giving way to primary 3D detection.

Advantages and disadvantages of CTC

- **Pros**
  - No sedation
  - Low-risk
  - Non-invasive
  - Certain visualization of entire colon length
  - High patient acceptance
  - Rapid
- **Cons**
  - Air insufflation uncomfortable
  - No biopsy capability
  - Radiation exposure
  - Can miss small and flat lesions
  - Wide range of provider interpretive skill
  - Not therapeutic (follow up optical colonoscopy often required)
  - Requires catharsis
  - Surveillance guidelines not established
  - Effectiveness for colorectal cancer reduction not established
  - Not always reimbursed

Practical Colonoscopy, First Edition. Jerome D. Waye, James Aisenberg, and Peter H. Rubin.
© 2013 John Wiley & Sons, Ltd. Published 2013 by John Wiley & Sons, Ltd.

CTC performance

There are no longitudinal studies that analyze either colorectal cancer incidence or reduction. In the absence of this gold standard, CTC studies analyze polyp detection rates, using optical colonoscopy as the reference standard. Overall, most studies suggest that in experienced hands CTC performs comparably to optical colonoscopy at detecting cancers and large polyps (>10 mm), with sensitivity and specificity rates above 90%. For smaller pedunculated or sessile polyps (5–9 mm), studies show more variable results, with detection rates ranging from 50 to 90%. During CTC, diminutive sessile lesions (<5 mm) are generally ignored. The widely cited American College of Radiology Imaging Network (ACRIN) Study, which involved a screening cohort of approximately 2500 patients across 15 institutions, showed a per patient sensitivity of 90% for large adenomas, although the specificity (86%) and positive predictive value (25%) for large adenomas were lower than in previous studies. Overall, the performance of CTC (like optical colonoscopy) is subject to considerable variability based on provider expertise. Improved software packages or fecal tagging ("prep-less") techniques will improve CTC performance and acceptance.

The relative benefits of virtual colonoscopy versus optical colonoscopy include the fact that it is less invasive and does not require pain control. Thus, patients can drive home or return to work afterward. The risk of perforation or bleeding is negligible. If a polyp is found, same-day or next-day optical colonoscopy can often be arranged, avoiding a second bowel preparation. Many patients prefer CTC to optical colonoscopy, and some individuals are unwilling to undergo optical colonoscopy but do accept CTC. CTC also detects lesions outside the bowel (e.g. solid tumors in adjacent organs); however, insignificant incidental findings may be reported and thereby trigger fruitless interventions.

The major drawbacks of CTC are that a cathartic bowel preparation is still needed, biopsy or polypectomy is not possible, and lesions less than 5 mm in diameter may not be noted. Flat lesions, such as sessile serrated adenomas, remain a diagnostic challenge, especially because they tend to flatten out completely when the colon is distended with gas. Although there is some debate over the clinical importance of polyps <5 mm and even of some flat polyps, clinical, genetic, and epidemiological data suggest that these polyps may possess malignant potential. CTC exposes patients to approximately 5 mSv of ionizing radiation (roughly equal to 1–2 years of typical background radiation). The rectal tube and distension of colon with air are moderately uncomfortable. The US Centers for Medicare and Medicaid Services determined in 2010 that CTC was not a covered service. This leads to variable coverage for diagnostic CTC.

Several studies have found that appropriately trained non-radiologists (e.g. gastroenterologists) can accurately interpret CTC. The American Gastroenterological Association has suggested that gastroenterologists become adept at reading these radiological images, as they will have a role in screening colonoscopy in the future.

Indications

When performed for failed colonoscopy, CTC is ideally performed on the same day as the incomplete colonoscopy, eliminating a repeat bowel cleansing. CTC may be advantageous in high risk patients—for example, those who are debilitated or elderly, have significant comorbidity, take systemic anticoagulants or have a bleeding diathesis, or are at significant risk for complications related to sedation. Some radiologists recommend CTC for surveillance of patients after polypectomy or colorectal cancer resection, but this indication remains uncertain. Radiologists suggest CTC surveillance of 6–9 mm polyps as an alternative to polypectomy; but most gastroenterologists argue that all polyps of this size require resection and examination by a pathologist.

Potential indications for CTC

- Incomplete optical colonoscopy
- Evaluation of suspected submucosal lesion
- Preexisting condition rendering optical colonoscopy high risk
- Contraindication to sedation/analgesia
- Technically difficult optical colonoscopy
- Surveillance of small unresected colorectal polyps
- Patient choice/unwillingness to undergo optical colonoscopy
- Unavailability of optical colonoscopy resources

Barium enema

In this procedure, a patient prepared with cathartics is given an enema containing a solution of radiopaque barium via a rectal tube. The radiologist views images on a fluoroscopic screen as barium is being infused. The patient evacuates, and air is instilled to provide contrast. In many communities, barium enema has been replaced by CTC. Barium enema often causes abdominal pain from the air insufflation. The dose of ionizing radiation from double contrast barium enema is approximately twice that from CTC.

Summary

CTC is a marked advance in radiologic imaging of the colon, approaching the diagnostic capability of optical colonoscopy. Studies show that CTC can diagnose colon cancer as accurately as optical colonoscopy. However, the rate of "interval" cancers after a CTC is not yet known, and the ability to find polyps by CTC is not at a point at which it is universally accepted as a screening modality. The interval for a repeat CTC when no polyps are detected is unknown. It is hoped that with improvements in imaging definition, the tagging of colon contents with special markers (so that cathartics can be eliminated), and the development of specific training guidelines for interpretation of the radiographic material, CTC will become an even more valuable adjunct to screening programs in the future.

Further reading

1. DeVaan MC, van Gelder RE, Graser A, Bipat S, Stoker J. Diagnostic value of CT-colonography as compared to colonoscopy in an asymptomatic screening population: a meta-analysis. *Eur Radiol* 2011;21: 1747–63.
2. Heresbach D, Djabbari M, Riou F, *et al.* Accuracy of computed tomographic colonography in a nationwide multicentre trial, and its relation to radiologist expertise. *Gut* 2011;60:658–65.
3. Johnson CD, Chen MH, Toledano AY, *et al.* Accuracy of CT colonography for detection of large adenomas and cancers. *N Engl J Med* 2008;359:1207–17.
4. Kim DH, Pickhardt PJ, Taylor AJ, *et al.* CT colonography versus colonoscopy for the detection of advanced neoplasia. *N Engl J Med* 2007;357:1403–12.
5. Neri E, Faggioni L, Cerri F, *et al.* CT colonography versus double-contrast barium enema for screening of colorectal cancer: comparison of radiation burden. *Abdom Imaging* 2010;35:596–601.
6. Pickhardt PJ, Hassan C, Halligan S, Marmo R. Colorectal cancer: CT colonography and colonoscopy for detection–systematic review and meta-analysis. *Radiology* 2011;259:393–405.
7. Pickhardt PJ, Hassan C, Laghi A, Zullo A, Kim DH, Morini S. Cost-effectiveness of colorectal cancer screening with computed tomographycolonography: the impact of not reporting diminutive lesions. *Cancer* 2007;109:2213–21.
8. Ray Q, Kim C, Scott T, *et al.* Gastroenterologist interpretation of CTC: pilot study demonstrating feasibility and similar accuracy compared to radiologists. *Gastroenterology* 2007;132:A92–3.
9. Rex DK. Colonoscopy is justified for any polyp discovered during computed tomographic colonography: PRO: Patients with polyps smaller than 1 cm on computed tomographic colonography should be offered colonoscopy and polypectomy. *Am J Gastroenterol* 2005;100:1903–5.
10. Von Wagner C, Smith S, Halligan S, *et al.* Patient acceptability of CT colonography compared with double contrast barium enema: results from a multicenter randomized controlled trial of symptomatic patients. *EurRadiol* 2011;21:2046–55.

CHAPTER 18

Advanced Imaging Techniques

Introduction

Ever since the first colonoscope was introduced in 1966, white light and conventional optics have been the standard way to image the lumen of the colon. However, this technology does not always reveal subtle mucosal abnormalities, and important pathology may be missed. Until recently, the only significant improvement was chromoendoscopy. But other enhanced optical technologies are entering colonoscopy practice.

Chromoendoscopy

Chromoendoscopy uses dyes to bring out mucosal elevations, irregularities, and depressions. Some lesions that appear flat before staining may subsequently appear depressed or elevated after chromoendoscopy. In several randomized studies, dye spraying has enhanced the detection of colonic intraepithelial neoplasms—of flat and small adenomas in particular. In addition, several studies have shown that chromoendoscopy with targeted biopsy may be practical and more accurate than random four-quadrant biopsy for detecting dysplasia during screening/surveillance in patients with chronic idiopathic colitis. The most commonly used stains are indigo carmine and methylene blue (applied in a concentration of about 0.1%), and crystal violet (0.05%). "Vital" stains, such as crystal violet and methylene blue, are actively absorbed by the epithelial cells of the colonic crypts, and are particularly useful for delineating the crypt orifices during magnification colonoscopy. "Contrast" stains, such as indigo carmine, are not absorbed but pool in the mucosal crevices and delineate subtle mucosal contours.

During chromoendoscopy, the dye can be applied on polyps, segments of the colon, or the entire colon. There are three methods of dye application: direct push through the working channel of the colonoscope; injection through a dye-spray catheter that has been passed through the working channel; and injection using the colonoscope's integrated water jet system. The mucosa must first be cleaned of debris. The direct push method is ideal for staining a small target, such as a single flat polyp. In this technique, 10 ml

Practical Colonoscopy, First Edition. Jerome D. Waye, James Aisenberg, and Peter H. Rubin.
© 2013 John Wiley & Sons, Ltd. Published 2013 by John Wiley & Sons, Ltd.

pre-diluted dye and 10 ml air are drawn up in a 20-ml syringe. The scope is pointed at the target and the syringe is emptied into the working channel; the air helps to push the dye through the scope channel. For more widespread staining, a catheter with a spray tip is used. The water-jet method facilitates widespread dye application. In this method, several ampoules of dye are added to the water-jet bottle (*caution*: do not insert dye into the water bottle that is used to clean the instrument lens and insufflate air). The dye is then pumped out of the scope's water jet while the tip of the scope is maneuvered to coat the mucosal surface. These dye-spraying techniques are relatively simple to master and are inexpensive.

Performing chromoendoscopy

- Dilute dye of choice in 1000 ml water
- Put solution in water-jet bottle and instill via water jet, or instill via a dedicated spray catheter (commercially available)
- Only worthwhile if the colon preparation is good to excellent
- Create a homogeneous, thin coating of mucosa
- Can use focally to dye individual segments of colon/lesions, or can use throughout colon

Chromoendoscopy

- **Pros**
  - May enhance
    - Detection of small polyps during routine surveillance and screening
    - Detection of polypoid dysplasia in chronic colitis
  - Low cost
  - Widely available
  - Technically straightforward
- **Cons**
  - Increases procedure time
  - Unproven cancer prevention benefit
  - Has not achieved widespread acceptance in most settings

Chromoendoscopy dyes

Dye	Dilution for use
Methylene blue	1:1000
Indigo carmine	1:1000
Crystal violet	1:2000

Water method of colonoscopy

During the water method of colonoscopy, the colonoscopist distends the colon with warm water and performs the examination with an "underwater view." The newer colonoscopes with an integral water jet permit rapid filling of the colon. It is postulated that the water load reduces the angulations of the sigmoid and relaxes the colonic musculature, so that intubation is mechanically easier. However, the process of water infusion is slower than gas insufflation, so the overall procedure time is increased. The water method has resulted in lower pain scores, higher cecal intubation rates, and a reduction in sedation drug demands. It is low cost. In some studies, the water method is associated with higher adenoma detection than gas insufflation, but this remains controversial. The benefits of the water method during colonoscopy under conventional sedation and in diverse patient populations are under study.

The water method

- **Pros**
  - May facilitate colon intubation
  - Less pain
    - Decreased sedative/analgesic requirement
    - Allows colonoscopy without sedation in some instances
  - Low cost
  - Water magnifies lesions
- **Cons**
  - Prolongs procedure
  - Not widely used
  - Benefit in diverse patient populations not established

New technologies

Most of the newest technologies are designed to improve the colonoscopist's ability to interpret the appearance of a lesion *after* the lesion has been detected, rather than to improve the ability to detect lesions in the first place. Some of these technologies provide a level of detail comparable to that seen under the microscope, and are termed "optical biopsy." The optical biopsy methods are expensive, and not currently adaptable to routine clinical use.

Magnifying colonoscopy

Magnifying colonoscopy requires a special "zoom" colonoscope containing a lens in the tip that instantly magnifies the image 75- or

Techniques designed to enhance discrimination of polyp characteristics

- Magnifying colonoscopy
- Narrow band imaging (NBI)
- Autofluorescence imaging (AFI)
- Endocytoscopy
- Confocal laser endomicroscopy
- Optical coherence tomography (OCT)
- Fujinon Intelligent Color Enhancement (FICE)
- iScan

100-fold. This magnification can disclose important mucosal characteristics, such as a central depression in a flat polyp. It is simple to use, but owing to cost and uncertain clinical role it is not widely utilized.

The best-studied application of magnification involves analyzing the micro-architecture of the mucosal crypts—the "pit pattern." In standard-view colonoscopy, the surface of the colon appears punctuated by myriad small dots, representing the crypt orifices, or pits. Dye-spraying and magnification enhance visualization of these pit patterns, which can be classified using a system developed by Kudo. Although this system's nomenclature is confusing to the uninitiated, it is not difficult to recognize the different visual patterns (Figs 18.1, 18.2, and 18.3). In normal mucosa (type I), the

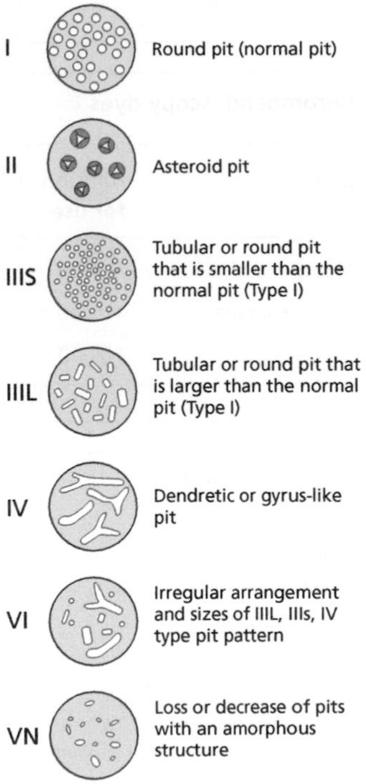

Fig 18.1 Pit pattern classification (schematic).

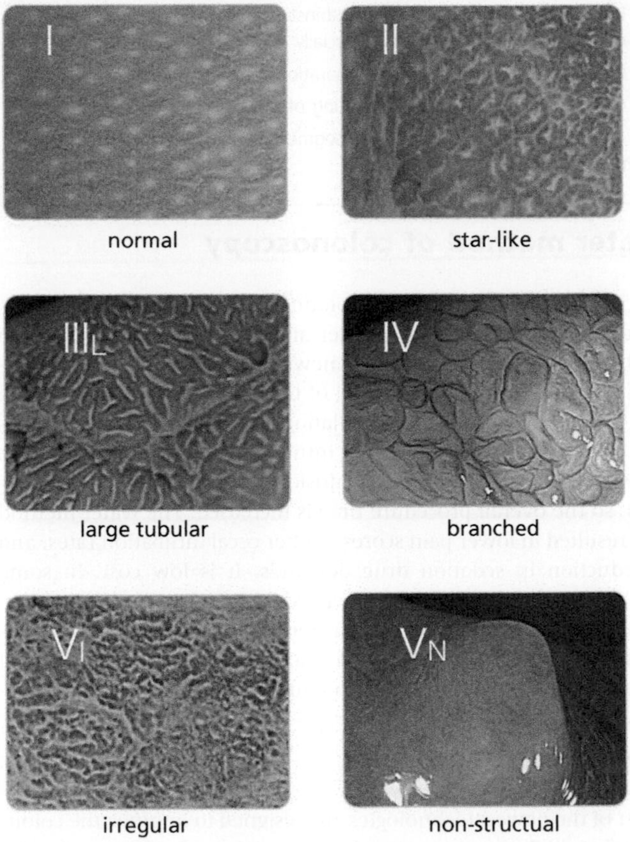

Fig 18.2 Pit pattern classification. In normal mucosa (type 1) the colonic pits (seen here as white circular dots) are round and arranged in a regular matrix. In hyperplastic mucosa (type II), the pits may be star-shaped but remain regular. In adenomatous polyps (types III and IV), the pits are often large and tubular, or branched, reflecting abnormal proliferation and growth. In colonic adenocarcinoma (type V) the pattern becomes irregular or nonstructural. Pit pattern analysis is typically performed with magnification endoscopy and chromoendoscopy, but the pit pattern is also visible to a lesser degree with standard high resolution video colonoscopy without magnification. (From *Colonoscopy: Principles and Practice*, 2nd edition.)

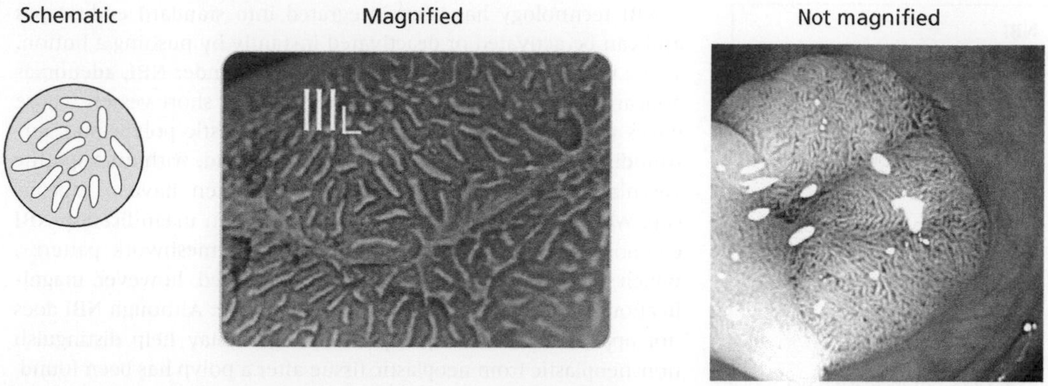

Fig 18.3 Pit pattern classification—adenoma. The pattern of type III pits, which are tubular, is common in adenomas. NBI may enhance pit pattern analysis.

pits are round and regular. The pits of hyperplastic polyps (type II) are larger, and are star-shaped or somewhat irregular, but like normal mucosa, appear in a regular matrix. Adenomas are comprised of pits that appear elongated and sometimes branched (type III or IV). The type V pit pattern, seen in cancers, is highly irregular or even absent ("non-structured"). Lesions that display type I or type II pit patterns are generally low risk and need not be removed. Overall, pit pattern analysis using dye and magnification differentiates between neoplastic and non-neoplastic colorectal polyps with 95.5% accuracy. Thus, accurate pit pattern interpretation can guide intraprocedural decision-making.

Classification of polyps by pit pattern

- **Kudo type I:** Normal; uniform, round crypts
- **Kudo type II:** Hyperplastic; uniform, larger, star-shaped crypts
- **Kudo types III,IV:** Adenoma; elongated, branched crypts
- **Kudo type V:** Cancer; highly irregular or absent crypts

Narrow band imaging

Narrow band imaging (NBI) is a novel optical technology that increases visualization of intramucosal vascular patterns (Video Clip 18.1). NBI is based on the hypothesis that characterization of lesions based on their micro-vessels can predict whether a lesion is normal, hyperplastic, dysplastic, or malignant. Neoplasms such as colon adenomas and carcinomas produce abnormal blood-vessel growth (angiogenesis), and therefore have vascular networks that look different from the vascular networks in normal or benign tissue.

During standard colonoscopy, the light source produces the full red–green–blue spectrum of visible white light (wavelength = 400–800 nm). In NBI, filters block the longer wavelengths, producing light that appears blue. Two bands of the color spectrum (415 and 540 nm) are unfiltered. These particular bands were chosen because they are within the hemoglobin absorption spectrum, thus enhancing visualization of surface microvascular structures during endoscopy. The wavelength of 415 nm provides information about the capillaries and pits of the surface mucosa, whereas the 540 nm light penetrates more deeply and provides information about the slightly deeper vessels in the submucosa.

> **NBI**
> - **Pros**
>   - Built into standard scope
>   - Instant on–off
>   - Does not prolong procedure
>   - No added cost
>   - May help discriminate hyperplastic from adenomatous polyps
> - **Cons**
>   - Manufacturer-specific
>   - Does not increase polyp detection (not "red-flag" technology)

NBI technology has been integrated into standard endoscopes and can be activated or deactivated instantly by pushing a button. There is no advanced preparation required. Under NBI, adenomas appear dark brownish, with a pattern of tiny, short vessels whose edges are well delineated, whereas hyperplastic polyps and surrounding mucosa appear pale brown and bland, without a specific vascular pattern. Sessile serrated polyps often have a mucous cap, which under NBI appears dark red. When magnification NBI colonoscopy is performed, specific capillary meshwork patterns, which correlate with lesion histology, are noted; however, magnification colonoscopies are not widely available. Although NBI does not appear to increase polyp detection, it may help distinguish non-neoplastic from neoplastic tissue after a polyp has been found. Recent studies suggest that the sensitivity, specificity, and accuracy of NBI for differentiating hyperplastic and adenomatous polyps range from 90 to 95%. NBI-based polyp analysis can be easily taught.

Several manufacturers have experimented with filters that alter the appearance of the endoscopic image after processing, as an alternative to NBI. In these systems, conventional white light illumination is used, and the modification is made to the final image. The Fujinon Intelligent Color Enhancement (FICE) system and the Pentax iScan are examples of such systems. Like NBI, these operate with the push of a button and require no preparation. Although they are included in some standard-issue colonoscopes, none of these systems has been shown to enhance routine colonoscopic diagnosis.

Autofluorescence imaging

When white light illuminates the surface of the colon, most of it is reflected; some enters the tissue, where it is scattered or absorbed by intramucosal structures; and some of the light photons are absorbed by fluorophores, which are molecules that emit light of a longer (fluorescent) wavelength when they absorb energy. During autofluorescence imaging (AFI), the natural (unenhanced) fluorescence emitted by an illuminated colonic wall is analyzed. The autofluorescence of the normal mucosal surface of the colon wall is relatively fixed, but in disease it is altered due to changes in blood flow, edema, biochemical composition, or other characteristics. These differences can be augmented by the administration of exogenous fluorophores intravascularly. Because neoplastic tissue autofluoresces differently from benign tissue, AFI can in theory enhance tumor detection. When viewed with an autofluorescence imaging scope, normal mucosa appears greenish, but neoplastic tissue appears reddish-violet. One advantage to AFI is that a wide field can be scanned in order to "red flag" lesions that require close inspection. Currently, AFI is an area of research but has not yet been commercialized.

Endocytoscopy

Endocytoscopy is a probe-based technology that requires a special endoscope. A target is stained with an absorptive contrast agent (methylene blue or toluidine blue) and then a high-power objective lens collects highly magnified images in order to visualize subcellular structures, such as nuclei. Endocytoscopy is useful for detection of dysplastic cells, but the scan is limited to the surface and provides no information about deeper structures or depth of penetration.

Confocal laser endomicroscopy

Confocal laser endomicroscopy (CLE) puts the power of a microscope at the tip of the colonoscope. A low-powered laser is focused through a lens at a tissue target, and the same lens is used to collect reflected light. The point of illumination and the point of detection and are at the same focal plane (hence the term "confocal"). The resolution is similar to that of a dissecting microscope, and CLE images show individual cells, their nuclei, and the relationships of abutting cells. The architecture of crypts, vessels, and lamina propria is evident, and a classification scheme has been created that distinguishes neoplastic from non-neoplastic tissues. The depth of penetration during CLE is only approximately 250 µm, which corresponds to the mucosal layer. This means that invasion through the muscularis mucosa cannot reliably be assessed. Because the area of imaging is small (about 0.5×0.5 mm) and relies on the probe touching the surface, CLE is used only to interrogate a known abnormality but not to search the larger colonic surface. A contrast agent is needed to highlight subcellular structures, in particular, nuclei. The most common contrast agents are acriflavine hydrochloride (applied topically) and fluorescein sodium (applied topically or intravenously). Acriflavine strongly labels the superficial epithelial cells, while intravenous fluorescein distributes throughout the mucosa. During routine colorectal cancer and polyp screening and surveillance, CLE discriminates neoplastic from non-neoplastic lesions with over 95% accuracy. Likewise, studies suggest that for dysplasia surveillance in chronic idiopathic colitis, pan-chromocolonoscopy followed by CLE-based interrogation of suspicious areas may provide an improvement over the current standard of care.

Confocal imaging has been integrated into some commercially available colonoscopes, and is also available as a probe-based system. The advantage of the latter system is that a disposable probe can be passed through the working channel of any colonoscope and produce CLE findings. While in vivo cellular analysis is a remarkable advance in endoscopy and the technology currently has considerable momentum, CLE remains costly and time-consuming, and the image interpretation is challenging to learn and observer-dependent. CLE requires the recognition of patterns or motifs during dynamic imaging. The current barriers to further adoption of this technology include training, standardization of imaging and interpretation, reimbursement, time, and cost.

Optical coherence tomography

Like endoscopic ultrasound, optical coherence tomography (OCT) enables cross-sectional imaging by a probe-based technique in near real time with high resolution (~10–20 μm). Instead of sound waves, the OCT images are formed by light reflected from tissues. In comparison with endoscopic ultrasound techniques, OCT has a high resolution but relatively poor depth of tissue penetration. OCT remains an investigative tool.

Comparison of different image enhancing technologies

	Field size		Depth of imaging		Push button
	Point	Wide	Surface	Deeper	
Chromoendoscopy		✓	✓		
Change in light wavelength (NBI, FICE, iSCAN)		✓	✓		✓
AFI		✓		✓	✓
Endocytoscopy	✓		✓		
Confocal	✓			✓	✓
OCT	✓			✓	✓

Summary

Numerous advanced optical colonoscopic techniques are currently under investigation. Some are commercially available. To date, many of the technologies are geared toward close analysis of a single point or lesion rather than broad mucosal scanning. For scanning, chromoendoscopy, an older technique, is potentially advantageous, but its disadvantages have curtailed acceptance. NBI appears to be most useful for discriminating hyperplastic from dysplastic polyps, and may help prevent unnecessary tissue acquisition or pathology costs. "High-tech" strategies such as CLE achieve spectacular mucosal detail, but for the foreseeable future will probably be performed by experts in specialized referral centers.

Further reading

1. Aguirre AD, Sawinski J, Huang SW, Zhou C, Denk W, Fujimoto JG. High speed optical coherence microscopy with autofocus adjustment and a miniaturized endoscopic imaging probe. *Opt Express* 2010;18:4222–39.
2. Imaizumi K, Harada Y, Wakabayashi N, *et al*. Dual-wavelength excitation of mucosal autofluorescence for precise detection of diminutive colonic adenomas. *Gastrointest Endosc* 2012;75:110–7.
3. Kiesslich R, Goetz M, Hoffman A, Galle PR. New imaging techniques and opportunities in endoscopy. *Nat Rev Gastroenterol Hepatol* 2011;8: 547–53.

4. Kuiper T, van den Broek FJ, Naber AH, *et al.* Endoscopic trimodal imaging detects colonic neoplasia as well as standard video endoscopy. *Gastroenterology* 2011;140:1887–94.
5. Kuiper T, van den Broek FJ, van Eeden S, *et al.* New classification for probe-based confocal laser endomicroscopy in the colon. *Endoscopy* 2011;43:1076–81.
6. Leung FW, Leung JW, Mann SK, Friedland S, Ramirez FC. The water method significantly enhances patient-centered outcomes in sedated and unsedated colonoscopy. *Endoscopy* 2011;43:816–21. Epub 2011 May 24.
7. Nass JP, Connolly SE. Current status of chromoendoscopy and narrow band imaging in colonoscopy. *Clin Colon Rectal Surg* 2010;23:21–30.
8. Neumann H, Fuchs FS, Vieth M, *et al.* Review article: in vivo imaging by endocytoscopy. *Aliment Pharmacol Ther* 2011;33:1183–93.
9. Sato R, Fujiya M, Watari J, *et al.* The diagnostic accuracy of high-resolution endoscopy, autofluorescence imaging and narrow-band imaging for differentially diagnosing colon adenoma. *Endoscopy* 2011;43:862–8.
10. Shahid MW, Buchner AM, Heckman MG, *et al.* Diagnostic accuracy of probe-based confocal laser endomicroscopy and narrow band imaging for small colorectal polyps: a feasibility study. *Am J Gastroenterol* 2012;107:231–9. Epub 2011 Nov 8.
11. Waye JD, Heigh RI, Fleischer DE, *et al.* A retrograde-viewing device improves detection of adenomas in the colon: a prospective efficacy evaluation (with videos). *Gastrointest. Endosc* 2010;71:551–556.
12. Waye JD, Rex DK, Williams CB, editors. *Colonoscopy: Principles and Practice*. 2nd ed. Chichester: Wiley-Blackwell; 2009.

Chapter video clip

Video Clip 18.1 Narrow band imaging

Narrow band imaging is used extensively to enhance visualization during resection of this minimally elevated adenoma.

CHAPTER 19

The Future of Colonoscopy

Introduction

Just a few decades ago, colonoscopy was performed with a clumsy, fiber-optic instrument and a few low-tech accessories. The colonoscopist viewed the mucosa through an eyepiece, and screwed an extension lens onto the end of the scope if an assistant or student wanted to view the findings. The image itself was small, and interrupted with black dots that resulted from broken optical fibers.

Today, colonoscopes are durable, responsive, and agile; they obtain high-resolution images for projection onto large, high-definition flat-screens; they accommodate a versatile armamentarium of accessories and specialized optics, such as narrow band imaging (NBI).

Yet colonoscopy, while still the gold standard for examining the large intestine, remains imperfect. For patients, the procedure is inconvenient, unpleasant, provides imperfect protection from cancer, and incurs risk. From a societal standpoint, colonoscopy is expensive, and because it is so resource-intensive, demand for colonoscopy currently outstrips supply. For the endoscopist, it is arduous, and the majority of screening and surveillance exams do not culminate in significant findings.

What advances could improve colonoscopy during the next decade?

Toward a therapeutic procedure

The majority of colonoscopy is performed for colorectal cancer screening and surveillance, and most screening exams are negative. This creates cost to society, inefficient deployment of a finite colonoscopy workforce, unnecessary risk of complications, and patients who ask "Did I really need to undergo that exam?" The cancer risk stratification guidelines that drive screening and surveillance intervals—based on family history, previous polyps, and patient age—provide a crude approximation of cancer risk. The risk pool, namely all persons over 50 years old, is enormous. The uncontestable advantage of optical colonoscopy over all other modalities is

Practical Colonoscopy, First Edition. Jerome D. Waye, James Aisenberg, and Peter H. Rubin.
© 2013 John Wiley & Sons, Ltd. Published 2013 by John Wiley & Sons, Ltd.

that it allows for immediate tissue sampling and removal. In the future, diagnostic screening and risk stratification may be performed by noninvasive means such as genetic testing, stool DNA sampling, or radiological imaging, and only patients with pathology or with high risk will be referred to the colonoscopist for polyp resection, or tissue diagnosis.

Toward a better catharsis

A better prep would improve adherence to guidelines, as well as the experience of the procedure. Current preps are distasteful to most patients. The ideal prep for optical colonoscopy is inexpensive, safe, palatable, and convenient (e.g. a few pills or a small, tasty potion taken within a few hours of the colonoscopy), and would result in high-level colonic cleansing. Such a breakthrough remains in the domain of research.

Toward less or no anesthesia

A sedation-less colonoscopy would: require fewer staff and supplies, and less recovery space; reduce patient (and escort) lost time from work; and essentially eliminate the risk of adverse cardiopulmonary events. Sedation-free optical colonoscopy will require a leap into a new technology platform, such as capsule or robotic colonoscopy (see below). Computed tomography colonography (CTC) is a procedure that requires no sedation, but it is not therapeutic.

Anesthesia requirement during tube-based colonoscopy can be decreased by better conventional scopes and better procedural technique. It is hoped that new teaching tools will enhance the technique of colonoscopists. Improvements in push-scope technology will help minimize pain. Water-method colonoscopy can be performed without the need for sedation, and this is gaining increasing interest.

Toward simpler tissue sampling

In patients who require multiple biopsies, the physician must pass the biopsy forceps back and forth through the working channel numerous times. It would be more convenient to deploy a single-pass device that allows for segmental sampling of mucosa throughout the colon or an electronically controlled built-in biopsy device that at the push of the button emerges from the scope tip and retrieves the tissue sample. Such ancillaries are as yet unavailable.

Toward decreasing the polyp miss rate

The "miss rate" for pre-cancerous polyps during routine colonoscopy is estimated to be 10–20%. It is hoped that educational efforts,

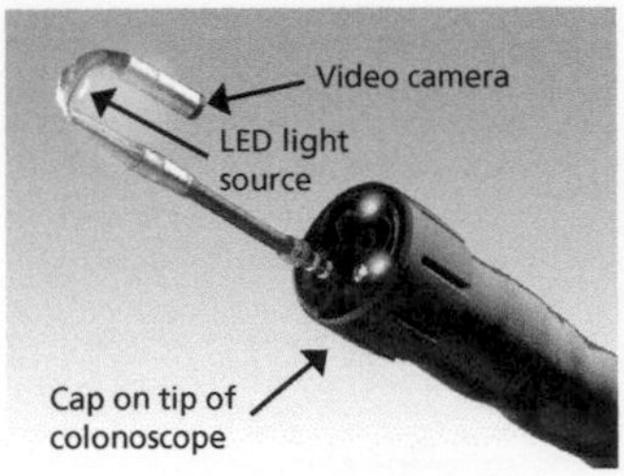

Fig 19.1 Third eye retroscope.

widespread adoption of split-dose bowel preparations, and routine assessment of practitioner quality will help improve performance. Improved magnification, high-definition screens and NBI, available on many recent colonoscopes are already improving polyp detection. Further advances in scope technology can be expected. A tiny endoscope is currently available that can be passed through the accessory channel of a colonoscope and flexed 180 to view the proximal aspect of haustral folds (Fig 19.1). Development is proceeding with colonoscopes offering ever-wider angle of view and "rear viewing."

A technology that "flags" hyperproliferative tissue would also simplify screening and surveillance. Such a technology must be sensitive, practical, efficient, and cost-effective. In its current incarnation, chromoendoscopy is cumbersome to perform and not widely practiced. Areas of ongoing research include metabolic or fluorescence-based biolabeling of pre-cancerous epithelial cells, and the use of endoscopes with specially enhanced optics.

Decreasing the interval cancer rate: Strategies

1. Improve quality of bowel cleansing
2. If bowel preparation is substandard, schedule repeat procedure
3. Improve recognition of flat lesions
4. Decrease incomplete polypectomy rate
5. Encourage meticulous, standardized mucosal examination technique
6. Improve scope technology
7. Encourage adherence to surveillance guidelines
8. Measure quality indicators

Toward decreasing incomplete resection

Unlike gross surgical specimens, endoscopic specimens often do not allow reliable assessment of margins. If the polyp is flat, the boundary between abnormal tissue and normal tissue may be difficult to appreciate endoscopically. Some experts remove a "collar" of normal tissue around a flat polyp during snare resection, whereas others biopsy the margin of a resection site. It will be important to focus colonoscopists on the hazard of incomplete polyp resection and to promote techniques to avoid it. Enhanced imaging technologies will enable better identification of the transition from abnormal to normal mucosa.

Toward "resect and discard"

Many experts advocate a "resect and discard" strategy, whereby low-risk diminutive polyps are resected, but not submitted to pathology. This saves time and pathology costs. This strategy relies on reliable gross morphological interpretation. New scope technologies such as NBI and high-resolution optics and magnification allow accurate "real-time" histology in over 95% of cases in expert hands. In the future, "optical biopsy" technology may eliminate the bulk of colonoscopy-related pathology costs.

Toward better identification of resectable malignant polyps

In the upper gastrointestinal tract and rectum, endoscopic ultrasonography (EUS) is currently used to determine the depth of invasion of neoplastic lesions. EUS permits inspection of all layers of the intestinal wall, as well as adjacent lymph nodes. It also adds fine needle aspiration capability. Colonoscope-based ultrasound technologies will help to determine which colonic polyps can be effectively removed via endoscopic techniques and which require full-thickness resection.

Toward tube-less colonoscopy

During the last decade we have witnessed the waxing and waning of computed tomographic colonography (CTC). CTC may gain wider acceptance if stool subtraction ("fecal tagging") technology permits it to be accomplished without catharsis.

A capsule colonoscope, akin to current generation of small bowel "pill" enteroscopes, has performed reasonably well in recent clinical trials (Fig 19.2). The disadvantages of current generation "pill colonoscopes" are the need for an intensive bowel preparation, the absence of maneuverability or biopsy capability, and a polyp detection rate that does not equal that of optical colonoscopy. Orally administered colon capsules, controlled remotely using extracorporeal magnets, are under study. The colon capsule of the future may discover neoplastic growths, mark them, biopsy them, or even remove them.

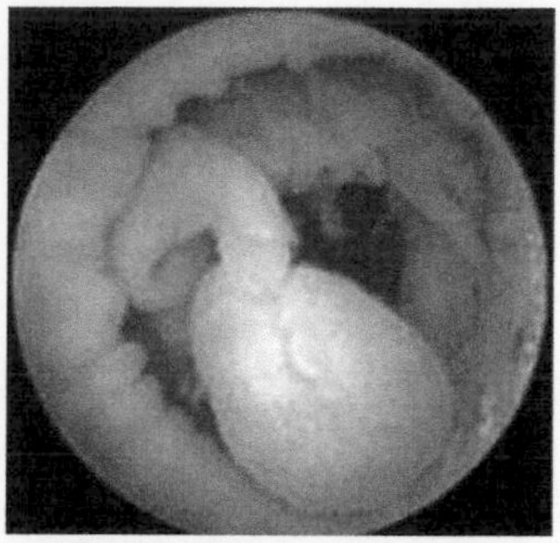

Fig 19.2 Pedunculated polyp seen at capsule colonoscopy. The lumen is filled with fluid, and the polyp appears to be "suspended" in it.

In gastroenterology, miniaturized robotic technology is under investigation: for example, rectally administered, hands-free, externally controlled devices self-propel through the colon using inchworm-like actions, and have the capability of reorienting to view different colonic surfaces, and to sample mucosa. Robotic technology could also enhance the action of tube-based scopes: for example, remote-controlled robotic arms at the tip of the scope could be utilized to push away haustral folds.

Toward transmural surgery

The field of natural orifice translumenal endoscopic surgery (NOTES) represents an important organized foray across the wall of the viscera. NOTES obviates the need for a skin incision. The colon represents a reasonable portal of entry, although it raises the concern of translumenal bacterial contamination. The future of transcolonic NOTES will depend on development of reliable tissue-closure devices, such as endoscopic suturing. Full-thickness mural biopsy, with sampling of the enteric nervous system, may become a useful diagnostic procedure in patients with functional colonic disorders.

Toward other novel therapies

Recently, several studies have shown that allogeneic fecal transplantation via colonoscopy may be a successful treatment option for refractory *Clostridium difficile* colitis. Manipulation of the fecal micro flora might also be used to treat functional or inflammatory bowel disorders. Manipulation of the colonic nervous system—for example, with a pacemaker, akin to that used for gastroparesis—may one day be used to treat severe constipation. Finally medical treatments such as chemotherapy or anti-inflammatory or immunomodulatory agents may be injected directly into abnormal mucosa under colonoscopic guidance.

Summary

Colonoscopy remains a technology in development. It is hoped that advances in provider education and performance, colonoscope technology, genetically based patient selection, epithelial cell biolabeling, and noninvasive screening will make colonoscopy safer, more versatile, more effective, and more cost-effective.

Further reading

1. Ahlquist DA, Zoo H, Domenici M, *et al.* Next-generation stool DNA test accurately detects colorectal cancer and large adenomas. *Gastroenterology* 2012;142:248–56.
2. Coe SG, Wallace MB. Colonoscopy: new approaches to better outcomes. *Curr Opin Gastroenterol* 2012;28:70–5.
3. Krier MJ, Pasricha PJ. Not your father's colonoscopy: a high-tech future for screening and surveillance of colorectal cancer. *Gastrointest Endosc Clin N Am* 2008;18:607–17, xi.
4. Kupier T, Dekker E, Van den Broek FJ, *et al.* Feasibility and accuracy of confocal endomicroscopy in comparison with narrow band imaging and chromoendoscopy for the differentiation of colorectal lesions. *Am J Gastroenterol* 2012;107:543–550.
5. Rex DK, Kahi C, O'Brien M, *et al.* The American Society for Gastrointestinal Endoscopy PIVI (Preservation and Incorporation of Valuable Endoscopic Innovations) on real-time endoscopic assessment of the histology of diminutive colorectal polyps. *Gastrointest Endosc* 2011;73: 419–22.
6. Riccioni ME, Urgesi R, Cianci R, Bizzotto A, Spada C, Costamagna G. Colon capsule endoscopy: advantages, limitations and expectations. Which novelties? *World J Gastrointest Endosc* 2012;4:99–107.
7. Roberts-Thomson IC, Singh R, Teo E, Nguyen NQ, Lidums I. The future of endoscopy. *J Gastroenterol Hepatol* 2010;25:1051–7.
8. Shergill AK, McQuaid KR, Deleon A, McAnanama M, Shah JN. Randomized trial of standard versus magnetic endoscope imaging colonoscopes for unsedated colonoscopy. *Gastrointest Endosc* 2012;75:1031–1036. e1. Epub 2012 Mar 3.
9. Spada C, Hassan C, Galmiche JP, *et al.* Colon capsule endoscopy: European Society of Gastrointestinal Endoscopy (ESGE) Guideline. *Endoscopy* 2012;44:527–36.
10. Winawer SJ, Pasricha PJ, Schmiegel W, *et al.* The future role of the gastroenterologist in digestive oncology: an international perspective. *Gastroenterology* 2011;141:e13–21. Epub 2011 Aug 24.

Subject Index

Note:
Page numbers in *italics* refer to figures

A
abdominal distension 19, 22, 67
  post-procedure management 22
  abdominal pressure 18
  loop formation prevention 53, 59
accessories, endoscope *see* endoscopic accessories
adenocarcinoma of colon
  biopsies 69
  colon obstruction, therapeutic colonoscopy 140–142
  colonoscopic findings 69
  debulking, endoscopic 141
  pit patterns 180, 181
  see also colorectal cancer
adenoma(s) 102
  "advanced" 101
  detection 102–103
    CT colonography 176
    narrow band imaging 181, 182
    rate, colonoscopy quality end point 162
  malignancy arising 133, *137*, 138
  pit patterns 180, 181
  prevalence 100
  sessile serrated *see under* polyp(s)
  traditional serrated (TSAs) 101
  tubular 99, 100
  tubulovillous 100, *101*
  villous 99, 100
  see also polyp(s)
adhesions, intra-abdominal 54, 149
advanced imaging techniques 178–185
  autofluorescence imaging 182
  confocal laser endomicroscopy 183
  endocytoscopy 182–183
  magnifying colonoscopy 179–181
  optical coherence tomography 183–184
  water method 51, 179, 187
air aspiration 50, 67
  flat/sessile polyp removal 109, 127–128
air expellation, post-procedural 22, 156
air insufflation *see* insufflation of air
air/water failure, troubleshooting 21
amebiasis 78, 79
American College of Radiology Imaging Network (ACRIN) study 176
American Society of Anesthesiology (ASA), physical status classification system 41
amyloidosis, submucosal biopsy 86
anal carcinoma, colonoscopic findings 70
analgesia 39
  quality end point 162
  safety optimization 43
anal lesions/abnormalities 70
anastomotic stricturing, TTS balloon dilatation 142
anesthesia
  decrease in need for 187
  general 28, 39
anesthesiologist 42–43, 148
anoscopy 70
antibiotic prophylaxis 31
anticoagulants 30–31
antiemetic agents 34
antiplatelet agents 30–31
anxiety, pre-procedural 3, 40
appendiceal orifice *59*, 60
appendix, polyp involving, removal 129
argon plasma coagulation (APC) 96–97
arrhythmias 31, 148
arteriography, with embolization 155
ascending colon
  back sides of folds 64
  intubation 59
  polyps, methods to increase detection 66, 67
aspiration (stomach contents) 148
aspirin 30
atrial fibrillation 31
autofluorescence imaging 182

B
"backwash ileitis" 73
balloon dilatation, benign colonic obstruction 142
barium enema, CT colonography 177
benzodiazepines 39–40, 40–41
biopsy 83–87
  anticoagulants and 30
  complications
    bleeding 153
    perforation 151
  flexible sigmoidoscopy with 29
  four-quadrant 25, 178
  inflammatory bowel disease, timing 25
  malignant polyp, colonoscopic resection after 138
  normal (macroscopically) mucosa 85
  "optical" 179, 188
  possibly malignant polyps 134
  protocol adherence, quality end point 162
  "well biopsy" 85, 86

Practical Colonoscopy, First Edition. Jerome D. Waye, James Aisenberg, and Peter H. Rubin.
© 2013 John Wiley & Sons, Ltd. Published 2013 by John Wiley & Sons, Ltd.

biopsy forceps 83–84, 151
advantages for use 104
bleeding after use 153
polypectomy 104
bleeding 153–155
causes 71, 153
coagulation of vessels 94–95
see also electrocautery
colonoscopy indication 24
complication of colonoscopy 153–155
management 154–155
prevention 154
diverticular 70–71
immediate postpolypectomy, management 154
non-thermal treatment 145
postpolypectomy *see* polypectomy
prevention, detachable loops use 13
radiation injury causing 72
rectal *see* rectal bleeding
risks in colonoscopy 30, 153
solitary rectal ulcer 72
vascular ectasia 78, 97
blind spots 64, *65*
polyp detection missed 64–65, 102
bow and arrow sign 60
bowel preparation 32–34
cardiopulmonary complications due to 148
children and infants 28
complications 156
"difficult-to-prepare" patient 33–34
future prospects 187
inadequate 33, 34, 63
large colorectal cancer and 69
quality end point 163
"split-dose" approach 32
bright red blood per rectum (BRBPR) 24
burns, electrosurgery 92
full thickness 152–153
perforation due to 151

C

cancer *see* colorectal cancer
cancer risk stratification guidelines 186
cap-assisted resection 129–130
capnography 41
capsule colonoscopy 188
carbon dioxide, insufflation 67, 156
carcinoid tumors 101
rectal 70
cardiopulmonary complications 148–149
cardiopulmonary function, monitoring during colonoscopy 44
catharsis
improving 187
see also bowel preparation
cathartic agents 32–33
additional, inadequate cleaning of mucosa 63
hypertonic phosphate-based 33, 156
"split-dose" approach 32
cauterization
argon plasma *see* argon plasma coagulation (APC)
"hot biopsy" forceps *83*, 84, 104
see also electrocautery
cecal intubation 59
caput cecum 60, *61*
colonoscopy quality measure 162
prevention by looping 54
"cecal patch" 73
cecum
barotrauma 150
"blow-out" perforation 50, 150
caput *61*, 64
difficult polyps in 116–117
intubation 60
identification criteria 59
length of scope to reach 55
nonmucosal elevated lesions, removal 130
perforation, in pseudo-obstruction 143
polyp detection missed 64
retroflexion *59*, *66*
volvulus 142–143
see also ileocecal valve
charge-coupled device (CCD) 7–8, 8–9
children, colonoscopy 28
chromoendoscopy 25, 74, 178–179
dyes 178, 179
application methods 178–179
circular muscles, colon 49, *58*
cleaning of colon *see* bowel preparation
cleaning of endoscopes 163
cleaning of mucosa 55, 56, 63–64
inadequate 63
see also bowel preparation
clips 13
applicators 13
indications 145
perforation/lesion closure 144, 151, 152
Clostridium difficile colitis 189–190
coagulation
argon plasma *see* argon plasma coagulation (APC)
in electrosurgery 92
see also electrocautery; hemostasis
"cobble-stoning" 73
cold snare technique 104–105
bleeding after 154
see also snare polypectomy
colectomy, ileal pouch-anal anastomosis (IPAA) 77
colitis
biopsy for 86
chronic, colon cancer risk 26
Clostridium difficile 189–190
collagenous 80
colonoscopy, reporting 76
diversion 72–73
diverticular 71
idiopathic 25
infectious *see* infectious colitis
ischemic 71–72
microscopic 80, 86
polypectomy in 76
pseudomembranous 79
ulcerative *see* ulcerative colitis (UC)
collagenous colitis 80
colocolonic anastomosis 77
colonic inertia 25, 143
colonic obstruction, acute, relief 140–143
benign obstruction 142
malignant obstruction 140–142
volvulus 142–143
colonic perforation (colonoscopy complication) 25, 149–152
air pressure causing 25, 50, 150
causes 50, 54, 149
cecal "blow-out" 50, 150
incidence 149
large polyp removal 119, 150
localized, closure by endoscopic clips 144, 151
management 152
pain due to 152
post-polypectomy syndrome 151
risk factors 149
risk from polypectomy 120
reduced by submucosal fluid injection 122–124
risk in electrosurgery 92, 151
submucosal saline injection to reduce *94*, 122

risk in severe colitis 74
risk reduction 151
symptoms/signs 149, 152
timing 149
types 149–151
colonic surgery, mortality 136
colonic volvulus 142–143
colonoscope 6–10, 7
advancing, assistance with 18, 47–48, 53
auxiliary, in difficult polypectomies 126–127
cleaning 163
control section 8
handling technique 47
developments 186
disinfection and sterilization 163
handle grip 47
head, holding 47, 56
holding, by assistant 18, 47–48
holding technique 46–48
insertion *see* intubation (colonoscopy)
length inserted 55
light source 7, 8, 9, 10, 181
magnification 10
pediatric 28, 63, 119
positioning in snare polypectomy 107
reprocessing and infection control 163
suction port 55
see also intubation (colonoscopy)
colonoscopic findings *see individual conditions*
colonoscopist
mid-career, continuing education 167, 171–172
requirements/abilities 168
training *see* training (colonoscopy)
colonoscopy *see specific topics/aspects*
colonoscopy assistant *see* endoscopy assistant
colonoscopy complications *see* complications of colonoscopy
colonoscopy report *see* reports (colonoscopy)
colonoscopy room *see* procedure rooms
colonoscopy technique 46–68
ergonomics, optimization 48
holding the scope 46–48
intubation *see* intubation
patient position *see* patient positioning
preparation for scope insertion 46
see also pre-colonoscopy tasks
reports 165
visualization increased, methods 65–67
decompression of colon 67
retroflexion *see* retroflexion
colopathy, radiation 72
colorectal cancer
colonoscopic findings 69, 70
detection by CT colonography 176
"interval" *see* "interval" cancer
post-resection surveillance 27
recurrence after malignant polyp resection 135, 136
recurrence after resection 27
risk
in chronic colitis 25, 26
in inflammatory bowel disease 25, 74
risk stratification guidelines 186
screening 26
clinical quality end points 161
colonoscopy indication 186
guidelines 26
size/length, estimating 69
"tattooing" sites 69
see also adenocarcinoma of colon; malignancy
colostomy
diverting, colitis after 72–73
purgative agent administration 34
complications of colonoscopy 147–157
bowel preparation causing 156
cardiopulmonary 148–149
as clinical quality end point 161
hemorrhage 153–155
see also bleeding
perforation *see* colonic perforation
postpolypectomy coagulation syndrome 92, 152–153
risk factors 147
computed tomographic colonography (CTC) 175–177, 187, 189
2D *vs* 3D 175
advantages/disadvantages 175, 176
indications 69, 176
procedure 175
radiation exposure 176
computer-based simulation 172
confocal laser endomicroscopy (CLE) 183
constipation
chronic, bowel preparation 33–34
colonoscopy indication 25
continuing education 167, 171–172
continuous quality improvement (CQI) programs 161
contraindications for colonoscopy 24
absolute and relative 28
"contre coup" burn 125–126
CQI programs 161
critical devices, sterilization 163
Crohn's disease 25
benign colonic obstruction 142
biopsy 85
colonoscopic findings 73
fistulas, and closure of 145
post-operative recurrence, colonoscopy for 25
ulcerative colitis differentiation 73
crystal violet 178, 179
CTC *see* computed tomographic colonography (CTC)
cytomegalovirus (CMV) colitis 78

D
debulking tumors
endoscopic 141
laser use 97–98
decompression of colon 67
acute colonic obstruction 140
malignant obstruction 140–142
pseudo-obstruction 143–144
sigmoid volvulus 143
decompression tube, transanal placement 141
detachable loops 13
devitalization of tissue 92, 151
diabetes, preparation for colonoscopy 32
diarrhea
bloody 24
chronic non-bloody 24–25
colonoscopy indication 24–25
persistent, biopsy for 85
diazepam 39–40
diet, liquid, bowel preparation 32
Dieulafoy lesions 80
disinfection, "high-level" 163
diversion colitis 72–73
diverticular bleeding 70–71
diverticular colitis 71

diverticular disease, sigmoid
  blind spots and 64
  colonoscopic findings 70–71
  insertion of scope into sigmoid colon 57, 58
  location of lumen and 49–50
diverticulitis, acute 71
drugs
  analgesic/sedative 39–40
    adverse effects 148
    benzodiazepines 39–40, 40–41
    narcotic/benzodiazepine antagonists 40
    opioids 39, 40–41
    pharmacology 39–40
    propofol 40
  colonoscopic abnormalities due to 80
  intralesional injection 144
dual antiplatelet therapy 30–31
dyes
  application methods 178–179
  chromoendoscopy 178, 179
dysplasia 25, 99
  adenomatous polyps 99, 100, 102
  colitis-associated 25
    detection, criteria for 75
    lesion characteristics 74
    management 76
    sporadic dysplasia *vs* 75, 76
  detection 26, 75
  high-grade 101
  pedunculated polyp *137*
  screening, pediatric 29
  sessile polyp *137*
  sporadic, colitis-associated *vs* 75, 76
  surveillance, biopsy protocols 86
  see also adenoma(s)

E
electrical current 93
  coagulation current 92
  cutting current 91, 92, 125
  high-frequency 91, 95
  snare cautery polypectomy 111
electrocardiography (ECG) 42
electrocautery
  bipolar probes 93, 94–95
  bleeding vessels 94–95
  common uses 94–95
  general precautions 95, 96
  heater probes 93, 94
  high-frequency 91, 95
  monopolar 91
  multipolar probes (MPEC) 93
  in polypectomy 94, 104, 106, 110–111
  see also electrosurgery
electronic colonoscopy report 165
electrosurgery 91–96
  general precautions 95–96
  instruments 91, 93
  monopolar accessories 93
  technique and recommendations 98
  thermal effects during 92–93
  see also electrocautery
electrosurgical unit (ESU) 91, 92, 95
endoloop 105
endoscopic accessories 10–14, 13
  clips and applicators *see* clips
  detachable loops 13
  for electrosurgery 93
  injection needles 13
  overtubes 14
  polypectomy snares *see* polypectomy snares
  polyp retrieval devices *see* polyp(s), retrieval devices
  specimen traps *see* specimen traps
  spray catheters 13
  transparent caps 14
endoscopic clips *see* clips
endoscopic mucosal resection (EMR) 122–124
endoscopic mucosal resection (EMR) expert 118
endoscopic submucosal dissection (ESD) 128–129
endoscopic ultrasonography (EUS) 188–189
endoscopy assistant 16–23
  additional personnel in endoscopy room 22, 169
  diagnostic biopsy assistance 84–85
  intra-colonoscopy tasks 17–22
    snare cautery polypectomy 106
    snare polypectomy 106, 107, 108, 110
    submucosal fluid injection 123
    troubleshooting 21
  post-procedure tasks 22
  pre-colonoscopy tasks 17, 43, 46
  sedation and 17–18, 43
endoscopy report *see* reports (colonoscopy)
endoscopy unit 3–6
  efficient, requirements 168
  resources for difficult polypectomy 117–118
enema
  barium 177
Entamoeba, colitis 78, 79
epinephrine 122, 126, 154, 155
ergonomics, optimization 48
Escherichia coli, colitis due to 78

F
failed colonoscopy 103, 176
falls, prevention 156
familial colorectal cancer syndrome 26
fecal impaction, management 142
fentanyl 39
"field defect" 86
fistulas, closure 145
flat lesions, colorectal 69
  see also polyp(s)
flexible sigmoidoscopy
  with biopsy 29
  sigmoid volvulus 143
fluids
  electrolyte-containing, bowel preparation 32
  intraluminal, suctioning *55*, 55–56
  submucosal injection *see* submucosal fluid injection
flumazenil 40
fluoroscopy 54
foreign body, removal 145

G
gallstone ileus 145
gastroscope use 63, 69
  in difficult polypectomies 126–127
  in rectum, for polyp removal 127
graft-*versus*-host disease 78

H
heart valves, prosthetic 30
heater probes 93, 94
hematochezia 71
hemorrhoids 24, 71
hemostasis
  argon plasma coagulation 96, 97
  difficult polypectomy 125–126
  electrosurgery instruments for 92, 93
  postpolypectomy bleeding *154*, 154–155
hepatic flexure
  blind spot 65, *65*
  intubation 58–59
hereditary non-polyposis colon cancer (HNPCC) 26

Hirschsprung's disease, biopsy 86
hot forceps (biopsy) 83, 84, 104
advantages for use 104
"hot" polypectomy *see* polypectomy
hyperplastic rectosigmoid polyps 100
see also polyp(s)
hypotension during colonoscopy 44, 148
hypoventilation, primary 42, 148

I
idiopathic colitis 25
ileal intubation 60–62
ileal pouches, endoscopy of 76–77
ileitis 77
"backwash" 73
pre-pouch 77
ileocecal valve *59*
abnormalities 81
intubation 61
difficulties 60
orifice
intubation tips 60
landmarks 62
polyp involving, removal 130
polyps concealed behind 64
ulceration 73
ileocolic anastomosis 61
ileosigmoid fistula 73
ileum, distal *see* terminal ileum
incomplete examination 59
incomplete polypectomy *see* polypectomy
indications for colonoscopy 24–28
colorectal cancer screening 26, 186
quality end point 162
indigo carmine 178, 179
infections
colonoscopy complication 156
prevention, endoscope reprocessing 163
infectious colitis
colonoscopic findings 78–79
inflammatory bowel disease
colon cancer risk and surveillance 74
colonoscopic findings 73–76
colonoscopy indication 25
pediatric colonoscopy 29
see also Crohn's disease; ulcerative colitis (UC)
informed consent 17, 34
quality end point 162
injection (tissue), indications 13
injection catheter, assistant's role in preparing 20–21
injection needles, for use during colonoscopy 13
insufflation of CO_2 67, 156
insulin 32
"interval" cancer 101, 161, xi
causes 101
as clinical quality end point 161
decreasing rate, strategies 188
intestinal tuberculosis 79
intralesional drug injection 144
intraluminal gas, immediate post-procedural pain 156
intraperitoneal gas 152
intubation
aborting, criteria for 54
advancing scope, assistance with 18, 47–48, 53
difficulties 50, 62–63
right colon and cecum 59, 60
in diverticular disease of sigmoid colon 57, 58
efficient, keys to 48–56
"impossible" colon 62–63
length of scope inserted 55
reintubation after "unpleating" of colon 64
repeating 103
scope holding technique for 46–48
scope shape during 54
segment by segment 56–63
techniques 48–56
water method 51, 179, 187
see also colonoscope; colonoscopy technique
iron-deficiency anemia 24
irrigation system 8, 18
irritable bowel syndrome 24
ischemic colitis, colonoscopic findings 71–72

J
"jumbo" forceps (biopsy) 83

K
Kock pouch (KP) 76–77
intubation difficulties 77
Kudo's system, pit pattern classification 180–181

L
landmarks, intubation 55
ileocecal valve orifice 62
lumen (of colon) 50
laryngospasm 148
laser, confocal laser endomicroscopy (CLE) 183
laser (neodymium-YAG) 97–98
laxatives 63
learning
process 168
simulation-based 172
see also training (colonoscopy)
ligatures, bleeding prevention 13
light, wavelengths, narrow band imaging 10, 181
light reflections, reading 49
light source, colonoscope 7, 8, 9, 10, 181
lipoma 86, 101
looping of scope *52*
causes/reasons 51–52
cecal intubation prevention 54
external, resolving 53
pain 51
paradoxical tip movement from 51, *51*
perforation due to 149–150
prevention of formation of 53–54
sigmoid loop 57
"push through" 52
reducing/eliminating 52–53
in sigmoid colon 57
suspected, being alert to 51–52
lubrication
adequacy 54
technique 55
lumen (of colon) *58*
knowing position 49–50
sigmoid diverticular disease 49–50
landmarks 50
lymphocytic colitis 80
lymphonodular hyperplasia, pediatric colonoscopy 29

M
magnifying colonoscopy 10, 179–181
malignancy
autofluorescence imaging 182
narrow band imaging 182
pit patterns, magnifying colonoscopy 180, 181
see also colorectal cancer
malignant obstruction, of colon 140–142
malignant polyps 132–139
adverse outcome 138
biopsy 134, 138
colonoscopic resection after biopsy 138

decision-making after resection 135–136
definition 132
flat *132*, 133
gross appearance 133–134
localization problems 135
management options
colonoscopic approach 134, 135, 136, 138
surgical resection 135, 136
pathology report 133
pedunculated *132*, 133, *137*
polypectomy indication 134
prognostic features (favourable) 138
recurrence of malignancy 136
resectable, better identification, methods 188–189
resection margin 138
sessile *132*, 133, *137*
resection 134
with/without invasion *137*
spread, risk of 136–137
suspected, resection 134–135
marking site 135
unsuspected, resection 135
Mayo Colonoscopy Skills Assessment Test 173
medical history 30
melanosis coli 25
meperidine 39
mesenteric attachments 51, 57
metallic clip, "hot" polypectomy and 105
methylene blue 178, 179
microscopic colitis 80, 86
midazolam 40
"mini-snare" 104–105, 126
MiraLax 32, 156
"miss rate" (polyps) 63, 101
decreasing 187–188
monitor (video), positioning 5, 47
monitoring during endoscopy
of abdomen 19
cardiopulmonary function 44
clinical signs 18
post-polypectomy 30
monitoring during recovery 41
mortality
from cardiopulmonary complications 148
colonic surgery 136
"Mount Fuji effect" 104
mucosa
enhancing inspection, by endoscopy assistant 18–19
hyperplastic, pit patterns 180, 181
normal
autofluorescence imaging 182
"collar", in snare polypectomy 108, 125, 134, 188
pit patterns 180
resection, polypectomy *see* polypectomy, difficult
mucosal biopsy 85, 86
mucosal bridges 76
mucosal crypts, magnifying colonoscopy 179–181
mucosal imaging 10
mucosal scarring 76
mucus, over sessile serrated adenomas 103
muscularis mucosa *132*
delayed perforation and *151*
dysplastic crypts invading *132*
muscularis propria 108, *132*, *151*
musculoskeletal injuries 47

N
naloxone 40
narcotic drugs 39
antagonists 40
narrow band imaging (NBI) 10, 100, 181–182
nasal cannula 42
natural orifice translumenal endoscopic surgery (NOTES) 189
neoplasia *see* colorectal cancer; malignancy
neostigmine 144
"no-look" transfer of ancillary devices 19
"non-lifting sign" 123–124, 134
non-steroidal anti-inflammatory drugs (NSAIDs) 30
NOTES (natural orifice translumenal endoscopic surgery) 189
novel therapies 189–190
number of colonoscopy cases
for training 173
undertaken per annum xi
nurse charting, quality end point 162

O
Ogilvie syndrome 143–144
"open access" colonoscopy 34
opioids 39, 40–41
antagonists 40
"optical biopsy" 179, 188
optical coherence tomography (OCT) 183–184
oral hypoglycemic agents 32
overinsufflation 69
oversedation 40
overtubes 14, 57
oximeters 42
oxygen, supplemental 42

P
pain 40, 43
abdominal, post-procedure 43, 152
colonic perforation causing 152
during colonoscopy 43
colonoscopy complication 43, 152, 155
immediate post-procedural, intraluminal gas 43, 156
intubation of sigmoid colon 57, *57*
stretching mesenteric attachments 51, 57
paradoxical insertion tube movement
from looping 51
right colon retroflexion 66
Paris criteria, polyps 99–100
pathology requisition form, biopsy 85
patient(s)
circular flow in endoscopy unit 4
instructions for bowel preparation 33
safety, training and 168
satisfaction, quality end point 162
patient positioning 46
intubation of ascending colon 59
post-procedure, to expel air 22, 156
repositioning
endoscopy assistant's role 18
indications 67
patient record, storage 6
patient stretcher 4, 46, 47
pediatric colonoscopy 28–29
pre-procedural issues 28
personal protective equipment 16–17
personnel
ancillary 22, 169
colonoscopic sedation 40, 41, 42–43
see also endoscopy assistant

phosphate-based bowel preparations 33, 156
piecemeal polypectomy 120
bleeding after 154
conditions favouring 120
ensuring complete polypectomy 125
large sessile polyps 120
procedure 120
"pillow sign" 84
pinworm infection 29, 79
"pit pattern", classification 180, *181*
polyethylene glycol (PEG) 3350 32, 156
polyp(s) 99
adenomatous 99, 100, 102
pit patterns 180, 181
surveillance guidelines 26
see also adenoma(s)
advanced 133
see also malignant polyps
appearance *99*, 99–100
broad-based sessile, polypectomy 120
classification 101, 102
detection 101–103
blind spots for missing 64–65, 102
endoscopic assistant's role 18
flat polyps 103
miss rate *see* "miss rate"
sessile serrated adenomas/polyps 103
small polyps 14
withdrawal phase 63–65, 102–103
difficult, management options 116
see also polypectomy, difficult
diminutive 100
"resect and discard" 188
elevation by submucosal fluid *see* submucosal fluid injection
flat 69, *99*, 99–100
CT colonography for 176
detection 103
malignant *132*, 133
removal 127–128
snare polypectomy 109, *111*, 112
histopathology 100–101, 102
hyperplastic 101
detection by narrow band imaging 182
of rectum 100
inflammatory 76
lesion characteristics 74
large
detection by CT colonography 176
removal *see* polypectomy, difficult
location 100
difficult polypectomy 116–117
malignant *see* malignant polyps
pedunculated *99*, 100
capsule colonoscopy 188
malignant *132*, 133
polypectomy *see* polypectomy
removal
avulsion 104
biopsy of surrounding mucosa after 86
during intubation 54, 104
see also polypectomy
retrieval devices 11–12, *12*
serrated 100, 101, 102
adenomas *vs*, polypectomy 117
detection rate, quality end point 162
elevation, submucosal fluid injection *124*
surveillance guidelines 27
traditional serrated adenomas 101
sessile *101*
broad-based, polypectomy 120
large, polypectomy *see* polypectomy, difficult
malignant *132*, 133
snare polypectomy 109
sessile serrated adenomas (SSAs) 99, 100, 101, 103
detection by narrow band imaging 182
polypectomy 117
"tenting" 104, 105, 112
see also adenoma(s)
polypectomy 99–115
advanced, equipment 117
ambulatory 119
argon plasma coagulation (APC) after 97
bleeding after 106, 124, 153
control, electrocautery 94, 104, 106
delayed *see below*
early *vs* late 153
immediate, management 154, *154*
management 153, 154–155
prevention 153, 154
bleeding during 153
complete removal of polyp 117
debulking giant polyps 126
delayed bleeding 31, 153
management 153, 154–155
thermal techniques increasing risk 93
electrocautery use in 94, 104, 106
follow-up after 27
general principles 104
"hot" 94, 104
goals 94
recommendations 105
safety precautions 105
incomplete 117, 129
avoidance in suspected malignant polyps 134
decreasing, new methods 188
large defect after, closure by clips 144
large polyps 110, 113
see also polypectomy, difficult
malignant polyps 133, 134–135
pedunculated polyps 114
bleeding prevention 154
ensuring complete removal 112
safety precautions 105
perforation after 150
delayed 151
right colon, bleeding management 154–155
scar 135
serrated lesion *vs* adenoma 117
small polyps 104–114
cold snare resection 104–105
"hot biopsy forceps" use 104, 105
snare cautery 106, 110–111
location/finding 112
"lost", finding 112, 114
retrieval *112*, 113
suctioning 113, 114
surveillance guidelines after 26–27
polypectomy, difficult 116–131
colonoscopes 119
endoscopic mucosal resection 122–124
mucosal defect after 124
endoscopic submucosal dissection 128–129, 151
flat polyps 127–128
air aspiration 127–128
giant polyps 126, 129
hospital *vs* outpatient unit 119
incomplete removal 129
tattooing 120, *122*

large sessile polyps 117, 125
closing snare, cautery and 125
elevation *see* submucosal fluid injection
perforation due to 150
piecemeal polypectomy 120, *121*
recommendations 126
snare resection 119–122
polyp involving appendix 129
preparation 118–119
residual fragments of adenoma 129
in retroflection 127
technique 119–126
to ensure complete polypectomy 125
thermal techniques 125–126
polypectomy snares 10–11
adjustment of position, assistant's role 19
handle, marking 20
loop configuration 10–11, *109*
"mini-snare" 104–105, 126
"no-look" transfer technique 19
small polyp removal 104–105
positioning
of endoscopist, snare polypectomy 111
of patients *see* patient positioning
of trainers/instructors 170–171
post-colonoscopy management (clinical) 41
post-polypectomy
bleeding *see under* polypectomy
surveillance guidelines 26–27
post-polypectomy syndrome 92, 151
post-procedure tasks
endoscopy assistant 22
reports 165
pouchitis 77
pre-colonoscopy management 41
pediatric patients 28
pre-colonoscopy tasks
of endoscopy assistant 17, 43, 46
reporting 165
pregnancy, colonoscopy during 28
preparation for colonoscopy 30–35
informed consent *see* informed consent
medication management 30–31
for scope insertion 46
pre-procedure area 6
pre-procedure assessment, by endoscopy assistant 17
procedure report 165
procedure rooms 4–5
area/size 4, *5*, 41–42
arrangement of equipment 4, *5*, 41–42, 47
resuscitation equipment 42
sedation equipment 41–42
setting up by endoscopy assistant 17
proctopathy, radiation 72
propofol 40, 41, 42–43
"balanced propofol sedation" 41
pseudomembranous colitis 79
pseudo-obstruction 143
predisposing factors 143
treatment 143–144

Q
quality (colonoscopy) 161–166
endoscope reprocessing/infection control 163
high-quality 161
metrics/measurement 161–163, 164
quality-improvement programs
continuous (CQI) 161

R
radiation proctopathy 72
recovery area 5–6
recovery beds, capacity/number 6
recovery room 22
rectal bleeding 72, 153, 154
etiology 71
radiation injury causing 72
see also bleeding
rectal cancer
surgical resection, follow-up 27
rectal folds (valves of Houston), blind spots 65, 102
rectal polyps 116, 136
rectal ulcer, solitary 72
rectum
distal, malignant polyps 136
foreign body removal 145
radiation injury 72
retroflexion 65, 102
renal failure, bowel preparations associated 33, 156
reporting system, endoscopic 5
reports (colonoscopy) 165
contents 165
quality 162
"resect and discard" strategy 188
resuscitation equipment 42
retroflexion 65–67
anus 70
cecum *59*, *66*
difficult polypectomy 127
rectal 65, 102
right colon 66, 67, 102
retroscope, third eye 67, *189*
rigid sigmoidoscopy, sigmoid volvulus 143
risk of colonoscopy, informed consent and 34
robotic technology 189
Roth Net 11

S
safety belt 17, 18
saline, submucosal fluid injection *94*, 122, 124, 134
scheduling, time required for colonoscopy 118, 169
"Scope Guide" 54
screening
colorectal cancer *see* colorectal cancer
see also surveillance recommendations
sedation 39–45, 46
approaches for colonoscopy 40–41
drugs for 39–40, 40–41, 43
see also drugs
endoscopy assistant role 17–18, 43
equipment for 41–42
history-taking for 41
pediatric 28
propofol 40, 41, 42–43
quality end point 162
staffing for 40, 41, 42–43
self-expanding metallic stents (SEMS)
benign anastomotic strictures 142
indications 142
malignant colonic obstruction 141–142
sigmoid colon
diverticular disease *see* diverticular disease, sigmoid
insertion of scope into 57
lacerations due to diagnostic colonoscopy 144
looping of scope 57
perforation due to 150
volvulus 142–143
sigmoidoscopy, flexible *see* flexible sigmoidoscopy
snare polypectomy
5 o'clock positioning 107, 113
angle for approach 108
cautery 106, 110–111

choice of snare 105
endoscopist position 111
flat or sessile polyps 109, *111*, 112
large polyps 110, 113
malignant polyp 133, 134–135
perforation due to 150
"tenting" of polyp 104, 105, 112, 128
transecting polyp 110–111, *112*
snares *see* polypectomy snares
specimen
biopsy, handling 84–85
polypectomy *see* polypectomy
specimen traps 12
types 12
Spider Net 11
spike forceps 83–84
splenic flexure
blind spot 65
intubation 58
splenic rupture/hemorrhage 155
staining, chromoendoscopy 178, 179
stents
designs, for malignant colonic obstruction 141–142
self-expanding metallic (SEMS) *141*, 141–142
stretcher 4, 46, 47
strictures, colonic 76
ileo-anal anastomosis 77
TTS balloon dilatation 142
submucosal fluid injection
cancer cell tracking 124
disadvantages 124
method 122, 123
non-lifting sign and 123–124, 134, *134*
polyp elevation by *94*, 105, 122–124
cancerous polyp 124
serrated polyp *124*
suspected malignant polyp 134
volume 123
suction/suctioning 63
failure, troubleshooting 21
polyp retrieval after polypectomy 113, 114
suprapubic pressure 53, 57
surgical approach
malignant polyp resection 135, 136
perforation management 152
surveillance recommendations
colorectal cancer 26, 186
inflammatory bowel disease 74
post-resection 27
malignant polyp
resection 135–136
post-polypectomy 26–27

T
tamponade of vessels 145, 154
tandem colonoscopy 63, 101
tattooing
incomplete polypectomy of large sessile polyp 120, *122*
site of colorectal cancer 69
site of suspected malignant polyp 135
teaching/training *see* training (colonoscopy)
terminal ileum 25
abnormalities 81
Crohn's disease 73
entering 60, 62
intubation 60–62
tips for 60–61
mucosa, appearance 62
orifice 60, 61
see also ileocecal valve
therapeutic colonoscopy 140–146, 186–187
bleeding after 153
contraindications 140
foreign body removal 145
pediatric 29
perforation/lesion closure *144*, 144–145, 151
polyp removal *see* polypectomy
thermal techniques 91–98
devices used in colonoscopy 95
see also electrosurgery
third eye retroscope 67, *189*
through-the-scope (TTS) balloon, benign colonic obstruction 142
through-the-scope (TTS) stents *141*, 141–142
tissue retrieval
polypectomy specimen *112*, 113
torque
clockwise *vs* counterclockwise *48*, 48–49
to reduce loops 52
trainees 170, 171
trainers 170
positioning 170–171
training (colonoscopy) 167–174
challenges 167
competence assessment 172–173
of endoscopic assistant 16–17
methods 172
of mid-career colonoscopists 167, 171–172
patient safety as priority 168
technical proficiency 173
transparent caps 14
transverse colon
intubation 58–59
TTS balloon 142

U
ulcer(s), mucosal, biopsy 86
ulcerative colitis (UC)
biopsy 85
colonoscopic findings 73
Crohn's disease differentiation 73
ultrasonography, endoscopic (EUS) 188–189
unsedated colonoscopy 40

V
vascular ectasia
colonoscopic findings 78
hemostasis by argon plasma coagulation 97
videotaping, colonoscopy 161
"virtual" colonoscopy *see* computed tomographic colonography (CTC)
"vital" stains 178
volvulus, colonic 142–143

W
waiting area 5–6
warfarin 30, 31
washing and suction 55–56, 63
polyp detection 102
water instillation 51, 62
difficult polypectomy 119
water-jet method, dye application 179
water method (of colonoscopy) 51, 179, 187
pros and cons 179
withdrawal of scope 63–65
blind spots 64–65, 102
cleaning mucosa 63–64
guiding principles 64
non-thermal treatment of bleeding 145
perforation detection 150
polyp detection 102–103
technique, quality end point 162
time taken 64, 103

Printed and bound by CPI Group (UK) Ltd, Croydon, CR0 4YY
09/10/2024
14571433-0001